Drug-Induced Ocular Side Effects and Drug Interactions

Drug-Induced Ocular Side Effects and Drug Interactions

F. T. FRAUNFELDER, M.D.

Professor and Chairman
Department of Ophthalmology
Oregon Health Sciences University
Portland, Oregon

Associate Editor

S. MARTHA MEYER, B.S.

Research Associate
Department of Ophthalmology
Oregon Health Sciences University
Portland, Oregon

Second Edition

Lea & Febiger   Philadelphia, 1982

Lea & Febiger
600 Washington Square
Philadelphia, Pa. 19106
U.S.A.

First Edition, 1976
Reprinted, 1979
Second Edition, 1982

Library of Congress Cataloging in Publication Data

Fraunfelder, Frederick T.

    Drug-induced ocular side effects and drug interactions.
    Bibliography: p.
    Includes index.
    1. Ocular pharmacology. 2. Drugs—Side effects. 3. Drug interactions. I. Title.
[DNLM: 1. Drug interactions—Outlines. 2. Drug therapy—Adverse effects—Out-
lines. 3. Iatrogenic disease—Outlines. 4. Eye—Drug effects—Outlines. WW 18
F845d]

RE994.F7 1982	615'.78	82-146
ISBN 0-8121-0850-7		AACR2

Printed in the United States of America

Print Number: 3 2 1

To
  Yvonne, Yvette, Helene Jean,
  Nina, Ricky, and Nicholas

Preface

The clinician is overwhelmed by the volume of ocular toxicology in the medical literature and is in need of a reference book that "boils it down." It is for the busy practitioner that this book is designed. The subject of our work is the *probable* medication-induced ocular side effects and the *possible* interactions of drugs prescribed by the ophthalmologist with those the patient is already taking. These areas are of increasing importance to the clinician, and possibly only in presentations of this type can he efficiently make use of the volume of data available. If a patient receiving medication has ocular signs or symptoms, these are not necessarily drug-related. *It is the physician's experience, his knowledge, and previous reports on the effects of a particular drug that will lead him to suspect a drug relationship.* In a controlled experimental environment it is often difficult to prove that a sign or symptom is drug related; in clinical practice, with multiple variables, it may in many instances be impossible. The clinician, however, needs to remember that there is no active drug known which is without undesirable side actions. It is the intent of this book to compile and organize "previous reports" into a format useful to the physician. This second edition is markedly changed, especially since the advent of the National Registry of Drug-Induced Ocular Side Effects which has accumulated much new data over the past six years. The Registry has served as the foundation for data in updating this edition. As in the first edition, no animal data have been included, since ocular toxicologic studies, except in primates, have had limited clinical correlation. Owing to the nature of this book and the volume of material covered, errors, omissions, and misemphasis are inevitable. In the hope of improving future editions, we welcome suggestions or corrections.

Data in this book have been accumulated by innumerable physicians and scientists who have suspected adverse reactions secondary to drug therapy and reported their suspicions to the Registry. Our sincere thanks to Bridget Hanson, Sherri Zurcher, Dianne Van Alstine, and Helene Fraunfelder for their expert assistance.

Portland, Oregon   F. T. Fraunfelder, M.D.
                                      S. Martha Meyer, B.S.

Instructions to Users

The basic format used in each chapter for each drug or group of drugs in this book includes

Class: The general category of the primary action of the drug is given.

Generic Name: The United States National Formulary name of each drug is listed. A name in parentheses following the National Formulary name is the international generic name if it differs from the one used in the United States.

Proprietary Name: The more common trade names are given. In a group of drugs, the number before a generic name corresponds to the number preceding the proprietary drug. This is true for both the systemic and ophthalmic forms of the drug. If a proprietary name differs from that of the United States, the country is given in parentheses after that particular proprietary name. Combination drugs are seldom included.

Primary Use: The type of drug and its current use in the management of various conditions are listed.

Ocular Side Effects:

A. Systemic Administration — Ocular side effects as reported from oral, nasal, intravenous, intramuscular, or intrathecal administration.
B. Local Ophthalmic Use or Exposure — Ocular side effects as reported from topical ocular application or subconjunctival, retrobulbar, or intracameral injection.
C. Inadvertent Ocular Exposure — Ocular side effects as reported due to accidental ocular exposure from any form of the drug.
D. Systemic Absorption from Topical Application to the Skin — Ocular side effects as reported secondary to topical dermatologic application.

The ocular side effects are listed in probable order of importance. The determination of importance is based on incidence of significance of the side effect. Side effects of inadequate documentation or current debate are followed by (?). The name of a drug in parentheses adjacent to an adverse reaction indicates that this is the only agent in the group reported to have caused this side effect.

Clinical Significance: A concise overview of the general importance of the ocular side effects produced is given to the clinician.

Interactions with Other Drugs:
  A. Effect of This Drug on Activity of Other Drugs
  B. Effect of Other Drugs on Activity of This Drug
  C. Synergistic Activity
  D. Cross Sensitivity
  E. Contraindications — specific

The amount of data in this area is voluminous. To make its use practical, only drugs which ophthalmologists might commonly prescribe are listed. If no interactions are listed, then none of major significance to the ophthalmologist have been reported. The symbol ($\uparrow$) means enhanced or increased effect on the activity of a drug while ($\downarrow$) means decreased effect on the activity of a drug. When ($\uparrow\downarrow$) is used, this means a variable response, in some cases increased, in others decreased.

References: References have been limited to either the best articles, the most current, or to those with the most complete bibliography. Since references for drug interactions are even more extensive, to save space they have not been included; however, a majority of the references are cited in Martin, E. W.: Drug Interactions Index 1978/79. Philadelphia, J. B. Lippincott Co., 1978 and Hansten, P. D.: Drug Interactions. 4th Ed., Philadelphia, Lea & Febiger, 1979.

Index of Side Effects: The lists of adverse ocular side effects due to drugs are intended in part to be indexes in themselves. The adverse ocular reactions are not separated in this index as to route of administration; however, this can be obtained by going to the text.

Index: The index includes both the drugs' generic and proprietary names. In addition, classification group names have also been added. The index is the primary source of entry into this book. This is a necessity since many drugs are in groups and would otherwise be missed. No indexing of drug interactions has been done, but this can be obtained by looking up the specific drug.

In the following section, the services of the National Registry of Drug-Induced Ocular Side Effects are outlined. The intent of this Registry is to make available data of possible drug-induced ocular side effects and to provide a central agency where possible adverse ocular drug reactions can be reported.

National Registry of Drug-Induced Ocular Side Effects

Rationale:

Collecting clinical data of drug-induced side effects for any organ system is still in its infancy. Reporting systems, registries, and surveys are currently being used along with costly prospective studies; however, none of these are being extensively used in ophthalmology. In a specialized area such as ophthalmology, seldom does a practitioner or even a group of practitioners see the patient volume necessary to make a correlation between possible cause and effect of drug-related or drug-induced ocular disease. A national registry to correlate this type of data may be of value, since this task would be difficult to carry out by any other method. If a number of these "possible" associations are found with a particular drug, then definitive controlled studies could be undertaken to obtain valid data. It is hoped that future editions of this book will present data with greater scientific significance, in part due to the reports of possible drug-induced ocular side effects which physicians will send to the Registry.

Objectives:

To establish a national center where possible drug-induced ocular side effects can be accumulated.

To review possible drug-induced ocular side effect data collected through the FDA Form 1639 and the FDA total community studies.

To compile the data in the world literature on reports of possible drug-induced ocular side effects.

To make available this data to physicians who feel they have a possible drug-induced ocular side effect.

Format:

The cases of primary interest are those adverse ocular reactions not previously recognized and those that are rare, severe, serious, or unusual. Data, to be of value, should be complete and follow the basic format as shown below.

Age:

Sex:

Suspected drug — trade name:

Suspected reaction — date of onset:

Route, dose and when drug started:

Improvement after suspected drug stopped — if restarted, did adverse reaction recur:

Other drugs taken at time of suspected adverse reaction:

Comments — optional: (Your opinion if drug-induced, probably related, possibly related, or unrelated.)

Your name and address — optional:

We are expanding the Registry from only drugs to include chemicals and other substances which may have potential ocular toxicology. We welcome all case reports and any impressions even without specific cases. To ensure confidentiality, no names of patients or physicians are used in any files or reports. This will protect you and the Registry from legal interference.

Send to:

Ms. Martha Meyer, Associate Director
National Registry of Drug-Induced Ocular Side Effects
Oregon Health Sciences University
3181 S.W. Sam Jackson Park Rd.
Portland, Oregon 97201

Phone: (503) 225-8456

Abbreviations

($\uparrow$) — Increase
($\downarrow$) — Decrease
($\uparrow\downarrow$) — Variable response — increased or decreased
Arg. — Argentina
Austral. — Australia
Aust. — Austria
Belg. — Belgium
Braz. — Brazil
Canad. — Canada
Cz. — Czechoslovakia
Denm. — Denmark
Fin. — Finland
Fr. — France
G.B. — Great Britain
Germ. — Germany
Ind. — India
Ire. — Ireland
Isr. — Israel
Ital. — Italy
Jap. — Japan
Neth. — Netherlands
Norw. — Norway
N.Z. — New Zealand
Pol. — Poland
Port. — Portugal
S. Afr. — South Africa
Scand. — Scandinavian
Span. — Spanish
Swed. — Sweden
Switz. — Switzerland
U.S.S.R. — Union of Soviet Socialist Republics

Contents

I
Anti-infectives

Class: Amebicides

Generic Name: 1. Amodiaquine; 2. Chloroquine; 3. Hydroxychloroquine. See under *Class: Antimalarial Agents.*

Generic Name: 1. Broxyquinoline; 2. Iodochlorhydroxyquin; 3. Iodo-quinol (Diiodohydroxyquinoline)

Proprietary Name: 1. Colipar (Fr.), Fenilor (Belg., Germ.); 2. Budo-form (Austral.), Chinoform (G.B.), Clioquinol (G.B.), Enteroquin (Austral.), Enteritan (Ital.), Entero-Valodon (G.B.), Entero-Vioform (G.B.), Iodochlorhydroxyquinoline (Ind.), Vioform; 3. Diiodohydroxy-quin, Diodoquin, Direxiode (Austral., Fr.), Embequin (G.B.), Flora-quin, Florequin (Swed.), Ioquin (Fr.), Moebiquin, Panaquin, Vaam-DHQ (Austral.), Yodoxin

Primary Use: These amebicidal agents are effective against *Entamoeba histolytica.*

Ocular Side Effects:
  A. Systemic Administration
    1. Decreased vision
    2. Optic atrophy
    3. Optic neuritis — subacute myelo-opticoneuropathy (SMON)
    4. Nystagmus
    5. Toxic amblyopia
    6. Macular edema
    7. Macular degeneration
    8. Diplopia
    9. Absence of foveal reflex
    10. Problems with color vision
      a. Dyschromatopsia
      b. Purple spots on white background

11. Corneal opacities (?)
12. Loss of eyelashes or eyebrows (?)

Clinical Significance: Major toxic ocular effects may occur with long-term oral administration of these amebicidal agents. Since they are given orally for *Entamoeba histolytica*, most reports are from the Far East. Data suggest that these amebicides may cause subacute myelo-opticoneuropathy (SMON). This neurologic disease has a 19 percent incidence of decreased vision and a 2.5 percent incidence of toxic amblyopia. Possibly iodoquinol causes fewer side effects since less is absorbed through the gastrointestinal tract than with iodochlorhydroxyquin. It has been suggested in patients being treated for acrodermatitis enteropathica, a disease of inherited zinc deficiency, optic atrophy may be secondary to zinc deficiency instead of iodochlorhydroxyquin or iodoquinol.

References:

Behrens, M. M.: Optic atrophy in children after diiodohydroxyquin therapy. JAMA 228:693, 1974.
Berggren, L. and Hansson, O.: Treating acrodermatitis enteropathica. Lancet 1:52, 1966.
Etheridge, J. E., Jr., and Stewart, G. T.: Treating acrodermatitis enteropathica. Lancet 1:261, 1966.
Nakae, K., Yamamoto, S., and Igata, A.: Subacute myelo-optico-neuropathy (SMON) in Japan. Lancet 2:510, 1971.
Strandvik, B., and Zetterström, R.: Amaurosis after broxyquinoline. Lancet 1:922, 1968.
Sturtevant, F. M.: Zinc deficiency. Acrodermatitis enteropathica, optic atrophy, SMON, and 5, 7-dihalo-8-quinolinols. Pediatrics 65:610, 1980.
Van Balen, A. T. M.: Toxic damage to the optic nerve caused by iodochlorhydroxy-quinoline (Enterovioform). Ophthalmologica 163:8, 1971.
Warshawsky, R. S., et al.: Acrodermatitis enteropathica. Corneal involvement with histochemical and electron micrographic studies. Arch. Ophthalmol. 93:194, 1975.

Generic Name: Emetine

Proprietary Name: Emetine

Primary Use: This alkaloid is effective in the treatment of acute amebic dysentery, amebic hepatitis, and amebic abscesses.

Ocular Side Effects:

A. Systemic Administration
   1. Nonspecific ocular irritation
      a. Lacrimation
      b. Hyperemia
      c. Photophobia

2. Pupils
    a. Mydriasis
    b. Absence of reaction to light
3. Paralysis of accommodation
4. Decreased vision
5. Eyelids or conjunctiva
    a. Urticaria
    b. Purpura
    c. Eczema
6. Visual fields
    a. Scotomas — central
    b. Constriction
B. Inadvertent Ocular Exposure
    1. Irritation
        a. Lacrimation
        b. Hyperemia
        c. Photophobia
    2. Eyelids or conjunctiva
        a. Allergic reactions
        b. Conjunctivitis — nonspecific
        c. Edema
        d. Blepharospasm
    3. Keratitis
    4. Corneal ulceration
    5. Iritis
    6. Corneal opacities

Clinical Significance: Systemic emetine occasionally causes adverse ocular effects; however, discontinuation of the drug returns the eyes to normal within a few days to weeks. Topical ocular exposure may cause a severe irritative response lasting from 24 to 48 hours. Typically, this ocular discomfort does not occur until 4 to 10 hours after the initial contact. Only one case of permanent blindness secondary to corneal opacities has been reported from inadvertent ocular exposure of emetine.

References:

Blue, J. B.: Emetin: A warning. (Correspondence). JAMA 65:1297, 1915.
Duke-Elder, S.: Systems of Ophthalmology. St. Louis, C. V. Mosby, Vol. XIV, Part 2, 1972, p. 1187.
Grant, W. M.: Toxicology of the Eye. 2nd Ed., Springfield, Charles C Thomas, 1974, pp. 445–446.
Jacovides: Troubles visuels a la suite d'injections fortes d'emetine. Arch. Ophtalmol. (Paris) 40:657, 1923.
Lasky, M. A.: Corneal response to emetine hydrochloride. Arch. Ophthalmol. 44:47, 1950.

Porges, N.: Tragedy in compounding. (Letter). J. Am. Pharm. Assoc. Pract. Pharm. 9:593, 1948.
Torres Estrada, A.: Ocular lesions caused by emetine. Bol. Hosp. Oftal. NS Luz. (Mex.) 2:145, 1944 (Am. J. Ophthalmol. 28:1060, 1945).
Wade, A. (Ed.): Martindale: The Extra Pharmacopoeia. 27th Ed., London, Pharmaceutical Press, 1977, pp. 343–351.

Class: Anthelmintics

Generic Name: 1. Antimony Lithium Thiomalate; 2. Antimony Potassium Tartrate; 3. Antimony Sodium Tartrate; 4. Antimony Sodium Thioglycollate; 5. Sodium Antimonylgluconate; 6. Stibocaptate; 7. Stibogluconate; 8. Stibophen

Proprietary Name: 1. Anthiomaline (G.B.); 2. Antimonial Wine (G.B.); 3. Antimony Sodium Tartrate; 4. Antimony Sodium Thioglycollate; 5. Sodium Antimonylgluconate; 6. Astiban (G.B.); 7. Pentostam; 8. Fantorin (Ind.), Fuadin

Primary Use: These trivalent antimony compounds are used in the treatment of schistosomiasis and filariasis.

Ocular Side Effects:

A. Systemic Administration
  1. Eyelids or conjunctiva
     a. Edema
     b. Urticaria
  2. Yellow discoloration of skin or sclera
  3. Decreased vision
  4. Pupils
     a. Mydriasis
     b. Absence of reaction to light
  5. Papilledema
  6. Optic atrophy
  7. Toxic amblyopia
  8. Subconjunctival or retinal hemorrhages secondary to drug-induced anemia

Clinical Significance: Since antimonials are rarely used in developed countries, only limited data on their complete toxicologic effects are available. While the preceding adverse reactions have been reported, few are well documented. Serious adverse ocular reactions have been seen, although infrequently.

References:

D'Amino, D.: Considerazioni sopra un caso di cecita instantanea bilaterale da avvelenamento per tartaro stibiato nella cura del Kala-azar. Lett. Oftalmol. 8:474, 1931.

Gilman, A. G., Goodman, L. S., and Gilman, A. (Eds.): The Pharmacological Basis of Therapeutics. 6th Ed., New York, Macmillan, 1980, pp. 1028–1031, 1074–1075.

Grant, W. M.: Toxicology of the Eye. 2nd Ed., Springfield, Charles C Thomas, 1974, p. 150.

Wade, A. (Ed.): Martindale: The Extra Pharmacopoeia. 27th Ed., London, Pharmaceutical Press, 1977, pp. 1371–1373, 1377–1379.

Generic Name: Diethylcarbamazine

Proprietary Name: Banocide, Carbilazine (Austral.), Ethodryl (G.B.), Franocide, Hetrazan, Notezine (Fr.)

Primary Use: This antifilarial agent is particularly effective against *W. bancrofti, W. malayi, O. volvulus,* and *Loa loa.*

Ocular Side Effects:

A. Systemic Administration
1. Eyelids or conjunctiva
   a. Allergic reactions
   b. Conjunctivitis—nonspecific
   c. Edema
   d. Urticaria
   e. Nodules
2. Uveitis
3. Visual field defects
4. Retinal pigmentary changes
5. Loss of eyelashes or eyebrows
6. Toxic amblyopia

Clinical Significance: Adverse ocular reactions to diethylcarbamazine may occur, but primarily only indirectly. After the filaria has been killed by the drug, an allergic reaction due to the release of foreign protein from the dead larvae or adult worms may occur. Nodules may form in the area of the dead worm with a resultant inflammatory reaction. This reaction in the eye may be so marked that toxic amblyopia follows.

References:

AMA Drug Evaluations. 4th Ed., New York, John Wiley & Sons, 1980, pp. 1416–1417.
American Hospital Formulary Service. Washington, D.C., American Society of Hospital Pharmacists, Vol. I, 8:08, 1978.
Bird, A. C., et al.: Visual loss during oral diethylcarbamazine treatment for onchocerciasis. Br. Med. J. 2:46, 1979.
Dralands, L.: Les anthelminthiques. Bull. Soc. Belge Ophtalmol. 160:436, 1972.
Duke, B. O. L.: Medicine in the tropics. Onchocerciasis. Br. Med. J. 4:301, 1968.
Dukes, M. N. G. (Ed.): Meyler's Side Effects of Drugs. Amsterdam, Excerpta Medica, Vol. IX, 1980, p. 540.
Gray, H. H.: Alopecia totalis after diethylcarbamazine treatment of loiasis. Trans. R. Soc. Trop. Med. Hyg. 59:718, 1965.

Generic Name: Piperazine

Proprietary Name: Adipalit (Ital.), Ancazine (Canad.), Antelmina (Fr.), Antepar, Antivermine (Pol.), Ascalix (G.B.), Bryrel, Citrazine (Austral.), Dietelmin (Fr.), Divermex (Austral.), Entacyl (G.B.), Eraverm (Germ.), Helmezine (G.B.), Lumbrioxyl (Fr.), Multifuge, Oxucide, Oxypel (Canad.), Paravermin (Germ.), Perin, Pinsirup, Pin-Tega, Pipenin (Jap.), Piperasol (Pol.), Piperol (Fr.), Piperzinal (Canad.), Pipril, Piprosan (Austral.), Razine, Stavermol (Germ.), Tasnon (Germ.), Ta-Verm, Uvilon (Germ.), Vermago, Vermicompren (Germ.), Vermolina (Austral.)

Primary Use: This anthelmintic agent is used in the treatment of ascariasis and enterobiasis.

Ocular Side Effects:

A. Systemic Administration
1. Decreased vision
2. Problems with color vision—dyschromatopsia
3. Paralysis of accommodation
4. Miosis
5. Nystagmus
6. Visual hallucinations
7. Paralysis of extraocular muscles
8. Visual sensations
   a. Flashing lights
   b. Entopic light flashes
9. Eyelids or conjunctiva
   a. Allergic reactions
   b. Edema
   c. Photosensitivity

      d. Urticaria

      e. Purpura

      f. Erythema multiforme

      g. Eczema

  10. Lacrimation

  11. Subconjunctival or retinal hemorrhages secondary to drug-induced anemia

  12. Cataracts (?)

Clinical Significance: While a number of ocular side effects have been attributed to piperazine, they are rare, reversible, and usually of little clinical importance. Adverse ocular reactions generally occur only in instances of overdose or in cases of impaired renal excretion. Only a few cases of well-documented extraocular muscle paralysis have been reported. Data on the cataractogenic potential of this drug are unproved; however, there are increasing data to suggest photosensitizing drugs have this potential.

References:

AMA Drug Evaluations. 4th Ed., New York, John Wiley & Sons, 1980, pp. 1420–1421.

American Hospital Formulary Service. Washington, D.C., American Society of Hospital Pharmacists, Vol. I, 8:08, 1978.

Bomb, B. S., and Bebi, H. K.: Neurotoxic side-effects of piperazine. Trans. R. Soc. Trop. Med. Hyg. 70:358, 1976.

Brown, H. W., Chan, K. F., and Hussey, K. L.: Treatment of enterobiasis and ascariasis with piperazine. JAMA *161*:515, 1956.

Combes, B., Damon, A., and Gottfried, E.: Piperazine (Antepar) neurotoxicity. Report of a case probably due to renal insufficiency. N. Engl. J. Med. 254:223, 1956.

Mezey, P.: The role of piperazine derivates in the pathogenesis of cataract. Klin. Monatsbl. Augenheilkd. *151*:885, 1967.

Walsh, F. B., and Hoyt, W. F.: Clinical Neuro-Ophthalmology. 3rd Ed., Baltimore, Williams & Wilkins, Vol. III, 1969, pp. 2637–2638.

Generic Name: Quinacrine (Mepacrine)

Proprietary Name: Atabrine, Tenicridine (Fr.)

Primary Use: This methoxyacridine agent is effective in the treatment of tapeworm infestations and in the prophylaxis and treatment of malaria.

Ocular Side Effects:

  A. Systemic Administration

      1. Decreased vision

      2. Visual fields

         a. Scotomas

         b. Enlarged blind spot

3. Optic neuritis
4. Corneal edema
5. Yellow, white, clear, brown, blue, or grey punctate deposits
    a. Conjunctiva
    b. Cornea
    c. Nasolacrimal system
6. Problems with color vision
    a. Dyschromatopsia
    b. Objects have yellow, green, blue, or violet tinge
    c. Colored haloes around lights—mainly blue
7. Subconjunctival or retinal hemorrhages secondary to drug-induced anemia
8. Eyelids or conjunctiva
    a. Blue-black hyperpigmentation
    b. Yellow discoloration
    c. Urticaria
    d. Exfoliative dermatitis
    e. Eczema
9. Photophobia
10. Paresis of extraocular muscles
11. Retinal pigmentary changes (?)
12. Ocular teratogenic effects (?)
B. Inadvertent Ocular Exposure
    1. Blue haloes around lights
    2. Eyelids, conjunctiva, or cornea
        a. Edema
        b. Yellow discoloration
    3. Irritation
        a. Lacrimation
        b. Ocular pain

Clinical Significance: Adverse ocular reactions due to quinacrine are common but seldom of clinical significance. Nearly all are reversible and fairly asymptomatic. Topical ocular application has been used for self-inflicted ocular damage; however, it has been apparently fairly devoid of any permanent ocular damage. Corneal deposits will disappear with time once the drug is discontinued; skin pigmentation will likewise diminish and often disappears as well.

References:

Abbey, E. A., and Lawrence, E. A.: The effect of Atabrine suppressive therapy on eyesight of pilots. JAMA 130:786, 1946.
American Hospital Formulary Service. Washington, D.C., American Society of Hospital Pharmacists, Vol. I, 8:08, 1978.

Chamberlain, W. P., and Boles, D. J.: Edema of the cornea precipitated by quinacrine (Atabrine). Arch. Ophthalmol. 35:120, 1946.

Dame, L. R.: The effects of Atabrine on the human visual system. Am. J. Ophthalmol. 29:1432, 1946.

Ferrara, A.: Optic neuritis from high doses of Atebrin. Rass. Ital. Ottalmol. 12:123, 1943.

Mann, I.: "Blue haloes" in Atebrin workers. Br. J. Ophthalmol. 31:40, 1947.

Generic Name: Suramin. See under *Class: Antiprotozoal Agents.*

Generic Name: Thiabendazole

Proprietary Name: Mintezol, Minzolum (Germ.)

Primary Use: This benzimidazole compound is used in the treatment of enterobiasis, strongyloidiasis, ascariasis, uncinariasis, trichuriasis, and cutaneous larva migrans. It has been advocated as an antimycotic in corneal ulcers.

Ocular Side Effects:

A. Systemic Administration
   1. Decreased vision
   2. Problems with color vision
      a. Dyschromatopsia
      b. Objects have yellow tinge
   3. Abnormal visual sensations
   4. Eyelids or conjunctiva
      a. Allergic reactions
      b. Hyperemia
      c. Angioneurotic edema
      d. Erythema multiforme
      e. Stevens-Johnson syndrome
      f. Exfoliative dermatitis
      g. Lyell's syndrome
   5. Keratoconjunctivitis sicca
   6. Subconjunctival or retinal hemorrhages secondary to drug-induced anemia

Clinical Significance: While thiabendazole is one of the more potent therapeutic agents known, it has surprisingly few reported ocular or systemic toxic side effects. Ocular side effects are transitory, reversible, and seldom of clinical importance. However, a mother and daughter after only a few doses developed keratoconjunctivitis sicca, xerostomia, cholangiostatic hepatitis, and pancreatic dysfunction. This is apparently an immunologic response, and the drug possibly acted as a hapten. These cases, as with practolol and one case due to penicillamine, may be the first instance of an oral medication affecting the periocular tissue by this type of mechanism.

References:

AMA Drug Evaluations. 4th Ed., New York, John Wiley & Sons, 1980, pp. 1425–1426.
Drugs for parasitic infections. Med. Lett. Drugs Ther. *21*:105, 1979.
Fink, A. I., MacKay, C. J., and Cutler, S. S.: Sicca complex and cholestatic jaundice in two members of a family caused by thiabendazole. Trans. Am. Ophthalmol. Soc. 76:108, 1978.
Fraunfelder, F. T.: Interim report: National Registry of Drug-Induced Ocular Side Effects. Ophthalmology *86*:126, 1979.
Gilman, A. G., Goodman, L. S., and Gilman, A. (Eds.): The Pharmacological Basis of Therapeutics. 6th Ed., New York, Macmillan, 1980, pp. 1027-1028.

Class: Antibiotics

Generic Name: 1. Amoxicillin; 2. Ampicillin; 3. Carbenicillin; 4. Cloxacillin; 5. Dicloxacillin; 6. Hetacillin; 7. Methicillin; 8. Nafcillin; 9. Oxacillin

Proprietary Name: 1. Amoxil, Amoxycillin (G. B.), Clamoxyl (Germ., Jap.), Imacillin (Swed.), Larotid, Polymox, Pasetocin (Jap.), Robamox, Sawacillin (Jap.), Sumox, Trimox, Utimox, Ulymox; 2. Acillin, A-Cillin, Alpen, Amblosin (Germ.), Amcill, Amipenix (Jap.), Ampen (Canad.), Amperil, Ampexin (Canad.), Ampicin (Canad.), Ampilean (Canad.), Ampilum (Ital.), Ampilux (Ital.), Ampipenin (Swed.), Austrapen (Austral.), Binotal (Germ.), D-Amp, D-Cillin, Deripen (Germ.), Doktacillin (Swed.), Domicillin (Jap.), Omnipen, Pen A or A/N, Pen-Bristol (Germ.), Penbriten, Penbritine (Fr.), Penbrock (Germ.), Penicline (Fr.), Pensyn, Pentrex (S. Afr.), Pentrexyl (G.B.), Pfizerpen A, Polycillin, Principen, Ro-ampen, Roampicillin, SK-Ampicillin, Supen, Suractin (Germ.), Synpenin (Jap.), Totacillin, Totapen (Fr.), Vidopen (G.B.); 3. Anabactyl (Germ.), Carbapen (Austral.), Fugacillin (Swed.), Geocillin, Geopen, Microcillin (Germ.), Pyopen; 4. Austrastaph (Austral.), Clocillin (Jap.), Cloxapen, Cloxypen (Fr.), Ekvacillin (Swed.), Orbenin, Orbenine (Fr.), Prostaphlin-A (S. Afr.), Staphobristol (Germ.), Staphybiotic (Fr.), Tegopen; 5.

Constaphyl (Germ.), Dichlor-Stapenor (Germ.), Diclocil (Fr., S. Afr.), Diclocila (Swed.), Dycill, Dynapen, Pathocil, Stafopenin (Swed.), Veracillin; 6. Penplenum, Uropen, Versapen; 7. Azapen, Belfacillin (Swed.), Celbenin, Cinopenil (Germ.), Flabelline (Fr.), Lucopenin (Denm.), Metin (Austral.), Penistaph (Fr.), Staphcillin, Synticillin (Denm.); 8. Nafcil, Unipen; 9. Bactocill, Bristopen (G.B., Fr.), Cryptocillin (Germ.), Prostaphlin, Staphenor (Germ.)

Primary Use: Semisynthetic penicillins are primarily effective against staphylococci, streptococci, pneumococci, and various other gram-positive and gram-negative bacteria.

Ocular Side Effects:

A. Systemic Administration
  1. Eyelids or conjunctiva
     a. Allergic reactions
     b. Blepharoconjunctivitis—nonspecific
     c. Edema
     d. Photosensitivity
     e. Angioneurotic edema
     f. Urticaria
     g. Erythema multiforme
     h. Stevens-Johnson syndrome
     i. Exfoliative dermatitis
     j. Lyell's syndrome
  2. Subconjunctival or retinal hemorrhages secondary to drug-induced anemia
  3. Diplopia (?)
  4. Decreased pupillary reaction to light (?)
B. Local Ophthalmic Use or Exposure—Topical Application or Subconjunctival Injection
  1. Irritation—primarily with subconjunctival injection
     a. Hyperemia
     b. Ocular pain
     c. Edema
  2. Eyelids or conjunctiva
     a. Allergic reactions
     b. Angioneurotic edema
  3. Overgrowth of nonsusceptible organisms
  4. Corneal opacities (cloxacillin)—primarily with subconjunctival injection
  5. Conjunctival necrosis (nafcillin)—primarily with subconjunctival injection
  6. Problems with color vision—dyschromatopsia (?) (hetacillin)

C. Local Ophthalmic Use or Exposure—Intracameral Injection
  1. Uveitis (methicillin)
  2. Corneal edema (methicillin)
  3. Lens damage (methicillin)

Clinical Significance: Surprisingly few ocular side effects other than dermatologically or hematologically related conditions have been reported with the semisynthetic penicillins. The incidence of allergic skin reactions due to ampicillin, however, is quite high. Nafcillin has been reported to cause conjunctival necrosis with subconjunctival injections.

Interactions with Other Drugs:

A. Effect of Other Drugs on Activity of Semisynthetic Penicillins
  1. Salicylates ↑
  2. Sulfonamides ↑
  3. Antibiotics ↓
     (Chloramphenicol, Erythromycin, Tetracyclines)
B. Cross Sensitivity
  1. Other penicillins

References:

AMA Drug Evaluations. 4th Ed., New York, John Wiley & Sons, 1980, pp. 384–385, 1215–1227.

Brick, D. C., West, C., and Ostler, H. B.: Ocular toxicity of subconjunctival nafcillin. Invest. Ophthalmol. Vis. Sci. (Suppl.) 18:132, 1979.

Davidson, S. I.: Reports of ocular adverse reactions. Trans. Ophthalmol. Soc. U. K. 93:495, 1973.

Ellis, P. P.: Handbook of Ocular Therapeutics and Pharmacology. 5th Ed., St. Louis, C. V. Mosby, 1977, pp. 33, 40, 45, 141–142.

Gilman, A. G., Goodman, L. S., and Gilman, A. (Eds.): The Pharmacological Basis of Therapeutics. 6th Ed., New York, Macmillan, 1975, pp. 1141–1150.

Laroche, J., and Laroche, C.: Nouvelles recherches sur la modification de la vision des couleurs sous l'action des medicaments à dose thérapeutique. Ann. Pharm. Fr. 35:173, 1977.

Generic Name: Bacitracin

Proprietary Name: Baciguent (*Systemic* and *Ophthalmic*)

Primary Use: This polypeptide bactericidal agent is primarily effective against gram positive cocci, *Neisseria,* and organisms causing gas gangrene.

Ocular Side Effects:

A. Systemic Administration
   1. Myasthenic neuromuscular blocking effect
      a. Paralysis of extraocular muscles
      b. Ptosis
   2. Decreased vision
   3. Diplopia
   4. Eyelids or conjunctiva
      a. Allergic reactions
      b. Angioneurotic edema
      c. Urticaria
B. Local Ophthalmic Use or Exposure—Topical Application or Subconjunctival Injection
   1. Irritation
   2. Eyelids or conjunctiva
      a. Allergic reactions
      b. Blepharoconjunctivitis—nonspecific
      c. Edema
      d. Urticaria
   3. Keratitis
   4. Overgrowth of nonsusceptible organisms
C. Local Ophthalmic Use or Exposure—Intracameral Injection
   1. Uveitis
   2. Corneal edema
   3. Lens damage

Clinical Significance: Ocular side effects from either systemic or ocular administration of bacitracin are rare. However, with increasing use of "fortified" bacitracin solution (10,000 units per ml), marked conjunctival irritation and keratitis may occur, especially if the drops are used frequently. The potential of decreased wound healing with prolonged use is real. The myasthenic neuromuscular blocking effect is more commonly seen if bacitracin is used in combination with neomycin, kanamycin, polymyxin, or colistin. Severe ocular or periocular allergic reactions, while rare, have been seen due to topical ophthalmic bacitracin application.

References:

Gilman, A. G., Goodman, L. S., and Gilman, A. (Eds.): The Pharmacological Basis of Therapeutics. 6th Ed., New York, Macmillan, 1975, pp. 1231–1232.
McQuillen, M. P., Cantor, H. E., and O'Rourke, J. R.: Myasthenic syndrome associated with antibiotics. Arch. Neurol. 18:402, 1968.
Small, G. A.: Respiratory paralysis after a large dose of intraperitoneal polymyxin B and bacitracin. Anesth. Analg. 43:137, 1964.

Wade, A. (Ed.): Martindale: The Extra Pharmacopoeia. 27th Ed., London, Pharmaceutical Press, 1977, pp. 1078–1079.
Walsh, F. B., and Hoyt, W. F.: Clinical Neuro-Ophthalmology. 3rd Ed., Baltimore, Williams & Wilkins, Vol. III, 1969, p. 2680.

Generic Name: 1. Benzathine Penicillin G; 2. Hydrabamine Penicillin V; 3. Potassium Penicillin G (Benzylpenicillin Potassium); 4. Potassium Penicillin V (Phenoxymethylpenicillin Potassium); 5. Potassium Phenethicillin; 6. Procaine Penicillin G

Proprietary Name: 1. Ben-P (Canad.), Bicillin, Dibencil, Duapen (Canad.), Dulpecen-G (Austral.), Extencilline (Fr.), LPG (Austral.), Neolin (G.B.), Penidural (G.B.), Penilente-LA (S. Afr.), Permapen, Tardocillin (Germ.); 2. Abbocillin-V (Austral.), Flavopen (Austral.); 3. Abbocillin (Canad.), Abbocillin-G (Austral.), Arcocillin, Biotic-T, Burcillin-G, Cilloral, Cryspen, Crystapen (G.B.), Deltapen, Dymocillin (Canad.), Eskacillin 100 (G.B.), Falapen (G.B.), Fivepen (Canad.), Forpen (Canad.), G-Recillin-T, Hyasorb, Hylenta (Canad.), Ka-Pen (Canad.), K-Cillin, Kesso-Pen, K-Pen, Lanacillin, Lemicillin, Liquapen, Nece-Pen (Fr.), Neo-Pens (Canad.), Novopen (Canad., S. Afr.), P-50 (Canad.), Paclin G, Palocillin, Parcillin, Penalev, Pencitabs (Canad.), Penevan (Austral.), Penioral (Canad.), Peniset (Austral.), Pensol (Austral.), Pensorb, Pentids, Pfizerpen G, Pharmacillin (Germ.), Purapen G (G.B.), SK-Penicillin G, Solupen (G.B.), Specilline G (Fr.), Sugracillin, Tabillin (G.B.), Therapen-K (Canad.), Tu Cillin, Wescopen (Canad.); 4. Abbocillin VK (Austral.), Acocillin (Swed.), Apopen (Swed.), Apsin VK (G.B.), Arcasin (Germ.), Beromycin (Germ.), Betapen-VK, Biotic-V, Bopen V-K, Bramcillin (Austral.), Calciopen (Swed.), Calcipen (Austral., Norw.), Caps-Pen V (Austral.), Cilicaine-V or VK (Austral.), Cillaphen (Austral.), Co-Caps Penicillin V-K (G.B.), Cocillin V-K, Compocillin-VK, Corcillin V (S. Afr.), Crystapen V (G.B.), Crystapen-VK (Austral.), CVK (G.B.), CVL (Austral.), Darocillin (S. Afr.), Deltacillin (S. Afr.), Diacipen-VK (S. Afr.), Distaquaine V or V-K (G.B.), Dowpen VK, Econocil-VK (G.B.), Econopen V (G.B.), Falcopen V or VK (Austral.), Fenoxcillin (Denm.), Fenoxypen (Germ., S. Afr., Swed.), GPV (G.B.), Hi-Pen (Canad.), Ia-pen (G.B.), Icipen (G.B.), Isocillin (Germ.), Ispenoral (Germ.), Jatcillin (S. Afr.), Kabipenin (Germ.), Kavepenin (Swed.), Kesso-Pen-VK, Lanacillin VK, Ledercillin VK, LPV (Austral.), LV, Meropenin (Swed.), Nadopen-V (Canad.), Norcillin (G.B.), Novopen-V (Canad.), Nutracillin (S. Afr.), Oracilline (Fr.), Orapen (S. Afr.), Oratren (Germ.), Orvepen (Neth.), Ospen (Fr., Germ.), Ospeneff (G.B.), Paclin VK, Pancillen (Austral.), Penapar VK, Pencompren (Germ.), Pengen-VK,

Penicals (G.B.), Penicillin V-K (Austral.), Peni-Vee (K) (Austral.), Penoxyl VK (G.B.), Pen-Vee (Canad.), Pen-Vee K, Pfipen V (Austral.), Pfizerpen VK, Phenethicillin, P-Mega-Tablinen (Germ.), Propen-VK (Austral.), PVF K (Canad.), PVK (Austral.), PVO (Austral.), QIDpen VK, Repen-VK, Robicillin VK, Rocilin (Austral., Norw.), Ro-Cillin VK, Roscopenin (Swed.), Saropen-VK, SK-Penicillin VK, Stabillin V-K (G.B.), Suspen V (Austral.), Ticillin V-K (G.B.), Tikacillin (Swed.), Uticillin VK, V-Cil-K (G.B.), V-Cillin K, VC-K (Canad.), Veecillin (Austral.), Veekay (S. Afr.), Veetids, Vepen (Swed.), Viacillin (Swed.), Vicin (Austral.), Vikacillin (S. Afr.), Viraxacillin-V (Austral.), V-Pen, VPV (Austral.), Weifapenin (Scand.), Win-V-K (Canad.); 5. Bendralan (Norw., S. Afr.), Broxil (G.B.), Chemipen, Maxipen, Pen-200 (Germ.), Peniplus (Fr.), Pensig (Austral.), Ro-Cillin, Syncillin, Synthecilline (Fr.); 6. Almopen (S. Afr.), Aquacaine G (Austral.), Aquacillin (Austral.), Ayercillin (Canad.), Cilicaine (Austral.), Crysticillin AS, Depocillin, Depocilline (S. Afr.), Duracillin AS, Eskacillin (G.B.), Evacilin (Austral.), Flo-Cillin, Flocilline (Fr.), Francacilline (Canad.), Hostacillin (Austral.), Hydracillin (Swed.), Ibacillin (Canad.), Megapen (Austral.), Novocillin (S. Afr.), Parencillin, Penlator, Pentids-P, Pfizerpan-AS, Procillin (Austral., S. Afr.), Pro-Stabillin AS (G.B.), Suspenin (Swed.), Therapen (Canad.), Viraxacillin (Austral.), Wycillin

Primary Use: These bactericidal penicillins are effective against streptococci, *S. aureus*, gonococci, meningococci, pneumococci, *T. pallidum*, *Clostridium*, *B. anthracis*, *C. diphtheriae*, and several species of *Actinomyces*.

Ocular Side Effects:

A. Systemic Administration
   1. Mydriasis
   2. Decreased accommodation
   3. Diplopia
   4. Papilledema
   5. Decreased vision
   6. Visual hallucinations
   7. Visual agnosia
   8. Eyelids or conjunctiva
      a. Allergic reactions
      b. Erythema
      c. Blepharoconjunctivitis—nonspecific
      d. Edema
      e. Angioneurotic edema

       f. Urticaria

       g. Lupoid syndrome

       h. Stevens-Johnson syndrome

       i. Lyell's syndrome

    9. Subconjunctival or retinal hemorrhages secondary to drug-induced anemia

B. Local Ophthalmic Use or Exposure—Topical Application or Subconjunctival Injection

    1. Irritation

    2. Eyelids or conjunctiva—allergic reactions

    3. Overgrowth of nonsusceptible organisms

C. Local Ophthalmic Use or Exposure—Intracameral Injection

    1. Uveitis

    2. Corneal edema

    3. Lens damage

Clinical Significance: Systemic administration of penicillin only rarely causes ocular side effects; however, topical ocular administration results in a high incidence of allergic reactions. The incidence of allergic reactions is greater in patients with Sjögren's syndrome or rheumatoid arthritis than in other individuals. The most serious adverse ocular reaction is papilledema secondary to elevated intracranial pressure. Most other ocular side effects due to penicillin are transient and reversible.

Interactions with Other Drugs:

A. Effect of Other Drugs on Activity of Penicillin

    1. Analgesics ↑

    2. Bacitracin ↑

    3. Salicylates ↑

    4. Antacids ↓

    5. Antibiotics ↓
       (Chloramphenicol, Erythromycin, Kanamycin, Neomycin, Streptomycin, Tetracyclines)

B. Synergistic Activity

    1. Cephalosporins

    2. Erythromycin

    3. Kanamycin

    4. Other penicillins

    5. Streptomycin

    6. Sulfonamides (occasionally indifferent or inhibitory)

C. Cross Sensitivity

    1. Cephalosporins

References:

Alarcón-Segovia, D.: Drug-induced antinuclear antibodies and lupus syndromes. Drugs *12*:69, 1976.

Bjornberg, A.: Hallucinatory reactions in association with oral administration of Probenecid Penicillin. Acta Med. Scand. *165*:207, 1959.

Bjornberg, A., and Selstam, J.: Acute psychotic reaction after injection of Procaine Penicilline. Acta Dermatovener. *37*:50, 1957.

Crews, S. J.: Ocular adverse reactions to drugs. Practitioner *219*:72, 1977.

New, P. S., and Wells, C. E.: Cerebral toxicity associated with massive intravenous penicillin therapy. Neurology *15*:1053, 1965.

Paull, A. M.: Occurrence of the "L.E." phenomenon in a patient with a severe penicillin reaction. N. Engl. J. Med. *252*:128, 1955.

Utley, P. M., Lucas, J. B., and Billings, T. E.: Acute psychotic reactions to aqueous Procaine Penicillin (G). South. Med. J. *59*:1271, 1966.

Generic Name: 1. Cefazolin; 2. Cephalexin; 3. Cephaloglycin; 4. Cephaloridine; 5. Cephalothin; 6. Cephradine

Proprietary Name: 1. Ancef, Celmetin (Swed.), Kefzol; 2. Ceporex (G.B.), Ceporexine (Fr., Swed.), Keflex, Oracef (Germ.); 3. Kafocin, Kefglycin; 4. Ceporan (Austral., Canad., S. Afr., Swed.), Ceporin (G.B.), Keflodin (Fr.), Kefspor (Germ., Swed.), Loridine; 5. Cefalotine (Fr.), Cepovenin (Germ.), Keflin; 6. Anspor, Cefril (S. Afr.), Eskacef (G.B.), Sefril (Germ.), Velosef

Primary Use: Cephalosporins are effective against streptococci, staphylococci, pneumococci, and strains of *E. coli, P. mirabilis,* and *Klebsiella.*

Ocular Side Effects:

A. Systemic Administration
  1. Nystagmus
  2. Eyelids or conjunctiva
     a. Allergic reactions
     b. Erythema
     c. Angioneurotic edema
     d. Urticaria
     e. Exfoliative dermatitis
  3. Subconjunctival or retinal hemorrhages secondary to drug-induced anemia
  4. Visual hallucinations
  5. Diplopia (cephaloridine)
  6. Decreased vision (?)
  7. Papilledema (?) (cephaloridine)
  8. Retinal pigmentary changes (?) (cephaloridine)

B. Local Ophthalmic Use or Exposure—Topical Application or Subconjunctival Injection
   1. Irritation
      a. Hyperemia
      b. Ocular pain
      c. Edema
   2. Eyelids or conjunctiva
      a. Allergic reactions
      b. Angioneurotic edema
      c. Urticaria
   3. Overgrowth of nonsusceptible organisms

Clinical Significance: Few significant ocular side effects have been reported with these antibiotics. All reported adverse ocular reactions are transitory when use of these drugs is discontinued. Only with cephaloridine has one possible instance of toxic papilledema or retinal change been suspected.

Interactions with Other Drugs:

A. Cross Sensitivity
   1. Penicillins

References:

AMA Drug Evaluations. 4th Ed., New York, John Wiley & Sons, 1980, pp. 1229–1248.
Ballingall, D. L. K., and Trupie, A. G. G.: Cephaloridine toxicity (Letter to editor). Lancet 2:835, 1967.
Crosbie, R. B.: Cephaloridine toxicity. Lancet 1:422, 1968.
Gilman, A. G., Goodman, L. S., and Gilman, A. (Eds.): The Pharmacological Basis of Therapeutics. 6th Ed., New York, Macmillan, 1980, pp. 1150–1157.
Grant, W. M.: Toxicology of the Eye. 2nd Ed., Springfield, Charles C Thomas, 1974, p. 249.

Generic Name: Chloramphenicol

Proprietary Name: *Systemic*: Amphicol, Aquamycetin (Germ.), Bipimycetin (Ind.), Catilan (Germ.), Chlomin (Austral.), Chloramex (S. Afr.), Chloramol (Austral.), Chloramphycin (Ind.), Chloramsaar (Germ.), Chlorcetin, Chlorcol (S. Afr.), Chlornicol (S. Afr.), Chloromycetin, Clorfen (S. Afr.), Cylphenicol, Enicol (Canad.), Fenicol (Canad.), Gotimycin (Germ.), Jatcetin (S. Afr.), Kamaver (Germ.), Kemicetine, Lennacol (S. Afr.), Leukomycin (Germ.), Mychel, Mycinol (Canad.), Nevimycin (Germ.), Novochlorocap (Canad.), Oleomycetin (Germ.), Pantovernil (Germ.), Paraxin, Pentamycetin (Canad.), Sintomicetine (Fr.), Solnicol (Fr.), Tifomycine (Fr.), Troymycetin (S.

Afr.) *Ophthalmic*: Antibiopto, Chloromycetin, Cloroptic, Econochlor, Kemicetin (G.B.), Opclor (Austral.), Ophthochlor

Primary Use: This bacteriostatic dichloracetic acid derivative is particularly effective against *Salmonella typhi, H. influenzae meningitis,* rickettsia, the lymphogranuloma-psittacosis group, and is useful in the management of cystic fibrosis.

Ocular Side Effects:

A. Systemic Administration
   1. Decreased vision
   2. Visual fields
      a. Scotomas
      b. Constriction
   3. Retrobulbar or optic neuritis
   4. Optic atrophy
   5. Toxic amblyopia
   6. Problems with color vision
      a. Dyschromatopsia
      b. Objects have yellow tinge
   7. Eyelids or conjunctiva
      a. Allergic reactions
      b. Angioneurotic edema
   8. Paralysis of accommodation
   9. Pupils
      a. Mydriasis
      b. Absence of reaction to light
  10. Retinal pigmentary changes
  11. Retinal edema
  12. Subconjunctival or retinal hemorrhages secondary to drug-induced anemia
  13. Nystagmus (?)
  14. Strabismus (?)
  15. Papilledema (?)
B. Local Ophthalmic Use or Exposure—Topical Application or Subconjunctival Injection
   1. Irritation
   2. Eyelids or conjunctiva
      a. Allergic reactions
      b. Depigmentation
   3. Overgrowth of nonsusceptible organisms
C. Local Ophthalmic Use or Exposure—Intracameral Injection
   1. Uveitis
   2. Corneal edema
   3. Lens damage

Clinical Significance: Ocular side effects from systemic chloramphenicol administration are uncommon in adults, but occur often in children, especially if the total dose exceeds 100 g or if therapy lasts over 6 weeks. Topical ophthalmic application causes infrequent ocular side effects. Although chloramphenicol has fewer allergic reactions than neomycin, those due to chloramphenicol are often the more severe. Like other antibiotics, this agent may cause latent hypersensitivity which lasts for many years. Topical ocular chloramphenicol probably has fewer toxic effects on the corneal epithelium than any other antibiotic. Four cases of significant blood dyscrasia or aplastic anemia following topical ocular chloramphenicol have been reported in the literature and to the Registry. Whether there is a cause-and-effect relationship is unknown. Chloramphenicol is the drug most commonly associated with aplastic anemia. The risk of developing pancytopenia or aplastic anemia after oral chloramphenicol treatment is 13 times greater than the risk of idiopathic aplastic anemia in the general population. Two forms of hemopoietic abnormalities, idiosyncratic and dose-related, may occur following systemic chloramphenicol. Although the latter response is unlikely from topical ophthalmic use of the drug, the incidence of the idiosyncratic response is unknown and indeed an important topic at this point in time. Each physician must weigh the evidence and decide if there is a specific reason for topical ophthalmic use of chloramphenicol since aplastic anemia potentially could occur. The facts are the following: 1. chloramphenicol is a known agent that can cause aplastic anemia; 2. the response following topical ophthalmic chloramphenicol would appear to be more likely idiosyncratic rather than dose related; 3. seldom is chloramphenicol indicated in ophthalmology that it cannot be substituted by another antibiotic; and 4. aplastic anemia occurs in 1 out of every 30,000 to 50,000 patients exposed to systemic chloramphenicol. Because it would require 1.5 million observations of patients on this drug to make a statistical correlation, a study does not appear feasible at this point since no one is interested in funding it. Therefore, it seems unlikely that medical data in the near future will provide an answer to this question, and each physician will have to decide the potential benefit-risk.

Interactions with Other Drugs:

   A. Effect of Chloramphenicol on Activity of Other Drugs
      1. Analgesics ↑
      2. Barbiturates ↑
      3. Cephalosporins ↓
      4. Penicillins ↓
   B. Effect of Other Drugs on Activity of Chloramphenicol
      1. Barbiturates ↓

C. Synergistic Activity
1. Erythromycin
2. Sulfonamides

References:

Abrams, S. M., Degnan, T. J., and Vinciguerra, V.: Marrow aplasia following topical application of chloramphenicol eye ointment. Arch. Intern. Med. *140*:576, 1980.

Cocke, J. G., Brown, R. E., and Geppert, L. J.: Optic neuritis with prolonged use of chloramphenicol. J. Pediatr. *68*:27, 1966.

Cole, J. G., Cole, H. G., and Janoff, L. A.: A toxic ocular manifestation of chloramphenicol therapy. Am. J. Ophthalmol. *44*:18, 1957.

Davidson, S. I.: Systemic effects of eye drops. Trans. Ophthalmol. Soc. U. K. *94*:487, 1974.

Francois, J., and Mortiers, P.: The injurious effects of locally and generally applied antibiotics on the eye. T. Geneeskd. *32*:139, 1976.

Fraunfelder, F. T., Bagby, G. C., Jr., and Kelly, D. J.: Fatal aplastic anemia following topical administration of ophthalmic chloramphenicol. Am. J. Ophthalmol. *93*:356, 1982.

Joy, R. J. T., Scalettar, R., and Sodee, D. B.: Optic and peripheral neuritis. Probable effect of prolonged chloramphenicol therapy. JAMA *173*:1731, 1960.

Lamda, P. A., Sood, N. N., and Moorthy, S. S.: Retinopathy due to chloramphenicol. Scot. Med. J. *13*:166, 1968.

Rosenthal, R. L., and Blackman, A.: Bone marrow hypoplasia following use of chloramphenicol eyedrops. JAMA *191*:136, 1965.

Rylance, G. W.: Chloramphenicol and phenobarbitone—a drug interaction. Arch. Dis. Child. *54*:563, 1979.

Generic Name: 1. Chlortetracycline; 2. Demeclocycline; 3. Doxycycline; 4. Methacycline; 5. Minocycline; 6. Oxytetracycline; 7. Tetracycline

Proprietary Name: *Systemic*: 1. Aureomycin, Aureomycine (Fr.), Chlortet (Austral.), CTC, Topmycin (S. Afr.); 2. Declomycin, Ledermycin, Ledermycine (Fr.), Mexocine (Fr.); 3. Doxin (Austral.), Doxy-II, Doxychel, Idocyklin (Swed.), Vibramycin, Vibramycine (Fr.), Vibra-Tabs, Vibraveineuse (Fr.), Vibravenös (Germ.); 4. Adriamicina (Ital.), Megamycine (Fr.), Rondomycin; 5. Klinomycin (Germ.), Minocin, Minomycin (Austral., S. Afr.), Mynocine (Fr.), Ultramycin (Canad.), Vectrin; 6. Abbocin (G.B.), Berkmycen (G.B.), Biotet (S. Afr.), Bobbamycin (Austral.), Chemocycline (G.B.), Clinimycin (G.B.), Dalimycin, Galenomycin (G.B.), Imperacin (G.B.), Lenocycline (S. Afr.), Macocyn (Germ.), 0-4-cycline (S. Afr.), Oppamycin (G.B.), Otetryn, Oxamycen (Jap.), Oxlopar, Oxycycline (Austral.), Oxydon (G.B.), Oxy-Dumocyclin (Swed.), Oxyject, Oxy-Kesso-Tetra, Oxymycin (G.B.), Oxytetral (Swed.), Roxy (S. Afr.), Stecsolin (G.B.), Terramycin, Terravenös (Germ.), Tetlong (S. Afr.), Tetramel (S. Afr.), Tetramine, Tetra-Tablinen (Germ.), Unimycin (G.B.), Uri-Tet, Vendarcin (Austral., Germ., Neth., S. Afr.); 7. Achromycin, Ambramycin-P

(S. Afr.), Amer-Tet, Amtet, Austramycin (Austral.), Bicycline, Brista-cycline, Bristrex, Capcycline (S. Afr.), Cefracycline (Canad.), Centet, Chemcycline (Canad.), Co-Caps Tetracycline (G.B.), Cycline, Cyclo-par, Decabiotic (Canad.), Decycline (Canad.), Dema, Desamycin, Dumocyclin (Swed.), Economycin (G.B.), Fed-Mycin, Fermentmycin (S. Afr.), Florocycline (Fr.), Gene-Cycline (Canad.), G-Mycin, GT-250/500 (Canad.), GT-Liquid (Canad.), Hexacycline (Fr.), Hostacy-clin (Germ.), Hostacycline (Austral., S. Afr.), Hydracycline (Austral.), Kesso-Tetra, Lemtrex, Lexacycline, Maso-Cycline, Maytrex, Mericy-cline, Miriamycine (Fr.), Muracine (Canad.), Neo-tetrine (Canad.), Nor-Tet, Novotetra (Canad.), Oppacyn (G.B.), Paltet, Panmycin, Par-trex, Pexobiotic (Canad.), Phosmycine (S. Afr.), Piracaps, Polycycline, QIDtet, Quadcin (N.Z.), Quadracycline-V (Austral.), Quatrax (Aus-tral.), Retet, Rexamycin, Robitet, Ro-Cycline, Sanclomycine (Fr.), Sarocycline, Scotrex, Sifacycline (Fr.), SK-Tetracycline, Steclin, Sumy-cin, Supramycin N (Germ.), Sustamycin (G.B.), Svedocyklin (Swed.), T-125/250, T-Caps, Tet-Cy, Tetrabiotic (Canad.), Tetra-C, Tetracap (Austral., Canad.), Tetrachel, Tetracitro S (Germ.), Tetraclor, Tetra-Co, Tetracrine (Canad.), Tetracyn, Tetracyne (Fr.), Tetradecin Novum (Swed.), Tetral (Canad.), Tetralan, Tetralean (Canad.), Tetralution (Germ.), Tetram, Tetramax, Tetramykoin (Austral.), Tetrex, Tetrosol (Canad.), T-Liquid (Canad.), Totomycin (G.B.), Trexin, Triacycline (Canad.), T-Tabs (Canad.), U-Tet, Wintracin (Canad.) *Ophthalmic*: 1. Aureomycin; 7. Achromycin

Primary Use: These bacteriostatic derivatives of polycyclic naphthacene carboxamide are effective against a wide range of gram-negative and gram-positive organisms, mycoplasm, and members of the lymphogran-uloma-psittacosis group.

Ocular Side Effects:

A. Systemic Administration
   1. Myopia
   2. Papilledema secondary to pseudotumor cerebri
   3. Decreased vision
   4. Photophobia
   5. Diplopia (minocycline, tetracycline)
   6. Problems with color vision (chlortetracycline)
      a. Dyschromatopsia
      b. Objects have yellow tinge
   7. Eyelids or conjunctiva
      a. Erythema
      b. Edema

      c. Yellow discoloration (methacycline, tetracycline)

      d. Photosensitivity

      e. Angioneurotic edema

      f. Urticaria

      g. Lupoid syndrome

      h. Erythema multiforme

      i. Stevens-Johnson syndrome

      j. Lyell's syndrome

  8. Myasthenic neuromuscular blocking effect

      a. Paralysis of extraocular muscles

      b. Ptosis

  9. Subconjunctival or retinal hemorrhages secondary to drug-induced anemia

  10. Enlarged blind spot.

  11. Visual hallucinations

  12. Ocular teratogenic effects—cataracts (?)

  13. Loss of eyelashes or eyebrows (?) (minocycline, tetracycline)

B. Local Ophthalmic Use or Exposure—Topical Application or Subconjunctival Injection

  1. Irritation

  2. Eyelids or conjunctiva—allergic reactions

  3. Overgrowth of nonsusceptible organisms

  4. Yellow-brown corneal discoloration (with drug soaked hydrophilic lenses)

C. Local Ophthalmic Use or Exposure—Intracameral Injection

  1. Uveitis

  2. Corneal edema

  3. Lens damage

Clinical Significance: Systemic or ocular use of the tetracyclines rarely causes ocular side effects. While a large variety of drug-induced ocular side effects has been attributed to tetracyclines, most are reversible. There are increasing reports in the literature and to the Registry of this group of drugs causing pseudotumor cerebri. This is most commonly reported with tetracycline and minocycline. Minocycline possibly possesses greater lipoid solubility as it passes into the CSF more readily than other polycyclic naphthacene carboxamides. Increased intracranial pressure is not dose related and may occur as early as 4 hours after first taking the drug or even years later. The oldest case on record is in a 24-year-old male. Paresis or paralysis of extraocular muscles may occur secondary to pseudotumor cerebri. Tetracycline has been implicated in aggravating or unmasking of myasthenia gravis with its associated ocular findings. Transient color defects have been reported only with chlortetracycline. Methacycline has caused pigmentation of light-exposed skin and yellow-brown pigmentation of exposed conjunctiva with long-term therapy. This occurs in about 3 percent of patients taking 400 to 1,600 g of this agent. No permanent adverse effects are associated with these findings. A recent report has found a yellow-brown discoloration of the cornea when hydrophilic lens are presoaked in tetracycline prior to ocular application. This has been advocated by some in an attempt to increase ocular drug contact time. While there have been suggestions in humans and animals that congenital cataracts might occur in the offspring of mothers taking this group of drugs, only recently has intense topical ocular administration been suggested to cause lens opacities and coloration in young animals. It has been suggested that these lens changes may also occur with subconjunctival or intraocular injections of these agents. These data, however, are conjectural as far as human applicability is concerned. The lowest reported incidence of contact dermatitis due to commonly used antibiotics is with chlortetracycline.

Interactions with Other Drugs:

A. Effect of Tetracyclines on Activity of Other Drugs
  1. Penicillins ↓
B. Effect of Other Drugs on Activity of Tetracyclines
  1. Alcohol ↑
  2. Antacids ↓
  3. Riboflavin ↓
C. Synergistic Activity
  1. Streptomycin

References:

Argov, Z., and Mastaglia, F. L.: Disorders of neuromuscular transmission caused by drugs. N. Engl. J. Med. 301:409, 1979.

Dyster-Aas, K., et al.: Pigment deposits in eyes and light-exposed skin during long-term methacycline therapy. Acta Derm. Venereol. 54:209, 1974.

Edwards, T. S.: Transient myopia due to tetracycline. JAMA 186:69, 1963.

Giles, C. L., and Soble, A. R.: Intracranial hypertension and tetracycline therapy. Am. J. Ophthalmol. 72:981, 1971.

Koch-Weser, J., and Gilmore, E. B.: Benign intracranial hypertension in an adult after tetracycline therapy. JAMA 200:169, 1967.

Krejcí, L., and Brettschneider, I.: Yellow-brown cornea: A complication of topical use of tetracycline. Ophthalmic Res. 10:131, 1978.

Krejcí, L., Brettschneider, I., Tříska, J.: Tetracycline hydrochloride and lens changes. Ophthalmic Res. 10:36, 1978.

Minkin, W., Cohen, H. J., and Frank, S. B.: Fixed-drug eruption due to tetracycline. Arch. Derm. 100:749, 1969.

Monaco, F., Agnetti, V., and Mutani, R.: Benign intracranial hypertension after minocycline therapy. Eur. Neurol. 17:48, 1978.

Stuart, B. H., and Litt, I. F.: Tetracycline-associated intracranial hypertension in an adolescent: A complication of systemic acne therapy. J. Pediatr. 92:679, 1978.

Generic Name: 1. Clindamycin; 2. Erythromycin; 3. Lincomycin; 4. Vancomycin

Proprietary Name: *Systemic*: 1. Cleocin, Dalacin C (G.B.), Sobelin (Germ.); 2. Abboject (S. Afr.), Abboticin (Swed.), Abboticine (Fr.), Bristamycin, Chemthromycin (Canad.), E-Biotic, E.E.S., Emcinka (Canad.), EMU-V (Austral., S. Afr.), E-Mycin, Eratrex (Austral.), Eromel (S. Afr.), Eromycin (Austral.), Erostin (Austral.), Erycen (G.B.), Erycinum (Germ.), Erypar, Erythrocin, Erythromid (G.B.), Erythromycetine (Canad.), Erythroped (G.B.), Erythro-ST (Jap.), Ethril, Ethryn (Austral.), Ilosone, Ilotycin, Kesso-Mycin, Neo-Erycinum (Germ.), Novorythro (Canad.), Paediathrocin (Germ.), Pediamycin, Pfizer-E, Propiocine (Fr.), Retcin (G.B.), Robimycin, RP-Mycin, Rythrocaps (S. Afr.), SK-Erythromycin, Wyamycin; 3. Albiotic (Germ.), Cillimycin (Germ.), Lincocin, Mycivin (G.B.); 4. Vancocin *Ophthalmic*: 2. Ilotycin; 3. Lincocin

Primary Use: These bactericidal antibiotics are effective against gram-positive or gram-negative organisms.

Ocular Side Effects:

A. Systemic Administration
   1. Problems with color vision—dyschromatopsia, blue-yellow defect (erythromycin)
   2. Eyelids or conjunctiva
      a. Allergic reactions
      b. Hyperemia
      c. Photosensitivity
      d. Angioneurotic edema
      e. Urticaria
      f. Stevens-Johnson syndrome
      g. Exfoliative dermatitis
   3. Subconjunctival or retinal hemorrhages secondary to drug-induced anemia
B. Local Ophthalmic Use or Exposure—Topical Application or Subconjunctival Injection
   1. Irritation
      a. Hyperemia
      b. Ocular pain
      c. Edema
   2. Eyelids or conjunctiva
      a. Allergic reactions
      b. Angioneurotic edema

3. Overgrowth of nonsusceptible organisms
4. Subconjunctival hemorrhages (lincomycin)
5. Mydriasis (erythromycin)
C. Local Ophthalmic Use or Exposure—Intracameral Injection
   1. Uveitis (erythromycin)
   2. Corneal edema (erythromycin)
   3. Lens damage (erythromycin)
D. Local Ophthalmic Use or Exposure—Retrobulbar or Subtenon Injection
   1. Irritation (clindamycin)
   2. Optic neuritis (clindamycin)
   3. Optic atrophy (clindamycin)

Clinical Significance: Few adverse ocular reactions due to either systemic or ophthalmic use of these antibiotics are seen. Nearly all ocular side effects are transitory and reversible after the drug is discontinued. Most adverse ocular reactions are secondary to dermatologic or hematologic conditions. A well-documented rechallenged idiosyncratic response to topical ocular application of erythromycin causing mydriasis has been reported to the Registry.

Interactions with Other Drugs:

A. Effect of These Antibiotics on Activity of Other Drugs
   1. Clindamycin ↓
   2. Erythromycin ↓
   3. Lincomycin ↓
   4. Penicillins ↓
B. Effect of Other Drugs on Activity of These Antibiotics
   1. Clindamycin ↓
   2. Erythromycin ↓
   3. Lincomycin ↓

References:

AMA Drug Evaluations. 4th Ed., New York, John Wiley & Sons, 1980, pp. 1255–1264, 1302–1303.
Gilman, A. G., Goodman, L. S., and Gilman, A. (Eds.): The Pharmacological Basis of Therapeutics. 6th Ed., New York, Macmillan, 1980, pp. 1222–1231.
Kastrup, E. K., and Schwach, G. H. (Eds.): Facts and Comparisons. St. Louis, Facts and Comparisons, Inc., 1974, p. 423.
Physicians' Desk Reference. 35th Ed., Oradell, N.J., Medical Economics Co., 1981, pp. 831, 1098, 1805, 1824.

Generic Name: 1. Colistimethate; 2. Colistin

Proprietary Name: *Systemic*: 1. Colimycine (Fr.), Colistinat (Swed.), Colistin Sulphomethate (G.B.), Coly-Mycin (Austral.), Colomycin Injection (G.B.), Coly-Mycin M; 2. Colimycine (Fr.), Colomycin (G.B.), Coly-Mycin (Austral.), Coly-Mycin S *Ophthalmic*: 2. Coly-Mycin S

Primary Use: These bactericidal polypeptides are effective against *Aerobacter, E. coli, K. pneumoniae, Ps. aeruginosa, Shigella,* and *Salmonella.*

Ocular Side Effects:

A. Systemic Administration
 1. Nystagmus
 2. Myasthenic neuromuscular blocking effect
  a. Paralysis of extraocular muscles
  b. Ptosis
 3. Diplopia
 4. Mydriasis
B. Local Ophthalmic Use or Exposure—Topical Application or Subconjunctival Injection
 1. Irritation
 2. Eyelids or conjunctiva—allergic reactions
 3. Overgrowth of nonsusceptible organisms
C. Local Ophthalmic Use or Exposure—Intracameral Injection
 1. Uveitis
 2. Corneal edema
 3. Lens damage

Clinical Significance: Only a few cases of ocular side effects from systemic or ocular colistimethate or colistin therapy have been reported. These adverse ocular reactions are usually transitory, reversible, and of little clinical importance. In resistant cases with overgrowth of nonsusceptible organisms, *Proteus* has been the most common bacterial organism found. Unfortunately, Colimycin is also the name given to an antibiotic of the neomycin group available in the U.S.S.R.

Interactions with Other Drugs:

A. Effect of Colistimethate or Colistin on Activity of Other Drugs
 1. Antibiotics (apnea) ↑
  (Kanamycin, Neomycin, Polymyxin, Streptomycin)
 2. Anticholinesterases (apnea) ↑
 3. General anesthetics (apnea) ↑

B. Synergistic Activity
   1. Sulfonamides
C. Cross Sensitivity
   1. Gentamicin
   2. Kanamycin
   3. Polymyxin B
   4. Streptomycin

References:

Argov, Z., and Mastaglia, F. L.: Disorders of neuromuscular transmission caused by drugs. N. Engl. J. Med. *301*:409, 1979.
Gold, G. N., and Richardson, A. P.: An unusual case of neuromuscular blockade seen with therapeutic blood levels of colistin methanesulfonate. (Coly-Mycin). Am. J. Med. *41*:316, 1966.
Lund, M. H.: Colistin sulfate ophthalmic in the treatment of ocular infections. Arch. Ophthalmol. *81*:4, 1969.
McQuillen, M. P., Cantor, H. E., and O'Rourke, J. R.: Myasthenic syndrome associated with antibiotics. Arch. Neurol. *18*:402, 1968.
Wolinsky, E., and Hines, J. D.: Neurotoxic and nephrotoxic effects of colistin in patients with renal disease. N. Engl. J. Med. *266*:759, 1962.

Generic Name: Cycloserine. See under *Class: Antitubercular Agents.*

Generic Name: 1. Framycetin; 2. Neomycin

Proprietary Name: *Systemic*: 1. Framycetin; 2. Bykomycin (Germ.), Emelmycin (S. Afr.), Herisan Antibiotic (Canad.), Myacyne (Germ.), Mycifradin, Myciguent, Neobiotic, Neobram (Austral.), Neocin (Canad.), Neomate (Austral.), Neomin (G.B.), Neo Morrhuol (Austral.), Neopan (S. Afr.), Neopt (Austral.), Nivemycin (G.B.) *Ophthalmic*: 1. Framygen (G.B.), Soframycin (G.B.); 2. Myciguent, Nivemycin (G.B.)

Primary Use: These bactericidal aminoglycosidic agents are effective against *Ps. aeruginosa, Aerobacter, K. pneumoniae, P. vulgaris, E. coli, Salmonella, Shigella,* and most strains of *S. aureus.*

Ocular Side Effects:

A. Systemic Administration—Neomycin
   1. Myasthenic neuromuscular blocking effect
      a. Paralysis of extraocular muscles
      b. Ptosis
   2. Decreased or absent pupillary reaction to light

B. Local Ophthalmic Use or Exposure—Topical Application or Subconjunctival Injection
  1. Irritation
  2. Eyelids or conjunctiva
     a. Allergic reactions
     b. Erythema
     c. Conjunctivitis—follicular
     d. Urticaria
  3. Punctate keratitis
  4. Overgrowth of nonsusceptible organisms
C. Local Ophthalmic Use or Exposure—Intracameral Injection
  1. Uveitis (neomycin)
  2. Corneal edema (neomycin)
  3. Lens damage (neomycin)

Clinical Significance: It is rare for nontopical ophthalmic application to cause ocular side effects; however, there are well-documented reports of decreased or absent pupillary reactions due to application of neomycin to the pleural or peritoneal cavities during a thoracic or abdominal operation. Topical ocular application of neomycin has been reported to cause allergic conjunctival or lid reactions in 4 percent of patients using this drug. Elsewhere on the skin, it is from 1 to 6 percent, since the drug is a potent contact sensitizer. If neomycin is used topically for longer than 7 days on inflammatory dermatosis, the incidence of allergic reaction is increased thirteen-fold over matched controls. Neomycin preparations for minor infections rarely should be used over 7 days. Also, if the patient has been previously exposed to neomycin or is currently on this therapy for over 7 days, there is a significantly higher chance of an allergic response. In a recent series, neomycin was found to be one of the three more common drugs causing periocular allergic contact dermatitis. In addition, some feel that, of the more commonly used antibiotics, topical neomycin has the greatest toxicity to the corneal epithelium. It probably produces plasma membrane injury and cell death primarily of the superficial cell layers with chronic ocular exposure. After long-term ocular exposure to framycetin or neomycin, fungi superinfections have been reported. Nystagmus has been reported in a nine-year-old child following topical treatment of the skin with 1 percent neomycin in 11 percent dimethyl sulfoxide ointment.

Interactions with Other Drugs:

A. Effect of Framycetin or Neomycin on Activity of Other Drugs
  1. EDTA (apnea) ↑

    2. General anesthetics (apnea) ↑
    3. Other antibiotics (apnea) ↑
       (Bacitracin, Colistin, Gentamicin, Kanamycin, Polymyxin B, Streptomycin)
    4. Oral penicillins ↓
    5. Oral vitamin B_{12} ↓
  B. Effect of Other Drugs on Activity of Framycetin or Neomycin
    1. EDTA ↑
    2. Anticholinesterases ↓
  C. Synergistic Activity
    1. Bacitracin
  D. Cross Sensitivity
    1. Gentamicin
    2. Kanamycin
    3. Streptomycin

References:

Argov, Z., and Mastaglia, F. L.: Disorders of neuromuscular transmission caused by drugs. N. Engl. J. Med. *301*:409, 1979.

Ferrara, B. E., and Phillips, R. D.: Respiratory arrest following administration of intraperitoneal neomycin. Am. Surg. *23*:710, 1957.

Gordon, D. M.: Gentamicin sulfate in external eye infections. Am. J. Ophthalmol. *69*:300, 1970.

Herd, J. K., et al.: Ototoxicity of topical neomycin augmented by dimethyl sulfoxide. Pediatrics *40*:905, 1967.

McCorkle, R. G.: Neomycin toxicity. A case report. Arch. Pediat. *75*:439, 1958.

McQuillen, M. P., Cantor, H. E., and O'Rourke, J. R.: Myasthenic syndrome associated with antibiotics. Arch. Neurol. *18*:402, 1968.

Prystowsky, S. D., et al.: Allergic hypersensitivity to neomycin. Relationship between patch test reactions and "use" tests. Arch. Dermatol. *115*:713, 1979.

Stechishin, O., Voloshin, P. C., and Allard, C. A.: Neuromuscular paralysis and respiratory arrest caused by intrapleural neomycin. Can. Med. Assoc. J. *81*:32, 1959.

Generic Name: Gentamicin

Proprietary Name: *Systemic*: Cidomycin (G.B.), Garamycin, Garamycina (Swed.), Gentalline (Fr.), Genticin (G.B.), Geomycine (Belg.), Refobacin (Germ.), Sulmycin (Germ.), U-Gencin *Ophthalmic*: Garamycin, Genoptic, Genticin (G.B.)

Primary Use: This aminoglycoside is effective against *Ps. aeruginosa, Aerobacter, E. coli, K. pneumoniae,* and *Proteus.*

Ocular Side Effects:

  A. Systemic Administration
    1. Decreased vision

    2. Papilledema secondary to pseudotumor cerebri
    3. Loss of eyelashes or eyebrows
    4. Subconjunctival or retinal hemorrhages secondary to drug-induced anemia
    5. Myasthenic neuromuscular blocking effect
      a. Paralysis of extraocular muscles
      b. Ptosis
    6. Eyelids
      a. Photosensitivity
      b. Urticaria
B. Local Ophthalmic Use or Exposure—Topical Application or Subconjunctival Injection
    1. Irritation
    2. Eyelids or conjunctiva
      a. Allergic reactions
      b. Conjunctivitis—follicular
      c. Depigmentation (?)
    3. Overgrowth of nonsusceptible organisms

Clinical Significance: Surprisingly few drug-induced ocular side effects from systemic administration of gentamicin have been reported. However, there have been an increased number of allergic and irritative reactions reported to the Registry due to topical ocular administration of this agent. Gentamicin and neomycin may be the more irritative antibiotics to the corneal epithelium. There has been an occasional report of skin depigmentation in blacks when topical ocular gentamicin is applied under an eye pad. However, pseudotumor cerebri with secondary papilledema and visual loss has been well documented. Other adverse ocular effects are reversible and transitory after discontinued use of the drug.

Interactions with Other Drugs:

A. Effect of Gentamicin on Activity of Other Drugs
    1. General anesthetics (apnea) ↑
B. Effect of Other Drugs on Activity of Gentamicin
    1. Penicillins ↓
C. Cross Sensitivity
    1. Kanamycin
    2. Neomycin
    3. Streptomycin

References:

AMA Drug Evaluations. 4th Ed., New York, John Wiley & Sons, 1980, pp. 384, 1286–1290.

Argov, Z., and Mastaglia, F. L.: Disorders of neuromuscular transmission caused by drugs. N. Engl. J. Med. *301*:409, 1979.

Boe, R., and Conner, C. S.: Pseudotumor cerebri. JAMA *226*:567. 1973.

Dukes, M. N. G. (Ed.): Meyler's Side Effects of Drugs. Amsterdam, Excerpta Medica, Vol. IX, 1980, pp. 460–461.

Gordon, D. M.: Gentamicin sulfate in external eye infections. Am. J. Ophthalmol. *69*:300, 1970.

Kastrup, E. K., and Schwach, G. H. (Eds.): Facts and Comparisons. St. Louis, Facts and Comparisons, Inc., 1974, p. 347.

Generic Name: Kanamycin

Proprietary Name: *Systemic*: Kamycine (Fr.), Kanabristol (Germ.), Kanasig (Austral.), Kanmy (S. Afr.), Kannasyn (G.B.), Kantrex, Kantrox (Swed.), Klebcil *Ophthalmic:* Ophtalmokalixan (Fr.)

Primary Use: This aminoglycoside is effective against gram-negative organisms and in drug-resistant staphylococcus.

Ocular Side Effects:

  A. Systemic Administration
   1. Decreased vision
   2. Myasthenic neuromuscular blocking effect
      a. Paralysis of extraocular muscles
      b. Ptosis
   3. Eyelids or conjunctiva
      a. Allergic reactions
      b. Lyell's syndrome
   4. Optic neuritis (?)
  B. Local Ophthalmic Use or Exposure—Subconjunctival Injection
   1. Irritation
   2. Eyelids or conjunctiva—allergic reactions
   3. Overgrowth of nonsusceptible organisms

Clinical Significance: Systemic and ocular side effects due to kanamycin are quite rare, partially due to its poor gastrointestinal absorption. Myasthenic neuromuscular blocking effect occurs more frequently if kanamycin is given in combination with other antibiotics, such as neomycin, gentamicin, polymyxin B, colistin, or streptomycin. Adverse ocular reactions to this agent are reversible, transitory, and seldom have residual complications.

Interactions with Other Drugs:

A. Effect of Kanamycin on Activity of Other Drugs
   1. General anesthetics (apnea) ↑
   2. Other antibiotics (apnea) ↑
B. Effect of Other Drugs on Activity of Kanamycin
   1. EDTA (apnea) ↑
   2. Anticholinesterases (apnea) ↓
C. Synergistic Activity
   1. Cephalosporins
   2. Penicillins
D. Cross Sensitivity
   1. Gentamicin
   2. Neomycin
   3. Streptomycin

References:

Finegold, S. M.: Kanamycin. Arch. Intern. Med. *104*:15, 1959.
Finegold, S. M.: Toxicity of kanamycin in adults. Ann. N.Y. Acad. Sci. *132*:942, 1966.
Freemon, F. R., Parker, R. L., Jr., and Greer, M.: Unusual neurotoxicity of kanamycin. JAMA *200*:410, 1967.
McQuillen, M. P., Cantor, H. E., and O'Rourke, J. R.: Myasthenic syndrome associated with antibiotics. Arch. Neurol. *18*:402, 1968.
Walsh, F. B., and Hoyt, W. F.: Clinical Neuro-Ophthalmology. 3rd Ed., Baltimore, Williams & Wilkins, Vol. III, 1969, pp. 2655, 2680.

Generic Name: Nalidixic Acid

Proprietary Name: Cybis, NegGram, Negram (G.B.), Nogram (Germ.), Wintomylon (Jap., S. Afr.)

Primary Use: This bactericidal naphthyridine derivative is effective against *E. coli, Aerobacter,* and *Klebsiella;* however, its primary clinical use is against *Proteus.*

Ocular Side Effects:

A. Systemic Administration
   1. Visual sensations
     a. Glare phenomenon
     b. Flashing lights—white or colored
     c. Scintillating scotomas—may be colored
   2. Problems with color vision
     a. Dyschromatopsia
     b. Objects have green, yellow, blue, or violet tinge

3. Photophobia
4. Paresis of extraocular muscles
5. Papilledema secondary to pseudotumor cerebri
6. Decreased vision
7. Decreased accommodation
8. Diplopia
9. Mydriasis
10. Nystagmus
11. Eyelids or conjunctiva
    a. Photosensitivity
    b. Angioneurotic edema
    c. Urticaria
12. Subconjunctival or retinal hemorrhages secondary to drug-induced anemia
13. Retinal degeneration (?)
14. Ocular teratogenic effects—ptosis (?)

Clinical Significance: Numerous ocular side effects due to nalidixic acid have been reported. In fact, in a recent annual report of adverse ocular reactions of the United Kingdom, almost one-third of all case reports were due to this drug. The most common adverse ocular reaction is a curious visual disturbance, which includes brightly colored appearances of objects as the main feature. This often appears soon after the drug is taken. Temporary visual loss also occurs and lasts from half an hour to 72 hours. Probably the most serious ocular reaction is papilledema secondary to elevated intracranial pressure. This side effect is more frequent in the younger age groups. Most adverse ocular reactions due to nalidixic acid are transitory and reversible if the dosage is decreased or the drug is discontinued.

Interactions with Other Drugs:

A. Effect of Nalidixic Acid on Activity of Other Drugs
   1. Alcohol ↑
B. Effect of Other Drugs on Activity of Nalidixic Acid
   1. EDTA ↑
   2. Antacids ↓

References:

AMA Drug Evaluations. 4th Ed., New York, John Wiley & Sons, 1980, pp. 1324–1325.
Boreus, L. O., and Sundstrom, B.: Intracranial hypertension in a child during treatment with nalidixic acid. Br. Med. J. 2:744, 1967.
Cahal, D. A.: Adverse reactions to nalidixic acid. Lancet 2:441, 1965.
Davidson, S. I.: Reports of ocular adverse reactions. Trans. Ophthalmol. Soc. U. K. 93:495, 1973.

Fraser, A.G., and Harrower, A.D.B.: Convulsions and hyperglycaemia associated with nalidixic acid. Br. Med. J. *2*:1518, 1977.

Leopold, I. H.: New dimensions in ocular pharmacology, 1975. Trans. Am. Acad. Ophthalmol. Otolaryngol. *81*:19, 1976.

Marshall, B. Y.: Visual side effects of nalidixic acid. Practitioner *199*:222, 1967.

VanDyk, H. J. L., and Swan, K. C.: Drug-induced pseudotumor cerebri. *In* Leopold, I. H. (Ed.): Symposium on Ocular Therapy. St. Louis, C. V. Mosby, Vol. IV, 1969, pp. 71–77.

Walker, S. H., Salanio, I., and Standiford, W. E.: Nalidixic acid in childhood urinary tract infection; clinical and laboratory experience with 50 patients. Clin. Pediat. *5*:718, 1966.

Generic Name: Nitrofurantoin

Proprietary Name: Berkfurin (G.B.), Co-Caps Nitrofurantoin (G.B.), Cyantin, Dantafur, Fua-Med (Germ.), Furachel, Furadantin, Furadoine (Fr.), Furalan, Furaloid, Furan (G.B.), Furanex (Canad.), Furanite (Canad.), Furantoin, Furatine (Canad.), Ituran (Germ.), Ivadantin, Macrodantin, Nephronex (Canad.), Nifuran (Canad.), Nitrex, Nitrofor-50/100, Novofuran (Canad.), N-Toin, Parfuran, Sarodant, Trantoin, Urantoin (G.B.), Uro-Tablinen (Germ.), Urotoin

Primary Use: This bactericidal furan derivative is effective against specific organisms which cause urinary tract infections, especially *E. coli*, enterococci, and *S. aureus*.

Ocular Side Effects:

A. Systemic Administration
　1. Nonspecific ocular irritation
　　a. Lacrimation
　　b. Burning sensation
　2. Vertical diplopia
　3. Nystagmus
　4. Decreased vision
　5. Paresis or paralysis of extraocular muscles
　6. Eyelids or conjunctiva
　　a. Allergic reactions
　　b. Photosensitivity
　　c. Angioneurotic edema
　　d. Urticaria
　　e. Lyell's syndrome
　　f. Loss of eyelashes or eyebrows (?)
　7. Papilledema secondary to pseudotumor cerebri
　8. Subconjunctival or retinal hemorrhages secondary to drug-induced anemia

9. Problems with color vision (?)
   a. Dyschromatopsia
   b. Objects have yellow tinge

Clinical Significance: The most aggravating ocular side effects due to nitrofurantoin are the severe itching, burning, and tearing which may persist long after use of the drug is stopped in some patients. All adverse ocular reactions due to this drug have been transitory and reversible if use was discontinued. Only a few cases of paralysis of extraocular muscles have been reported. There have been two well-documented cases of pseudotumor cerebri associated with nitrofurantoin therapy. One case was in a 10-month-old infant and the other was in a 23-year-old obese woman.

Interactions with Other Drugs:

A. Effect of Other Drugs on Activity of Nitrofurantoin
   1. Antacids ↓
   2. Barbiturates ↓
   3. Carbonic anhydrase inhibitors ↓

References:

Delaney, R. A., Miller, D. A., and Gerbino, P. P.: Adverse effects resulting from nitrofurantoin administration. Am. J. Pharm. *149*:26, 1977.
Kastrup, E. K., and Schwach, G. H. (Eds.): Facts and Comparisons. St. Louis, Facts and Comparisons, Inc., 1974, pp. 382a–382b.
Mushet, G. R.: Pseudotumor and nitrofurantoin therapy. Arch. Neurol. *34*:257, 1977.
Peritt, R. A.: Eye complications resulting from systemic medication. Ill. Med. J. *117*: 423, 1960.
Sharma, D. B., and James, A.: Benign intracranial hypertension associated with nitrofurantoin therapy. Br. Med. J. *4*:771, 1974.
Toole, J. F., et al.: Neural effects of nitrofurantoin. Arch. Neurol. *18*:680, 1968.

Generic Name: Polymyxin B

Proprietary Name: *Systemic:* Aerosporin, Polmix (Austral.) *Ophthalmic:* Aerosporin

Primary Use: This bactericidal polypeptide is effective against gram-negative bacilli, especially *Ps. aeruginosa.*

Ocular Side Effects:

A. Systemic Administration
   1. Myasthenic neuromuscular blocking effect

      a. Paralysis of extraocular muscles
      b. Ptosis
   2. Decreased vision
   3. Diplopia
   4. Nystagmus
   5. Mydriasis
B. Local Ophthalmic Use or Exposure—Topical Application or Subconjunctival Injection
   1. Irritation—ocular pain
   2. Eyelids or conjunctiva—allergic reactions
   3. Overgrowth of nonsusceptible organisms
C. Local Ophthalmic Use or Exposure—Intracameral Injection
   1. Uveitis
   2. Corneal edema
   3. Lens damage

Clinical Significance: Although ocular side effects due to polymyxin B are well documented, they are quite rare and seldom of major clinical importance, except for topical ocular irritative or allergic reactions. The clinically important side effects are secondary to intracameral injections where permanent changes to the cornea and lens have occurred.

Interactions with Other Drugs:

A. Effect of Polymyxin B on Activity of Other Drugs
   1. General anesthetics (apnea) ↑
B. Effect of Other Drugs on Activity of Polymyxin B
   1. Other antibiotics (apnea) ↑
      (Colistin, Gentamicin, Kanamycin, Neomycin, Streptomycin)
   2. Anticholinesterases (apnea) ↑↓
C. Cross Sensitivity
   1. Colistin

References:

Francois, J., and Mortiers, P.: The injurious effects of locally and generally applied antibiotics on the eye. T. Geneeskd. *32*:139, 1976.

Gilman, A. G., Goodman, L. S., and Gilman, A. (Eds.): The Pharmacological Basis of Therapeutics. 6th Ed., New York, Macmillan, 1980, pp. 1228–1230.

McQuillen, M. P., Cantor, H. E., and O'Rourke, J. R.: Myasthenic syndrome associated with antibiotics. Arch. Neurol. *18*:402, 1968.

Pohlmann, G.: Respiratory arrest associated with intravenous administration of polymyxin B sulfate. JAMA *196*:181, 1966.

Small, G. A.: Respiratory paralysis after a large dose of intraperitoneal polymyxin B and bacitracin. Anesth. Analg. *43*:137, 1964.

Generic Name: Streptomycin

Proprietary Name: Darostrep (S. Afr.), Isoject-Streptomycin Injection, Novostrep (S. Afr.), Orastrep (G.B.), Strepolin (Austral., S. Afr.), Streptevan (Austral.), Strept-evanules (Austral.), Streptosol (Canad., S. Afr.), Strycin

Primary Use: This bactericidal aminoglycosidic agent is effective against *Brucella, Pasteurella, Mycobacterium,* and *Shigella.*

Ocular Side Effects:

A. Systemic or Intrathecal Administration
    1. Nystagmus
    2. Decreased vision
    3. Toxic amblyopia
    4. Myasthenic neuromuscular blocking effect
        a. Paresis or paralysis of extraocular muscles
        b. Ptosis
    5. Visual sensations
        a. Visual disturbance during motion
        b. Continuance of image after ocular movement
    6. Photophobia
    7. Problems with color vision
        a. Dyschromatopsia, blue or green defect
        b. Objects have yellow tinge
    8. Decreased accommodation
    9. Retrobulbar or optic neuritis
    10. Scotomas
    11. Optic atrophy
    12. Retinal vasospasm
    13. Eyelids or conjunctiva
        a. Allergic reactions
        b. Conjunctivitis—nonspecific
        c. Edema
        d. Angioneurotic edema
        e. Lupoid syndrome
    14. Subconjunctival or retinal hemorrhages secondary to drug-induced anemia
    15. Loss of eyelashes or eyebrows (?)
B. Local Ophthalmic Use or Exposure—Subconjunctival Injection
    1. Irritation
    2. Eyelids or conjunctiva—allergic reactions
    3. Overgrowth of nonsusceptible organisms

C. Local Ophthalmic Use or Exposure—Intracameral Injection
  1. Uveitis
  2. Corneal edema
  3. Lens damage
  4. Retinal damage (?)

Clinical Significance: Since more effective aminoglycosidic antibiotics exist, the clinical use of streptomycin is limited. Toxic visual effects are rare, usually transitory, and reversible with systemic administration; however, permanent blindness and optic atrophy have been reported with intrathecal injection. Nystagmus due to streptomycin can be produced without vestibular damage. Skin sensitization is common among medical personnel who handle this drug and may lead to dermatitis not infrequently associated with periorbital edema and conjunctivitis.

Interactions with Other Drugs:

A. Effect of Streptomycin on Activity of Other Drugs
  1. Colistin (apnea) ↑
  2. EDTA (apnea) ↑
  3. General anesthetics (apnea) ↑
  4. Penicillins ↑
B. Effect of Other Drugs on Activity of Streptomycin
  1. Oxygen ↑
  2. Anticholinesterases (apnea) ↓
C. Synergistic Activity
  1. Cephalosporins
  2. Chloramphenicol
  3. Erythromycin
  4. Penicillins
  5. Sulfonamides
  6. Tetracycline
D. Cross Sensitivity
  1. Gentamicin
  2. Kanamycin
  3. Neomycin

References:

AMA Drug Evaluations. 4th Ed., New York, John Wiley & Sons, 1980, pp. 1292–1293.
Sannella, L. S.: An early symptom of streptomycin neurotoxicity. Arch. Ophthalmol. 50:331, 1953.
Sykowski, P.: Streptomycin causing retrobulbar optic neuritis. Am. J. Ophthalmol. 34:1446, 1951.
Thomas, E. B.: Scotomas in conjunction with streptomycin therapy. Report of 11 cases. Arch. Ophthalmol. 43:729, 1950.

Wade, A. (Ed.): Martindale: The Extra Pharmacopoeia. 27th Ed., London, Pharmaceutical Press, 1977, pp. 1181–1185.
Walker, G. F.: Blindness during streptomycin and chloramphenicol therapy. Br. J. Ophthalmol. 45:555, 1961.

Generic Name: 1. Sulfacetamide; 2. Sulfachlorpyridazine; 3. Sulfacytine (Sulfacitine); 4. Sulfadiazine; 5. Sulfadimethoxine; 6. Sulfamerazine; 7. Sulfameter (Sulfametoxydiazine); 8. Sulfamethazine (Sulfadimidine); 9. Sulfamethizole; 10. Sulfamethoxazole; 11. Sulfamethoxypyridazine; 12. Sulfanilamide; 13. Sulfaphenazole; 14. Sulfapyridine; 15. Sulfasalazine; 16. Sulfathiazole; 17. Sulfisoxazole (Sulfafurazole)

Proprietary Name: *Systemic*: 1. Antebor (Fr.), Sebizon, Sulamyd, Sulf-10, Sulphacetamide (G.B.); 2. Cosulfa (Canad.), Cosulid, Nefrosul, Sonilyn, Sulphachlorpyridazine (G.B.), Vetisulid; 3. Renoquid; 4. Adiazine (Fr.), Coco-Diazine, Diazyl (Austral.), Microsulfon, Solu-Diazine (Canad.), Sulfadets (Canad.), Sulphadiazine (G.B.); 5. Agribon, Albon, Lensulpha (S. Afr.), Longisulf (S. Afr.), Madribon (G.B.), Madroxine (Pol.), Pansulph (S. Afr.), Sulfathox (S. Afr.), Sulfoplan (Denm.), Sulphadimethoxine (G.B.), Sulphribon (S. Afr.), Unisulph (S. Afr.); 6. Solumedine (Fr.), Sulphamerazine (G.B.); 7. Bayrena (Fr., Scand., S. Afr.), Durenat (Germ.), Durenate (G.B.), Kirocid (Austral.), Kiron (Fr., S. Afr.), Longasulf (Swed.), Sulla, Sulphamethoxydiazine (G.B.); 8. Diminsul (Austral.), Neotrizine, S-Dimidine (Austral.), Sulfadine (Canad.), Sulphadimidine (G.B.), Sulphamezathine (G.B.); 9. Bursul, Famet (Austral.), Lucosil (Scand.), Methisul (G.B.), Microsul, Proklar-M, Rufol (Fr.), Salimol (Jap.), S-Methizole (Austral.), Sulfametin (Swed.), Sulfasol, Sulfstat, Sulfurine, Sulphamethizole (G.B.), Thiosulfil, Urifon, Uri-Pak Urocydal (Jap.), Urolex (Austral.), Urolin (Austral.), Urolucosil (G.B.), Uroz (Austral.); 10. Gantanol; 11. Davosin (Germ.), Kynex, Lederkyn (G.B.), Midicel, Minikel (Belg.), SDM (Canad.), Sulphamethoxypyridazine (G.B.), Sultirene (Fr.); 12. Amindan (Germ.), Exoseptoplix (Fr.), Pyodental (Germ.), Sulphanilamide (G.B.), Tablamide (Fr.); 13. Orisul (Austral., Canad., Germ., Switz.), Orisulf (G.B), Sulfabid, Sulphaphenazole (G.B.); 14. Dagenan (Canad., Fr.), Eubasinum (Germ.), M&B 693 (G.B.), Septipulmon (Swed.), Sulphapyridine (G.B.); 15. Azulfidine, Salazopyrin, Salazopyrine (Fr.), Salicylazosulfapyridine, S.A.S.-500, S.A.S.P., Sulcolon, Sulphasalazine (G.B.); 16. Cibazol (Germ., Switz.), Sulfamul (Canad.), Sulphathiazole (G.B.), Thiazomide (Fr.); 17. Gantrisin, Gantrisine (Fr.), Lipo Gantrisin, Novosoxazole (Canad.), SK-Soxazole, Sosol, Soxomide, Sulfagen (Canad.), Sulfalar, Sulfizin, Sulfizole (Canad.), Sulphafurazole (G.B.), US-67 (Canad.) *Ophthalmic:*

1. Acetopt (Austral.), Ak-Sulf, Albucid (G.B.), Bleph-10, Cetamide, Isopto Cetamide, Op-Sulfa, Optamide (Austral.), Optiole S (Canad.), Sulfacel, Sulamyd, Sulphacalyre (G.B.), Sulphacetamide (G.B.), Vaso-sulf (G.B.); 9. Sulfamethizoli (G.B.); 17. Gantrisin

Primary Use: The sulfonamides are bacteriostatic agents effective against most gram-positive and some gram-negative organisms. Sulfonamides are the agents of choice for treatment of nocardiosis, chancroid, and toxoplasmosis.

Ocular Side Effects:

- A. Systemic Administration
    1. Decreased vision
    2. Myopia—with or without astigmatism
    3. Decreased depth perception—with or without decreased adduction at near
    4. Nonspecific ocular irritation
        a. Lacrimation
        b. Photophobia
    5. Keratitis
    6. Problems with color vision
        a. Dyschromatopsia
        b. Objects have yellow or red tinge
    7. Subconjunctival or retinal hemorrhages
    8. Visual fields
        a. Scotomas
        b. Constriction
    9. Optic neuritis
    10. Myasthenic neuromuscular blocking effect
        a. Paralysis of extraocular muscles
        b. Ptosis
    11. Periorbital edema
    12. Visual hallucinations
    13. Papilledema
    14. Cortical blindness
    15. Vivid light lavender colored retinal vascular tree
    16. Decreased anterior chamber depth—may precipitate narrow-angle glaucoma
    17. Eyelids or conjunctiva
        a. Allergic reactions
        b. Conjunctivitis—nonspecific
        c. Photosensitivity
        d. Urticaria

  e. Purpura
  f. Lupoid syndrome
  g. Erythema multiforme
  h. Stevens-Johnson syndrome
  i. Exfoliative dermatitis
  j. Lyell's syndrome
  k. Pemphigoid lesion with or without symblepharon
18. Uveitis
19. Toxic amblyopia (?)
20. Optic atrophy (?)
21. Hypermetropia (?)
B. Local Ophthalmic Use or Exposure—Topical Application
  1. Irritation
  2. Eyelids or conjunctiva
    a. Allergic reactions
    b. Conjunctivitis—follicular
    c. Deposits
  3. Overgrowth of nonsusceptible organisms
  4. Delayed corneal wound healing

Clinical Significance: While there are numerous reported ocular side effects from systemic sulfa medication, most are rare and reversible. Probably the most common ocular side effect seen in patients on systemic therapy is myopia. This is transient, with or without induced astigmatism, usually bilateral, and may exceed several diopters. This is most likely due to refractive changes within the lens. Since sulfa not infrequently causes dermatologic problems, associated conjunctivitis, keratitis, and lid problems may be seen. The ophthalmologist should be aware that anaphylactic reactions, Stevens-Johnson syndrome, and exfoliative dermatitis have all been reported, although rare, from topical ocular administration of sulfa preparations. Optic neuritis has been reported even in low dosages and is usually reversible with complete recovery of vision. Optic nerve and retinal disorders have been seen but are quite rare.

Interactions with Other Drugs:

A. Effect of Sulfonamides on Activity of Other Drugs
  1. Penicillins ↑
  2. Pyrimethamine ↑
  3. Ascorbic acid ↓
B. Effect of Other Drugs on Activity of Sulfonamides
  1. Analgesics ↑
  2. Ascorbic acid ↑

      3. Phenothiazines ↑
      4. Salicylates ↑
      5. Antacids ↓
      6. Local anesthetics ↓
      7. Mineral oil ↓
  C. Synergistic Activity
      1. Colistin
      2. Erythromycin
      3. Penicillin (occasionally indifferent or inhibitory)
  D. Cross Sensitivity
      1. Carbonic anhydrase inhibitors
      2. Other sulfonamides
  E. Contraindications
      1. Ophthalmic solutions containing silver or aminobenzoic acid

References:

Boettner, E. A., Fralick, F. B., and Wolter, J. R.: Conjunctival concretions of sulfa-diazine. Arch. Ophthalmol. 92:446, 1974.

Bucy, P. C.: Toxic optic neuritis resulting from sulfanilamide. JAMA 109:1007, 1937.

Haviland, J. W., and Long, P. H.: Skin and ocular reactions in sulfathiazole therapy. Bull. Johns Hopkins Hosp. 66:263, 1940.

Hornbogen, D. P.: Transient myopia during sulfanilamide therapy. Am. J. Ophthalmol. 24:323, 1941.

Newell, F. W., and Greetham, J. S.: Pemphigus conjunctivae. Am. J. Ophthalmol. 29:1426, 1946.

Rubin, Z.: Ophthalmic sulfonamide-induced Stevens-Johnson syndrome. Arch. Dermatol. 113:235, 1977.

Taub, R. G., and Hollenhorst, R. W.: Sulfonamides as a cause of toxic amblyopia. Am. J. Ophthalmol. 40:486, 1955.

Class: Antifungal Agents

Generic Name: Amphotericin B

Proprietary Name: Ampho-Moronal (Germ.), Fungilin (G.B.), Fungizone

Primary Use: This polyene fungistatic agent is effective against *Blastomyces, Histoplasma, Cryptococcus, Coccidiomyces, Candida,* and *Aspergillus.*

Ocular Side Effects:

A. Systemic Administration
   1. Decreased vision
   2. Paresis of extraocular muscles
   3. Retinal exudates
   4. Subconjunctival or retinal hemorrhages secondary to drug-induced anemia
   5. Diplopia
B. Local Ophthalmic Use or Exposure—Topical Application or Subconjunctival Injection
   1. Irritation
      a. Ocular pain
      b. Burning sensation
   2. Punctate keratitis
   3. Eyelids or conjunctiva
      a. Allergic reactions
      b. Ulceration
      c. Conjunctivitis—follicular
      d. Necrosis—subconjunctival injection
      e. Nodules—subconjunctival injection
      f. Yellow discoloration—subconjunctival injection
   4. Overgrowth of nonsusceptible organisms
   5. Uveitis
C. Local Ophthalmic Use or Exposure—Intracameral Injection
   1. Uveitis
   2. Corneal edema
   3. Lens damage

Clinical Significance: Seldom are significant ocular side effects seen from systemic administration of amphotericin B, except with intrathecal injections. In general, blurred vision is the most common, but this is usually transitory. Allergic reactions are so rare that initially it was felt they did not even occur. Topical ocular administration, however, can be quite irritating, with conjunctival and corneal changes being quite frequent but seldom permanent. There is evidence that this agent can affect cell membranes and allow increased penetration of other drugs into the cornea. There have been rare reports of marked iridocyclitis with small hyphemas occurring after each reapplication of topical ocular amphotericin B. Probably, the most significant adverse ocular effect besides those that occur from intraocular injection is the formation of salmon-colored raised nodules which can occur secondary to subconjunctival injection, especially if the dosage exceeds 5 mg. In addition, the injection of this agent can cause permanent yellowing of the conjunctiva. Some clinicians feel that amphotericin B is too toxic to the tissue to be given subconjunctivally; therefore, many advise against its use in this mode of delivery.

Interactions with Other Drugs:

A. Effect of Amphotericin B on Activity of Other Drugs
   1. Corticosteroids ↓

References:

AMA Drug Evaluations. 4th Ed., New York, John Wiley & Sons, 1980, pp. 385–386, 1355–1357.

Bell, R. W., and Ritchey, J. P.: Subconjunctival nodules after amphotericin B injection. Medical therapy for *Aspergillus* corneal ulcer. Arch. Ophthalmol. *90*:402, 1973.

Dukes, M. N. G. (Ed.): Meyler's Side Effects of Drugs. Amsterdam, Excerpta Medica, Vol. IX, 1980, pp. 475–476.

Lorber, B., Cutler, C., and Barry, W. E.: Allergic rash due to amphotericin B. Arch. Intern. Med. *84*:54, 1976.

Spickard, A., et al.: The improved prognosis of cryptococcal meningitis with amphotericin B therapy. Ann. Intern. Med. *58*:66, 1963.

Utz, J. P.: Current concepts in therapy. Chemotherapeutic agents for the systemic mycoses. N. Engl. J. Med. *268*:938, 1963.

Generic Name: Griseofulvin

Proprietary Name: Fulcin (G.B.), Fulvicin-P/G, Fulvicin-U/F, Grifulvin V, Grisactin, Grisefuline (Fr.), Grisovin (G.B.), Grisowen, Gris-PEG, Lamoryl (Swed.), Likuden M (Germ.)

Primary Use: This is the only commercially available oral antifungal agent effective against *Microsporum, Epidermophyton,* and *Trichophyton.*

Ocular Side Effects:

A. Systemic Administration
   1. Decreased vision
   2. Problems with color vision—objects have green tinge
   3. Macular edema
   4. Visual hallucinations
   5. Eyelids or conjunctiva
      a. Allergic reactions
      b. Hyperemia
      c. Edema
      d. Photosensitivity
      e. Angioneurotic edema

3

    f. Urticaria

    g. Lupoid syndrome

    h. Exfoliative dermatitis

6. Papilledema secondary to pseudotumor cerebri
7. Subconjunctival or retinal hemorrhages secondary to drug-induced anemia
8. Macular degeneration (?)
9. Paresis of extraocular muscles (?)

Clinical Significance: Griseofulvin rarely causes ophthalmic problems; however, it may cause severe allergic reactions with ocular involvement. Most of the above adverse ocular reactions are based on only a few cases. There have been a number of adverse effects due to this agent reported to the Registry. Pseudotumor cerebri with resultant papilledema and visual loss has been seen from this drug. A case of superficial corneal deposits resembling Meeman's corneal dystrophy has been reported to resolve after discontinuation of the drug. This agent is a photosensitizing drug, and a higher prevalence of eyelid and conjunctival reactions has been seen with increased light exposure. Posterior subcapsular cataracts in a 52-year-old patient were reported to the Registry following griseofulvin administration. After only a brief exposure, griseofulvin rarely induces systemic lupus erythematosus, probably on the basis of an allergic reaction. In general, serious adverse effects are rarely associated with griseofulvin; but they are more likely to occur if griseofulvin is given in high dosages or for prolonged periods.

Interactions with Other Drugs:

A. Effect of Griseofulvin on Activity of Other Drugs
    1. Alcohol ↑
    2. Barbiturates ↑
    3. Anticoagulants ↓
B. Effect of Other Drugs on Activity of Griseofulvin
    1. Antihistamines ↓
    2. Phenylbutazone ↓
    3. Sedatives and hypnotics ↓
C. Cross Sensitivity
    1. Penicillins

References:

Alarcón-Segovia, D.: Drug-induced antinuclear antibodies and lupus syndromes. Drugs *12*:69, 1976.

AMA Drug Evaluations. 4th Ed., New York, John Wiley & Sons, 1980, pp. 1360–1362.

Delman, M., and Leubuscher, K.: Transient macular edema due to griseofulvin. Am. J. Ophthalmol. *56*:658, 1963.

Dukes, M. N. G. (Ed.): Meyler's Side Effects of Drugs. Amsterdam, Excerpta Medica, Vol. IX, 1980, pp. 474–475.

Duverne, J., et al.: Accidents hallucinatoires repetes chez une enfant traitee par la grisefuline pour dermatophyties multiples. Lyon Med. *211*:1773, 1964.

Gilman, A. G., Goodman, L. S., and Gilman, A. (Eds.): The Pharmacological Basis of Therapeutics. 6th Ed., New York, Macmillan, 1980, pp. 1237–1238.

Generic Name: Nystatin

Proprietary Name: Candex, Candio-Hermal (Germ.), Canstat (S. Afr.), Diastatin (Austral.), Fungalex (S. Afr.), Fungistatin (S. Afr.), Korostatin, Moronal (Germ.), Mycostatin, Mycostatine (Fr.), Nilstat, Nystan (G.B.), Nystavescent (G.B.), O-V Statin

Primary Use: This polyene fungistatic and fungicidal agent is effective against *Candida.*

Ocular Side Effects:

A. Systemic Administration
   1. Optic neuritis
   2. Decreased vision
B. Local Ophthalmic Use or Exposure—Topical Application or Subconjunctival Injection
   1. Irritation
   2. Eyelids or conjunctiva—allergic reactions
   3. Overgrowth of nonsusceptible organisms

Clinical Significance: Ocular side effects from systemic or ocular nystatin administration are unusual. Most adverse ocular reactions due to it are reversible and transitory.

References:

Ellis, P. P.: Ocular Therapeutics and Pharmacology. 5th Ed., St. Louis, C. V. Mosby, 1977, pp. 148, 222–223.

Havener, W. H.: Ocular Pharmacology. 4th Ed., St. Louis, C. V. Mosby, 1978, pp. 141–144.

Physicians' Desk Reference. 35th Ed., Oradell, N.J., Medical Economics Co., 1981, p. 1717.

Saraux, H.: La nevrite optique par intoxication medicamenteuse. Communication Soc. Med. Milit. December 17, 1970.

Wasilewski, C.: Allergic contact dermatitis from nystatin. Arch Derm. *102*:216, 1970.

Generic Name: Thiabendazole. See under *Class: Anthelmintics.*

Class: Antileprosy Agents

Generic Name: Amithiozone. See under *Class: Antitubercular Agents.*

Generic Name: Clofazimine

Proprietary Name: Lamprene

Primary Use: This phenazine derivative is used in the treatment of leprosy.

Ocular Side Effects:

A. Systemic Administration
    1. Eyelids or conjunctiva
       a. Red discoloration
       b. Hyperpigmentation
    2. Corneal opacities
    3. Pigmentary changes
       a. Cornea
       b. Macula

Clinical Significance: This phenazine derivative can cause reversible reddish pigmentation of the skin and conjunctiva. Fine brownish subepithelial lines, not unlike those seen with chloroquine, have been described in patients receiving clofazimine. These corneal changes have not interfered with vision and disappear within a few months after the drug has been discontinued. While macular pigmentary changes have been reported and seem to persist, little is known regarding incidence, visual loss, or reversibility.

References:

AMA Drug Evaluations. 4th Ed., New York, John Wiley & Sons, 1980, pp. 1350–1351.
Davies, D. M. (Ed.): Textbook of Adverse Drug Reactions. New York, Oxford University Press, 1977, p. 297.
Ohman, L., and Wahlberg, I.: Ocular side effects of clofazimine. Lancet 2:933, 1975.
Wade, A. (Ed.): Martindale: The Extra Pharmacopoeia. 27th Ed., London, Pharmaceutical Press, 1977, pp. 1498–1499.
Walinder, P.-E., Gip, L., and Stempa, M.: Corneal changes in patients treated with clofazimine. Br. J. Ophthalmol. 60:526, 1976.

Generic Name: Dapsone

Proprietary Name: Avlosulfon

Primary Use: This sulfone is used in the treatment of all forms of leprosy.

Ocular Side Effects:

A. Systemic Administration
   1. Decreased vision
   2. Eyelids or conjunctiva
      a. Hyperpigmentation
      b. Urticaria
      c. Purpura
      d. Exfoliative dermatitis
   3. Optic atrophy—toxic states
   4. Subconjunctival or retinal hemorrhages secondary to drug-induced anemia

Clinical Significance: This sulfone has been reported to cause optic atrophy, but only when administered in massive doses. Otherwise, most adverse ocular reactions are seldom of clinical importance at normal dosages. Darkening of skin color may be due to iatrogenic cyanosis, as a slate gray discoloration is characteristic of drug-induced methemoglobinemia.

References:

Davies, D. M. (Ed.): Textbook of Adverse Drug Reactions. New York, Oxford University Press, 1977, p. 297.
Dukes, M. N. G. (Ed.): Side Effects of Drugs. Annual 4. Amsterdam, Excerpta Medica, 1980, p. 217.
Homeida, M., Babikr, A., and Daneshmend, T. K.: Dapsone-induced optic atrophy and motor neuropathy. Br. Med. J. *281*:1180, 1980.
Physicians' Desk Reference. 35th Ed., Oradell, N.J., Medical Economics Co., 1981, p. 951.
Wade, A. (Ed.): Martindale: The Extra Pharmacopoeia. 27th Ed., London, Pharmaceutical Press, 1977, pp. 1499–1503.

Generic Name: Ethionamide. See under *Class: Antitubercular Agents.*

Generic Name: Rifampin. See under *Class: Antitubercular Agents.*

Class: Antimalarial Agents

Generic Name: 1. Amodiaquine; 2. Chloroquine; 3. Hydroxychloroquine

Proprietary Name: 1. Basoquin (G.B.), Camoquin, Flavoquine (Fr.); 2. Aralen, Arechin (Pol.), Avoclor (G.B.), Chlorocon, Chlorquin (Austral.), Malaquin (Austral.), Malarex (Denm.), Malarivon (G.B.), Nivaquine (G.B.), Resochin (G.B.), Roquine, Siragan (Aust.), Tresochin (Swed.); 3. Ercoquin (Norw., Swed.), Plaquenil, Plaquinol (Port.), Quensyl (Germ.)

Primary Use: These aminoquinolines are used in the treatment of malaria, extraintestinal amebiasis, rheumatoid arthritis, and lupus erythematosus.

Ocular Side Effects:

A. Systemic Administration
1. Decreased vision
2. Cornea
    a. Whirl-like deposits
    b. Hudson-Stähli lines
    c. Edema
    d. Decreased reflex
    e. Aggravation of keratoconjunctivitis sicca (?)
3. Retinal or macular
    a. Pigmentary changes—pigmentary retinopathy, bull's eye, doughnut
    b. Vasoconstriction
    c. Decreased or absent foveal reflex
    d. Edema
    e. Abnormal ERG or EOG
4. Visual fields
    a. Scotomas—annular, central, or paracentral
    b. Constriction
    c. Hemianopsia
5. Problems with color vision
    a. Dyschromatopsia
    b. Objects have yellow, green, or blue tinge
    c. Colored haloes around lights
6. Extraocular muscles
    a. Paresis or paralysis
    b. Nystagmus

7. Lens
   a. Anterior subcapsular cataracts—snowflake opacities
   b. Posterior subcapsular cataracts—fleck type
8. Photophobia
9. Night blindness
10. Visual hallucinations
11. Diplopia
12. Flashing lights
13. Eyelids or conjunctiva
    a. Allergic reactions
    b. Photosensitivity
    c. Poliosis
    d. Ptosis
    e. Blepharoclonus
    f. Blepharospasm
    g. Erythema multiforme
    h. Stevens-Johnson syndrome
    i. Exfoliative dermatitis
    j. Loss of eyelashes or eyebrows (?)
14. Decreased accommodation
15. Oculogyric crises
16. Optic atrophy
17. Toxic amblyopia
18. Decreased dark adaptation
19. Subconjunctival or retinal hemorrhages secondary to drug-induced anemia
20. Ocular teratogenic effects (?)
21. Uveitis (?)

B. Inadvertent Ocular Exposure
   1. Corneal deposits

Clinical Significance: Significant ocular side effects, including blindness, have occurred due to these drugs. It is becoming increasingly apparent that hydroxychloroquine in daily dosages not exceeding 400 mg is a much safer drug compared to chloroquine as far as ocular side effects are concerned. Chloroquine alone appears to have more ocular side effects than if given with hydroxychloroquine. Although the incidence of hydroxychloroquine side effects seems significantly less, to date, the data in the Registry imply that any adverse effect reported for chloroquine can also be seen with hydroxychloroquine. Since amodiaquine is used comparatively infrequently, not enough data are available to make generalizations for this agent. In the United States, chloroquine is seldom used anymore, although this is not true for some other countries. In dosages below 250 mg, significant ocular side effects are rarely seen. However, if this dosage is maintained for over 6 months, significant adverse ocular effects have been reported. Corneal deposition has no direct relationship to posterior segment disease and is reversible. It may first appear as a Hudson-Stähli line or an increase in a preexisting Hudson-Stähli line. Probably more common is a whirl-like pattern known as "cornea verticillata." It has been recently shown that a number of drugs and diseases can cause this pattern, which morphologically, histologically, and electron microscopically are identical. "Amphophilic" drugs, such as chloroquine, amiodarone, and chlorpromazine, form complexes with cellular phospholipids, which cannot be metabolized by lysosomal phospholipases. Therefore, these intracellular deposits occur and are seen in the superficial portion of the cornea. Toxic maculopathy usually is reversible only in its earliest phases. If these drugs have caused skin, eyelid, or hair changes, this is an excellent indicator of possible drug-induced retinopathy. Since these agents are concentrated in pigmented tissue, macular changes have been thought to progress long after the drug therapy is stopped. This is now being questioned by some investigators. The "bull's eye" macula is not diagnostic for aminoquinoline-induced disease since a number of other entities can cause this same clinical picture. While retinal toxicity occurs in patients on hydroxychloroquine, the incidence is low. How to detect early toxic changes is still the subject of debate. In general, if the patient is visually symptom free (i.e., home visual acuity and color vision testing), semiannual ocular testing is probably adequate to catch reversible retinal toxicity. Every 6 months, the ophthalmologist should take a careful history and perform visual acuity, funduscope, visual field testing with both red and white targets, and red Amsler grids. Emphasis should be placed in the 4 to 6° area from fixation hunting for relative scotoma with a red test object. Electroretinographies, electro-oculographies, Farnsworth or similar color vision testing, and fluorescein angiograms may also be helpful. Fluorescein angiography shows a loss of pigment epithelium, a kind of window-type defect that allows fluorescein to show through more easily. The side effects of these drugs are variable, but include neuromuscular blockade which may cause abnormal extraocular muscle responses. They can also interreact to give a myasthenia gravis-like syndrome. The mechanism of retinal toxicity with this group of drugs is not fully understood, and an assessment of this toxicity is not as precise as one would like. The predictability of progression after the drug is discontinued as well as at what stage changes are reversible are still unknown and areas of clinical concern.

Interactions with Other Drugs:

    A. Effect of Other Drugs on Activity of Aminoquinolines
        1. Antacids ↑
        2. Monoamine oxidase inhibitors ↑

References:

Apt, L., and Gaffney, W. L.: Ocular teratogens: A commentary. J. Pediatr. 87:844, 1975.

Arden, G. B., and Kolb, H.: Antimalarial therapy and early retinal changes in patients with rheumatoid arthritis. Br. Med. J. 1:270, 1966.

Argov, Z., and Mastaglia, F. L.: Disorders of neuromuscular transmission caused by drugs. N. Engl. J. Med. 301:409, 1979.

Bernstein, H. N.: Chloroquine ocular toxicity. Surv. Ophthalmol. 12:415, 1967.

Burns, R. P.: Delayed onset of chloroquine retinopathy. N. Engl. J. Med. 275:693, 1966.

Kubota, Y., and Kuroda, N.: Chloroquine retinopathy. Long term follow up after discontinuation of chloroquine. Jap. J. Clin. Ophthalmol. 30:63, 1976.

Laaksonen, A.-L., Koskiahde, V., and Juva, K.: Dosage of antimalarial drugs for children with juvenile rheumatoid arthritis and systemic lupus erythematosus. Scand. J. Rheumatol. 3:103, 1974.

Lal, S., and Gupta, A. K.: Lenticular deposits associated with chloroquine keratopathy. Indian J. Ophthalmol. 22:34, 1974.

Lazar, M., Regenbogen, L., and Stein, R.: Anterior uveitis due to chloroquine. Ophthalmologica 146:411, 1963.

Mark, J. S.: Motor polyneuropathy and nystagmus associated with chloroquine phosphate. Postgrad. Med. 55:569, 1979.

Martin, L. J., Bergen, R. L., and Dobrow, H. R.: Delayed onset chloroquine retinopathy: Case report. Ann. Ophthalmol. 10:723, 1978.

Ogawa, S., et al.: Progression of retinopathy long after cessation of chloroquine therapy. Lancet 1:1408, 1979.

Percival, S. P. B., and Behrman, J.: Ophthalmological safety with chloroquine. Br. J. Ophthalmol. 53:101, 1969.

Pülhorn, G., and Thiel, H.-J.: Das ultrastrukturelle Bild der Chloroquine-keratopathie. Albrecht Von Graefes Arch. Klin. Exp. Ophthalmol. 201:89, 1976.

Rynes, R. I., et al.: Ophthalmologic safety of long-term hydroxychloroquine treatment. Arthritis Rheum. 22:832, 1979.

Seiler, K.-U., Thiel, H.-J., and Wassermann, O.: Die Chloroquinkeratopathie als Beispiel einer arzneimittelinduzierten Phospholipidosis. Klin. Monatsbl. Augenheilkd. 170:64, 1977.

Generic Name: Quinacrine (Mepacrine). See under *Class: Anthelmintics.*

Generic Name: Quinine

Proprietary Name: Bi-quinate (Austral.), Coco-Quinine, Dentojel (Canad.), Quinamm, Quinate (Austral.), Quinbisan (Austral.), Quine, Quinsan (Austral.)

Primary Use: This alkaloid is effective in the management of nocturnal leg cramps, myotonia congenita, and in resistant *P. falciparum.* It is also used in attempted abortions. Ophthalmologically, it is useful in the treatment of eyelid myokymia.

Ocular Side Effects:

A. Systemic Administration
    1. Decreased vision—all gradations of visual loss including toxic amblyopia
    2. Pupils
        a. Mydriasis
        b. Decreased or absent reaction to light
    3. Retinal or macular
        a. Edema
        b. Degeneration
        c. Pigmentary changes
        d. Exudates
        e. Vasodilatation followed by vasoconstriction
        f. Absence of foveal reflex
        g. Abnormal ERG
    4. Visual sensations
        a. Distortion due to flashing lights
        b. Distortion of images secondary to sensations of wave
    5. Optic nerve
        a. Papilledema
        b. Atrophy
    6. Problems with color vision
        a. Dyschromatopsia, red-green or blue-yellow defect
        b. Objects have red or green tinge
    7. Visual fields
        a. Scotomas
        b. Constriction
    8. Iris atrophy
    9. Eyelids or conjunctiva
        a. Allergic reactions
        b. Photosensitivity
        c. Angioneurotic edema
        d. Purpura
        e. Urticaria
        f. Erythema multiforme
        g. Stevens-Johnson syndrome
    10. Ocular teratogenic effects—optic nerve hypoplasia
    11. Night blindness
    12. Visual hallucinations
    13. Vertical nystagmus
    14. Subconjunctival or retinal hemorrhages secondary to drug-induced anemia

Clinical Significance: The use of quinine with the resultant adverse ocular side effects is on the rise. It has become increasingly used as a diluent for many of the "street drugs" and as a possible method to terminate a pregnancy; additionally, it is found in a number of proprietary medications for the previously described medical indications. While the primary adverse reactions are dose related and usually occur only with massive amounts, a number of reports show that some idiosyncratic reactions as well as chronic low dosage exposure may cause ocular side effects. In cases of massive exposure, visual loss may be sudden or progressive over a number of hours or days. In the worst cases, retinal arteriolar constriction, venous congestion, and retinal and papillary edema are pronounced. Complete loss of vision may occur, but most patients have some return of vision. Mild cases may only show minimal macular changes by Amsler grid, blurred vision, or some constriction of the visual field. The etiology of the toxic effect of quinine is unknown. Recent animal data do not support direct toxicity on the ganglion cells, and retinal arteriolar vasoconstriction does not seem to explain all the adverse effects seen. It is apparent that quinine can cause optic nerve hypoplasia and decreased vision, including blindness, in the offspring secondary to prenatal maternal ingestion, if taken in toxic doses. Therapy of this entity is also controversial. Suggested treatment includes stellate ganglion blocks, vasodilators, anterior chamber paracentesis, corticosteroids, vitamin B, and iodides. It is difficult to prove that any of these have significant clinical effects.

Interactions with Other Drugs:

A. Effect of Quinine on Activity of Other Drugs
1. Antibiotics (apnea) ↑
   (Kanamycin, Neomycin, Streptomycin)
2. Anticholinergics ↑
3. Anticholinesterases ↓

References:

Bard, L. A., and Gills, J. P.: Quinine amblyopia. Arch. Ophthalmol. 72:328, 1964.

Barsky, D.: Quinine idiosyncrasy and optic atrophy. J. Mich. St. Med. Soc. 60:612, 1961.

Behrman, J., and Mushin, A.: Electrodiagnostic findings in quinine amblyopia. Br. J. Ophthalmol. 52:925, 1968.

Braveman, B. L., Koransky, D. S., and Kulvin, M. M.: Quinine amaurosis. Am. J. Ophthalmol. 31:731, 1948.

Francois, J., De Rouck, A., and Cambie, E.: Retinal and optic evaluation in quinine poisoning. Ann. Ophthalmol. 4:177, 1972.

Knox, D. L., Palmer, C. A. L., and English, F.: Iris atrophy after quinine amblyopia. Arch. Ophthalmol. 76:359, 1966.

Maltzman, B., Sutula, F., and Cinotti, A. A.: Toxic maculopathy. Part I. A result of quinine usage. Ann. Ophthalmol. 7:1321, 1975.

McKinna, A. J.: Quinine induced hypoplasia of the optic nerve. Can. J. Ophthalmol. 1:261, 1966.

Pruzon, H., Kiebel, G., and Maltzman, B.: Toxic maculopathy. Part II: A result of quinine usage as demonstrated by fluorescein angiography and electroretinography. Ann. Ophthalmol. 7:1475, 1975.

Valman, H. B., and White, D. C.: Stellate block for quinine blindness in a child. Br. Med. J. 1:1065, 1977.

Class: Antiprotozoal Agents

Generic Name: Suramin

Proprietary Name: Moranyl (Fr.)

Primary Use: This nonmetallic polyanion is effective in the treatment of trypanosomiasis and as adjunctive therapy in onchocerciasis.

Ocular Side Effects:

  A. Systemic Administration
    1. Nonspecific ocular irritation
      a. Lacrimation
      b. Photophobia
    2. Eyelids or conjunctiva
      a. Edema
      b. Urticaria
    3. Subconjunctival or retinal hemorrhages secondary to drug-induced anemia
    4. Keratitis
    5. Iritis
    6. Optic atrophy

Clinical Significance: Suramin is available in the United States only from the Center for Disease Control. It can cause a variety of untoward reactions which vary in intensity and frequency with the nutritional status of the patient and reach rather serious proportions among the malnourished. Most of these ocular adverse reactions occur up to 24 hours after drug administration; however, some can occur even later. It is postulated that optic atrophy occurs secondary to an inflammatory response in the optic nerve from the dead microfilariae.

References:

Drugs for parasitic infections. Med. Lett. Drugs Ther. *21*:105, 1979.
Gilman, A. G., Goodman, L. S., and Gilman, A. (Eds.): The Pharmacological Basis of Therapeutics. 6th Ed., New York, Macmillan, 1980, pp. 1070–1071.
Thylefors, B., and Rolland, A.: The risk of optic atrophy following suramin treatment of ocular onchocerciasis. Bull. WHO 57:479, 1979.
Wade, A. (Ed.): Martindale: The Extra Pharmacopoeia. 27th Ed., London, Pharmaceutical Press, 1977, pp. 1580–1581.

Generic Name: Tryparsamide

Proprietary Name: Tryparsamide

Primary Use: This organic arsenical is used in the treatment of trypanosomiasis (African sleeping sickness).

Ocular Side Effects:

A. Systemic Administration
   1. Constriction of visual fields
   2. Decreased vision
   3. Visual sensations
     a. Smokeless fog
     b. Shimmering effect
   4. Optic neuritis
   5. Optic atrophy
   6. Toxic amblyopia

Clinical Significance: The most serious and common adverse drug reactions due to tryparsamide involve the eye. Incidence of ocular side effects vary from 3 to 20 percent of cases, with constriction of visual fields followed by decreased vision as the characteristic sequence. Almost 10 percent of individuals taking tryparsamide experience visual changes consisting of "shimmering" or "dazzling" which may persist for days or even weeks. If the medication is not immediately discontinued following these visual changes, the pathologic condition of the optic nerve may become irreversible and progress to blindness.

References:

Doull, J., Klaassen, C. D., and Amdur, M. O. (Eds.): Casarett and Doull's Toxicology. The Basic Science of Poisons. 2nd Ed., New York, Macmillan, 1980, pp. 301–302.
Gilman, A. G., Goodman, L. S., and Gilman, A. (Eds.): The Pharmacological Basis of Therapeutics. 6th Ed., New York, Macmillan, 1980, p. 1074.
Grant, W. M.: Toxicology of the Eye. 2nd Ed., Springfield, Charles C Thomas, 1974, pp. 1069–1070.

LeJeune, J. R.: Les oligo-elements et chelateurs. Bull. Soc. Belge Ophtalmol. *160*:241, 1972.
Walsh, F. B., and Hoyt, W. F.: Clinical Neuro-Ophthalmology. 3rd Ed., Baltimore, Williams & Wilkins, Vol. III, 1969, pp. 2594–2596.

Class: Antitubercular Agents

Generic Name: 1. Aminosalicylate (Para-Aminosalicylate); 2. Amino-salicylic Acid

Proprietary Name: 1. Neopasalate, Pamisyl (Canad.), Parasal, P.A.S., Pasalba (Austral.), Pasan (Austral.), Pasara, Pasdium, Solu-PAS (Germ.), Teebacin; 2. Para-Pas, Parasal, P.A.S., Pascorbic, PASNA, Teebacin Acid

Primary Use: These bacteriostatic agents are effective against *M. tuberculosis.*

Ocular Side Effects:

  A. Systemic Administration
   1. Decreased accommodation (?)
   2. Decreased vision (?)
   3. Optic neuritis (?)
   4. Scotomas (?)
   5. Optic atrophy (?)
   6. Eyelids or conjunctiva
      a. Allergic reactions (?)
      b. Blepharitis (?)
      c. Edema (?)
      d. Lupoid syndrome
      e. Stevens-Johnson syndrome (?)
      f. Exfoliative dermatitis (?)
   7. Subconjunctival or retinal hemorrhages secondary to drug-induced anemia (?)

Clinical Significance: Aminosalicylates are so seldom used by themselves that many, if not most, of the preceding ocular side effects may be due to other drugs. Even so, the total number of reported cases of possible adverse ocular reactions is low. Aminosalicylates have been shown to induce the lupus syndrome in an allergic type reaction.

Interactions with Other Drugs:

A. Effect of Aminosalicylates on Activity of Other Drugs
    1. Barbiturates ↑
    2. Sulfonamides ↓
    3. Vitamin B_{12} ↓
B. Effect of Other Drugs on Activity of Aminosalicylates
    1. Salicylates ↑
    2. Streptomycin ↑

References:

Alarcón-Segovia, D.: Drug-induced antinuclear antibodies and lupus syndromes. Drugs *12*:69, 1976.
AMA Drug Evaluations. 4th Ed., New York, John Wiley & Sons, 1980, pp. 1341–1342.
Dukes, M. N. G. (Ed.): Meyler's Side Effects of Drugs. Amsterdam, Excerpta Medica, Vol. IX, 1980, p. 531.
O'Hara, H.: Blepharitis squamosa occurred before dermatitis exfoliativa caused by PAS-Ca and streptomycin. J. Clin. Ophthalmol. (Tokyo) *10*:1421, 1956.
Pohjola, S., and Horsmanheimo, A.: Keratitis sicca after erythema exudativum multiforme caused by P.A.S. (Case report). Acta Ophthalmol. *44*:415, 1966.
Steiner, C.: Un cas d'intoxication par PAS et produits analogues. Bull. Soc. Ophtalmol. Fr. p. 527, April, 1951.

Generic Name: Amithiozone (Thiacetazone)

Proprietary Name: Thioparamizone (G.B.)

Primary Use: This tuberculostatic agent is effective against *M. tuberculosis* and *M. leprae*.

Ocular Side Effects:

A. Systemic Administration
    1. Decreased vision
    2. Nonspecific ocular irritation
        a. Photophobia
        b. Ocular pain
        c. Burning sensation
    3. Eyelids or conjunctiva
        a. Allergic reactions
        b. Hyperemia
        c. Blepharoconjunctivitis—nonspecific
        d. Erythema multiforme
        e. Stevens-Johnson syndrome
        f. Exfoliative dermatitis

4. Retinal edema
5. Subconjunctival or retinal hemorrhages secondary to drug-induced anemia
6. Loss of eyelashes or eyebrows (?)

Clinical Significance: Numerous adverse ocular reactions due to amithiozone have been seen. Skin manifestations have been the most frequent. Nearly all ocular side effects are reversible and of minor clinical significance. One instance of toxic amblyopia has been reported; however, the patient was also receiving aminosalicylic acid.

Interactions with Other Drugs:

A. Effect of Other Drugs on Activity of Amithiozone
  1. Corticosteroids ↓

References:

Jopling, W. H., and Kirwan, E. W. O'G.: Toxic amblyopia caused by TB3: A case record. Trans. R. Soc. Trop. Med. Hyg. 46:656, 1952.
Sarma, O. A.: Reactions to thiacetazone. Indian J. Chest Dis. 18:51, 1976.
Steiner, C.: Un cas d'intoxication par P.A.S. et produits analogues. Bull. Soc. Ophtalmol. Fr. p. 527, April 1951.
von Oettingen, W. F.: Poisoning. 2nd Ed., Philadelphia, W. B. Saunders, 1958.
Wade, A. (Ed.): Martindale: The Extra Pharmacopoeia. 27th Ed., London, Pharmaceutical Press, 1980, pp. 1603–1605.

Generic Name: Capreomycin

Proprietary Name: Capastat, Caprocin, Ogostal (Germ.)

Primary Use: This polypeptide tuberculostatic antibiotic is effective against *M. tuberculosis*. It is used when less toxic antitubercular agents have been ineffective.

Ocular Side Effects:

A. Systemic Administration
  1. Visual sensations
    a. Flickering vision
    b. Flashing lights
  2. Problems with color vision—objects have white tinge
  3. Eyelids or conjunctiva
    a. Angioneurotic edema
    b. Urticaria
  4. Decreased vision
  5. Visual hallucinations (?)

Clinical Significance: Adverse ocular reactions due to capreomycin are not common, and all ocular side effects are transitory and reversible. Decreased vision is usually of only short duration and reversible.

Interactions with Other Drugs:

A. Effect of Other Drugs on Activity of Capreomycin
   1. Antibiotics ↑
      (Kanamycin, Streptomycin, Viomycin)
   2. General anesthetics (apnea) ↑
   3. Anticholinesterases ↓
   4. Corticosteroids ↓

References:

Davidson, S. I.: Reports of ocular adverse reactions. Trans. Ophthalmol. Soc. U. K. 93:495, 1973.

Physicians' Desk Reference. 35th Ed., Oradell, N.J., Medical Economics Co., 1981, p. 1044.

Wade, A. (Ed.): Martindale: The Extra Pharmacopoeia. 27th Ed., London, Pharmaceutical Press, 1980, pp. 1585–1586.

Generic Name: Cycloserine

Proprietary Name: Closina (Austral.), Seromycin

Primary Use: This isoxazolidone is effective against certain gram-negative and gram-positive bacteria and *M. tuberculosis.*

Ocular Side Effects:

A. Systemic Administration
   1. Decreased vision
   2. Eyelids or conjunctiva
      a. Allergic reactions
      b. Photosensitivity
   3. Visual hallucinations
   4. Flickering vision
   5. Subconjunctival or retinal hemorrhages secondary to drug-induced anemia
   6. Decreased accommodation (?)
   7. Optic neuritis (?)
   8. Optic atrophy (?)

Clinical Significance: Even though ocular complications due to cycloserine are quite rare, this drug is primarily used in combination with other drugs so that to pinpoint cause for ocular side effects is most difficult. Optic nerve damage has been reported, but the data are not conclusive.

References:

AMA Drug Evaluations. 4th Ed., New York, John Wiley & Sons, 1980, pp. 1343–1344.
Gilman, A. G., Goodman, L. S., and Gilman, A. (Eds.): The Pharmacological Basis of Therapeutics. 6th Ed., New York, Macmillan, 1980, pp. 1210–1211.
Grant, W. M.: Toxicology of the Eye. 2nd Ed., Springfield, Charles C Thomas, 1974, pp. 345–346.
Physicians' Desk Reference. 35th Ed., Oradell, N.J., Medical Economics Co., 1981, p. 1093.
Walsh, F. B., and Hoyt, W. F.: Clinical Neuro-Ophthalmology. 3rd Ed. Baltimore, Williams & Wilkins, Vol. III, 1969, p. 2680.

Generic Name: Ethambutol

Proprietary Name: Dexambutol (Fr.), Etibi (Canad.), Miambutol (Ital.), Myambutol

Primary Use: Ethambutol is a tuberculostatic agent which is effective against *M. tuberculosis.*

Ocular Side Effects:

A. Systemic Administration
1. Decreased vision
2. Visual fields
   a. Scotomas—annular, central, or centrocecal
   b. Constriction
   c. Hemianopsia
   d. Enlarged blind spot
3. Optic nerve
   a. Retrobulbar or optic neuritis
   b. Papilledema
   c. Peripapillary atrophy
4. Photophobia
5. Problems with color vision—dyschromatopsia, red-green or blue-yellow defect
6. Retinal or macular
   a. Vascular
      1.) Hemorrhages
      2.) Dilatation
      3.) Spasms
   b. Edema
   c. Pigmentary changes
7. Paresis of extraocular muscles

8. Toxic amblyopia
9. Depressed visual evoked cortical responses

Clinical Significance: A large number of adverse ocular responses due to ethambutol are reversible, but there are some well-documented irreversible changes, including blindness, in the world literature and in the Registry. The "D" isomer of ethambutol is the form currently in use, since the "L" isomer caused significant toxic optic nerve effects. In general, the side effects of ethambutol are dose related; however, in rare instances, an adverse ocular response may occur after only a few weeks of therapy. There are histologic data both in primates and in humans that this drug can cause chiasmal demyelinization. The ethambutol daily dosage range of 15 mg/kg appears to be comparatively free from adverse ocular effects. However, between 1 and 2 percent of patients on 25 mg/kg or more will have a significant adverse ocular effect. While the onset of most adverse ocular reactions is abrupt, they may occasionally be insidious. There are two types of optic neuritis, axial and periaxial. The axial type is associated with a macular degeneration, decreased visual acuity and decreased color perception. The periaxial type is more often associated with visual field defects, paracentral scotomas with normal vision and normal color perception. With axial involvement, green color vision testing loss is more common than red loss. One author suggested that if the optic neuritis has not improved within two months after ethambutol, isoniazid should be suspected. While isoniazid may be a contributing factor, ethambutol alone can also cause irreversible optic nerve disease. The management of patients on or to be placed on ethambutol therapy should include the following: an ocular examination prior to starting therapy and informed patient consent if there is a history of optic atrophy or optic neuritis. Also, it is well documented that patients with renal disease have a much higher incidence of optic nerve toxicity because blood levels of ethambutol are elevated due to the inability of the body to rid itself of the drug. Patients should be instructed in home testing for visual acuity and color vision. If the dosage exceeds 15 mg/kg, screening the patient on 2- to 4-week intervals is recommended. If there is any significant change in the patients' vision, they should be instructed to stop the drug and immediately seek an ocular examination. Visual recovery is variable but usually occurs within 3 to 12 months, although in some instances no recovery is obtained. There are data to suggest that cases of optic nerve toxicity should be treated with 100 to 250 mg of oral zinc sulfate three times daily.

Interactions with Other Drugs:

A. Effect of Other Drugs on Activity of Ethambutol
   1. Corticosteroids ↓

References:

Barron, G. J., Tepper, L., and Iovine, G.: Ocular toxicity from ethambutol. Am. J. Ophthalmol. 77:256, 1974.

Boman, G., and Calissendorff, B.: A case of irreversible bilateral optic damage after ethambutol therapy. Scand. J. Resp. Dis. 55:176, 1974.

Brontë-Stewart, J., Pettigrew, A. R., and Foulds, W. S.: Toxic optic neuropathy and its experimental production. Trans. Ophthalmol. Soc. U.K. 96:355, 1976.

Carr, R. E., and Henkind, P.: Ocular manifestations of ethambutol. Arch. Ophthalmol. 67:566, 1962.

Deodati, F., et al.: Optic neuritis due to ethambutol. Rev. Otoneuroophtalmol. 46: 191, 1974.

Karmon, G., et al.: Bilateral optic neuropathy due to combined ethambutol and isoniazid treatment. Ann. Ophthalmol. 11:1013, 1979.

Leibold, J. E.: The ocular toxicity of ethambutol and its relation to dose. Ann. N.Y. Acad. Sci. 135:904, 1966.

Renard, G., and Morax, P. V.: Nevrite optique au cours des traitements antitubercu-leus. Ann. Oculist. 210:53, 1977.

Roussos, T., and Tsolkas, A.: The toxicity of myambutol on the human eye. Ann. Ophthalmol. 2:578, 1970.

Van Lith, G. H. M.: Electro-ophthalmology and side-effects of drugs. Doc. Ophthal-mol. 44:19, 1977.

Yonekura, Y., Mori, T., and Kondo, N.: Optic nerve complications of ethambutol. Folia Ophthalmol. Jap. 20:545, 1969.

Generic Name: Ethionamide

Proprietary Name: Trecator, Trescatyl (G.B.), Tubenamide (Jap.)

Primary Use: This isonicotinic acid derivative is effective against *M. tu-berculosis* and *M. leprae*. It is indicated in the treatment of patients when resistance to primary tuberculostatic drugs has developed.

Ocular Side Effects:

A. Systemic Administration
   1. Decreased vision
   2. Diplopia
   3. Eyelids or conjunctiva
      a. Allergic reactions
      b. Erythema
      c. Exfoliative dermatitis
   4. Photophobia
   5. Problems with color vision
      a. Dyschromatopsia
      b. Heightened color perception
   6. Optic neuritis
   7. Loss of eyelashes or eyebrows (?)

Clinical Significance: The incidence of adverse ocular effects due to ethionamide is quite small and seldom of clinical significance. While certain adverse effects occur at low dosage levels, they usually do not continue even if the dosage is increased.

Interactions with Other Drugs:

A. Effect of Ethionamide on Activity of Other Drugs
   1. Alcohol ↑
B. Effect of Other Drugs on Activity of Ethionamide
   1. Corticosteroids ↓

References:

Dukes, M. N. G. (Ed.): Meyler's Side Effects of Drugs. Amsterdam, Excerpta Medica, Vol. IX, 1980, p. 531.

Fox, W., et al.: A study of acute intolerance to ethionamide, including a comparison with prothionamide, and of the influence of a vitamin B-complex additive in prophylaxis. Tubercule *50*:125, 1969.

Gilman, A. G., Goodman, L. S., and Gilman, A. (Eds.): The Pharmacological Basis of Therapeutics. 6th Ed., New York, Macmillan, 1980, pp. 1208–1209.

Wade, A. (Ed.): Martindale: The Extra Pharmacopoeia. 27th Ed., London, Pharmaceutical Press, 1977, pp. 1587–1589.

Generic Name: Isoniazid

Proprietary Name: Cedin (Germ.), Cotinazin, Dinacrin, Dow-Isoniazid, Hydronsan (Jap., S. Afr.), Hyzyd, INH, Isobicina (Ital.), Isotamine (Canad.), Isotinyl (Austral.), Isozid (Germ.), Laniazid, Neoteben (Germ.), Niconyl, Nidaton, Nydrazid, Panazid, Rimifon (G.B.), Rolazid, Tb-Phlogin (Germ.), Teebaconin, Tibinide (Swed.), Triniad, Uniad

Primary Use: This hydrazide of isonicotinic acid is effective against *M. tuberculosis.*

Ocular Side Effects:

A. Systemic Administration
   1. Decreased vision
   2. Optic neuritis
   3. Optic atrophy
   4. Visual fields
      a. Scotomas
      b. Constriction
      c. Hemianopsia

   5. Papilledema
   6. Problems with color vision—dyschromatopsia, red-green defect
   7. Eyelids or conjunctiva
       a. Allergic reactions
       b. Angioneurotic edema
       c. Lupoid syndrome
       d. Stevens-Johnson syndrome
       e. Exfoliative dermatitis
   8. Pupils
       a. Mydriasis
       b. Absence of reaction to light
   9. Paralysis of accommodation
  10. Diplopia
  11. Paresis of extraocular muscles
  12. Keratitis
  13. Nystagmus
  14. Subconjunctival or retinal hemorrhages secondary to drug-induced anemia
  15. Toxic amblyopia
  16. Photophobia
  17. Visual hallucinations (?)

Clinical Significance: The true incidence or significance of isoniazid-induced ocular side effects is difficult to evaluate since they are seen most commonly in malnourished, chronic alcoholics and in individuals who are characteristically on multiple drugs. Many, if not almost all, of the neurologic side effects can be prevented by the daily administration of pyridoxine. Signs and symptoms other than the neuro-ophthalmic complications are usually insignificant and reversible. Recently, it has been shown that isoniazid can cause an antinuclear antibody in the majority of patients taking this drug; however, only a small percentage develop the lupus syndrome.

Interactions with Other Drugs:

   A. Effect of Isoniazid on Activity of Other Drugs
       1. Analgesics ↑
       2. Anticholinergics ↑
       3. Barbiturates ↑
       4. General anesthetics ↑
       5. Sedatives and hypnotics ↑
       6. Sympathomimetics ↑
       7. Tricyclic antidepressants ↑
   B. Effect of Other Drugs on Activity of Isoniazid

1. Salicylates ↑
2. Alcohol ↓
3. Corticosteroids ↓
4. Pyridoxine ↓
C. Synergistic Activity
   1. Streptomycin

References:

Alarcón-Segovia, A.: Drug-induced antinuclear antibodies and lupus syndromes. Drugs *12*:69, 1976.

Dixon, G. J., Roberts, G. B. S., and Tyrrell, W. F.: The relationship of neuropathy to the treatment of tuberculosis with isoniazid. Scot. Med. J. *1*:350, 1956.

Kalinowski, S. Z., Lloyd, T. W., and Moyes, E. N.: Complications in the chemotherapy of tuberculosis. A review with analysis of the experience of 3,148 patients. Am. Rev. Respir. Dis. *83*:359, 1961.

Karmon, G., et al.: Bilateral optic neuropathy due to combined ethambutol and isoniazid treatment. Ann. Ophthalmol. *11*:1013, 1979.

Kass, I., et al.: Isoniazid as a cause of optic neuritis and atrophy. JAMA *164*:1740, 1957.

Keeping, J. A., and Searle, C. W. A.: Optic neuritis following isoniazid therapy. Lancet *2*:278, 1955.

Money, G. L.: Isoniazid neuropathies in malnourished tuberculosis patients. J. Trop. Med. Hyg. *62*:198, 1959.

Sutton, P. H., and Beattie, P. H.: Optic atrophy after administration of isoniazid with P.A.S. Lancet *1*:650, 1955.

Generic Name: Rifampin (Rifampicin)

Proprietary Name: *Systemic:* Rifa (Germ.), Rimactane, Rifadin *Ophthalmic:* Rifampin

Primary Use: *Systemic:* This bactericidal as well as bacteriostatic agent is effective against *Mycobacterium,* many gram-positive cocci and some gram-negative, including *Neisseria* species and *Hemophilus influenzae.* *Ophthalmic:* This agent is used for treatment of ocular chlamydia infections.

Ocular Side Effects:

A. Systemic Administration
   1. Decreased vision
   2. Eyelids or conjunctiva
      a. Hyperemia
      b. Erythema
      c. Blepharoconjunctivitis
      d. Edema
      e. Yellow or red discoloration

        f. Angioneurotic edema
        g. Urticaria
        h. Purpura
        i. Stevens-Johnson syndrome
        j. Exfoliative dermatitis
        k. Pemphigoid lesion
    3. Lacrimation
    4. Problems with color vision—dyschromatopsia, red-green defect
    5. Tears and/or contact lenses stained orange
    6. Uveitis
    7. Subconjunctival or retinal hemorrhages secondary to drug-induced anemia
    8. Retrobulbar or optic neuritis (?)
  B. Local Ophthalmic Use or Exposure
    1. Irritation
        a. Lacrimation
        b. Hyperemia
        c. Ocular pain
        d. Edema

Clinical Significance: Ocular side effects from rifampin may occur in 5 to 15 percent of patients, depending on the frequency and amount of this drug. Reactions vary from conjunctival hyperemia, to a mild blepharoconjunctivitis, to a painful severe exudative conjunctivitis. The latter includes tender, markedly congested palpebral and bulbar conjunctiva with thick white exudates. Although not all patients secrete this drug or a byproduct in their tears, the Registry has received reports of orange staining of contact lenses and the inability to wear lenses while taking this drug. In general, these ocular side effects appear to occur more frequently during intermittent treatment than during daily treatment and have been reversible when the drug has been discontinued. Topical ocular use of 1 percent rifampin ointment has been reported to cause approximately a 10 percent incidence of adverse effects, which are primarily due to irritation and include discomfort, tearing, lid edema, and conjunctival hyperemia. The irritation, discomfort, and tearing usually last only 10 to 50 minutes after the application of the ointment.

Interactions with Other Drugs:

  A. Effect of Rifampin on Activity of Other Drugs
    1. Corticosteroids ↑
    2. Oral contraceptives ↓
  B. Effect of Other Drugs on Activity of Rifampin

1. Barbiturates ↓
2. Salicylates ↓

References:

Darougar, S., et al.: Topical therapy of hyperendemic trachoma with rifampicin, oxy-tetracycline, or spiramycin eye ointments. Br. J. Ophthalmol. *64*:37, 1980.
Fraunfelder, F. T.: Orange tears. Am. J. Ophthalmol. *89*:752, 1980.
Girling, D. J.: Ocular toxicity due to rifampicin. Br. Med. J. *1*:585, 1976.
Lyons, R. W.: Orange contact lenses from rifampin. N. Engl. J. Med. *300*:372, 1979.
Mangi, R. J.: Reactions to rifampin. N. Engl. J. Med. *294*:113, 1976.
Nyirenda, R., and Gill, G. V.: Stevens-Johnson syndrome due to rifampicin. Br. Med. J. *2*:1189, 1977.
Stewart, W. M.: Pemphigus et pemphigoide. Dermatologica *160*:217, 1980.

Generic Name: Streptomycin. See under *Class: Antibiotics.*

II

Agents Affecting the Central Nervous System

Class: Analeptics

Generic Name: Pentylenetetrazol (Pentetrazol)

Proprietary Name: Cardiazol, Leptazol (G.B.), Metrazol, Nelex, Nioric

Primary Use: This CNS stimulant is used to enhance the mental and physical activity of elderly patients.

Ocular Side Effects:

A. Systemic Administration
   1. Pupils
      a. Mydriasis
      b. Absence of reaction to light
      c. Hippus
   2. Problems with color vision
      a. Dyschromatopsia
      b. Objects have yellow tinge
   3. Blepharospasm
   4. Visual hallucinations
   5. Scintillating scotomas
   6. Extraocular muscles
      a. Abnormal conjugate deviations
      b. Strabismus

Clinical Significance: Ocular side effects due to pentylenetetrazol are rare when the drug is administered orally; however, they are not uncommon if the drug is given intravenously. Ocular side effects are transient, most are reversible, and recovery is rapid after use of the drug is discontinued.

References:

AMA Drug Evaluations. 4th Ed., New York, John Wiley & Sons, 1980, p. 345.

Grant, W. M.: Toxicology of the Eye. 2nd Ed., Springfield, Charles C Thomas, 1974, p. 797.

Lubeck, M. J.: Effects of drugs on ocular muscles. Int. Ophthalmol. Clin. *11*(2):35, 1971.

Reese, H. H., Vander Veer, A., and Wedge, A. H.: Effect of induced Metrazol convulsions on schizophrenic patients. J. Nerv. Ment. Dis. 87:570, 1938.

Walsh, F. B., and Hoyt, W. F.: Clinical Neuro-Ophthalmology. 3rd Ed., Baltimore, Williams & Wilkins, Vol. III, 1969, pp. 2626–2627.

Class: Anorexiants

Generic Name: 1. Amphetamine; 2. Dextroamphetamine (Dexamphetamine); 3. Methamphetamine; 4. Phenmetrazine

Proprietary Name: 1. Badrin (Austral.), Benzedrine; 2. Amphedex, Curban, Daro, Dexamed (G.B.), Dexamine (Austral.), Dexampex, Dexamphate (Austral.), Dexaspan, Dexedrine, Diphylets, Ferndex, Obotan, Oxydess, Phetadex (Austral.), Robese P, Spancap, Tidex; 3. Dee-10, Desoxyn, Desyphed, Methampex, Methylamphetamine (G.B.), Neodrine (Canad.), Pervitin (Germ.), Syndrox; 4. Anorex (Austral.), Apedine (Austral.), Melfiat, Preludin

Primary Use: These sympathomimetic amines are used in the management of exogenous obesity. Amphetamine, dextroamphetamine, and methamphetamine are also effective in narcolepsy and in the management of minimal brain dysfunction in children.

Ocular Side Effects:

A. Systemic Administration
1. Decreased vision
2. Pupils
   a. Mydriasis — may precipitate narrow-angle glaucoma
   b. Decreased reaction to light
3. Widening of palpebral fissure
4. Decreased accommodation
5. Decreased convergence
6. Visual hallucinations
7. Problems with color vision — objects have blue tinge (amphetamine)

8. Posterior subcapsular cataracts (phenmetrazine)
9. Loss of eyelashes or eyebrows (?)
10. Blepharospasm (?)
11. Retinal venous thrombosis (?)

Clinical Significance: Ocular side effects due to these sympathomimetic amines are seldom of consequence and are mainly seen in overdose situations. Blepharospasm and retinal venous thrombosis have only been reported at massive dosages in one instance. Probable posterior subcapsular cataracts were seen in two young females on phenmetrazine who were on a massive weight reduction program and were extensive enough to require cataract extraction. Alopecia has been reported due to this group of drugs.

Interactions with Other Drugs:

A. Effect of Sympathomimetics on Activity of Other Drugs
    1. Analgesics ↑
    2. Local anesthetics ↑
    3. Adrenergic blockers ↓
B. Effect of Other Drugs on Activity of Sympathomimetics
    1. Antacids ↑
    2. Carbonic anhydrase inhibitors ↑
    3. Diuretics ↑
    4. Local anesthetics ↑
    5. Monoamine oxidase inhibitors ↑
    6. Tricyclic antidepressants ↑
    7. Ascorbic acid ↓
    8. Phenothiazines ↓

References:

Bartholomew, A. A., and Marley, E.: Toxic response to 2-phenyl-3-methyl-tetrahydro-1, 4-oxazine hydrochloride "Preludin" in humans. Psychopharmacologia 1:124, 1959.
Fenske, N. A., and Johnson, S. A. M.: Major causes of alopecia with suggestions for history taking, workup, and therapy. Postgrad. Med. 60:79, 1976.
LeGrand, J., and Chevannes, H.: Les opacifications du cristallin dans les traitements contre l'obesité. Bull. Soc. Ophtalmol. Fr. 65:943, 1965.
McCormick, T. C., Jr.: Toxic reactions to amphetamines. Dis. Nerv. Syst. 23:219, 1962.
Waud, S. P.: The effects of toxic doses of benzyl methyl carbinamine (Benzedrine) in man. JAMA 110:206, 1938.

Generic Name: 1. Benzphetamine; 2. Chlorphentermine; 3. Diethylpropion (Amfepramone); 4. Fenfluramine; 5. Phendimetrazine; 6. Phentermine

Proprietary Name: 1. Didrex, Inapetyl (Fr.); 2. Chlorophen, Pre-Sate; 3. Danylen (Swed.), DEP-75, Dietil-Retard (Belg.), Dobesin (Swed.), Frekentine (Neth.), Nu-Dispoz, Prefamone (Fr.), Regenon Retard (Germ.), Ro-Diet, Tenuate, Tepanil; 4. Ponderal (Canad., Fr.), Ponderax (G.B.), Pondimin, Ponflural (Switz.); 5. Adphen, Anorex, Arcotrol, Bacarate, B.O.F., Bontril, Delcozine, Di-Ap-Trol, Dietabs, Di-Metrex, Elphemet, Ex-Obese, Limit, Melfiat, Minus, Obacin, Obalan, Obepar, Obesan-X (S. Afr.), Obe-Tite, Obex (S. Afr.), Obezine, Phen-70, Phenazine, Phendorex, Phentazine, Phenzine, Plegine, Prelu-2, Reducto, Robese, Ropledge, Slim-Tabs, SPRX, Statobex, Stim-35, Stodex, Tanorex, Trimstat, Trimtabs, Wehless-35, Weightrol; 6. Adipex, Duromine (G.B.), Fastin, Ionamin, Linyl (Fr.), Mirapront (Belg., Denm., Swed.), Netto Longcaps (Germ.), Parmine, Phentrol, Rolaphent, Tora, Unifast, Wilpo, Wilpowr

Primary Use: These sympathomimetic amines are used in the treatment of exogenous obesity.

Ocular Side Effects:

A. Systemic Administration
  1. Decreased vision
  2. Pupils
    a. Mydriasis — may precipitate narrow-angle glaucoma
    b. Absence of reaction to light (fenfluramine) — toxic states
  3. Rotary nystagmus (fenfluramine) — toxic states
  4. Decreased accommodation
  5. Eyelids or conjunctiva
    a. Erythema
    b. Urticaria
  6. Subconjunctival or retinal hemorrhages secondary to drug-induced anemia (fenfluramine)
  7. Loss of eyelashes or eyebrows (?)
  8. Retinal venous thrombosis (?)
  9. Retrobulbar or optic neuritis (?)

Clinical Significance: Ocular side effects due to these sympathomimetic amines are rare and seldom of clinical significance. Nystagmus and dilated nonreactive pupils are most common in fenfluramine overdose.

Interactions with Other Drugs:

A. Effect of Sympathomimetics on Activity of Other Drugs
  1. Adrenergic blockers ↓
B. Effect of Other Drugs on Activity of Sympathomimetics

1. Monoamine oxidase inhibitors ↑
2. Phenothiazines ↓

References:

Council on Drugs: Evaluation of an anorexiant drug chlorphentermine hydrochloride (Pre-Sate). JAMA *196*:165, 1966.
Grant, W. M.: Toxicology of the Eye. 2nd Ed., Springfield, Charles C Thomas, 1974, pp. 281, 384, 814.
Physicians' Desk Reference. 35th Ed., Oradell, N.J., Medical Economics Co., 1981, pp. 1871, 1877.
Riley, I., et al.: Fenfluramine overdosage. Lancet 2:1162, 1969.
Rubin, R. T.: Acute psychotic reaction following ingestion of phentermine. Am. J. Psychiatry *120*:1124, 1964.

Class: Antianxiety Agents

Generic Name: 1. Carisoprodol; 2. Meprobamate

Proprietary Name: 1. Caprodat (Swed.), Carisoma (G.B.), Flexartal (Fr.), Rela, Sanoma (Germ.), Soma, Somadril (Swed.); 2. Amosene, Aneural (Germ.), Cyrpon (Germ.), Dabrobamat (Germ.), Equanil, Kesso-Bamate, Lan-Dol (Canad.), Libiolan (Fr.), Meditran (Canad.), Mepavlon (G.B.), Meprate (G.B.), Mepriam, Meproban (Swed.), Meprocompren (Germ.), Mepromate (Austral.), Mepron (Austral.), Meprosa (Germ.), Meprospan, Meprotabs, Milonorm (G.B.), Miltaun (Germ.), Miltown, Neo-tran (Canad.), Novomepro (Canad.), Pantranquil (S. Afr.), Pimal (Austral.), Probal (Canad.), Protran, QID-bamate, Quaname (Belg., Neth., Switz.), Quanil (Ital.), Quietal (Canad.), Restenil (Germ., Swed.), SK-Bamate, Tised (G.B.), Trelmar (Canad.), Urbilat (Germ.), Vio-Bamate, Wescomep (Canad.)

Primary Use: These agents are used to treat skeletal muscle spasms. In addition, meprobamate is used as a psychotherapeutic sedative in the treatment of nervous tension, anxiety, and simple insomnia.

Ocular Side Effects:
A. Systemic Administration
1. Decreased accommodation
2. Decreased vision
3. Diplopia
4. Paralysis of extraocular muscles

5. Decreased corneal reflex
6. Constriction of visual fields
7. Periorbital edema
8. Eyelids or conjunctiva
   a. Allergic reactions
   b. Angioneurotic edema
   c. Urticaria
   d. Erythema multiforme
   e. Stevens-Johnson syndrome
   f. Exfoliative dermatitis
9. Nonspecific ocular irritation
10. Pupils
    a. Mydriasis
    b. Miosis
    c. Decreased or absent reaction to light
11. Nystagmus
12. Subconjunctival or retinal hemorrhages secondary to drug-induced anemia
13. Random ocular movements
14. Decreased intraocular pressure (?)

Clinical Significance: Significant ocular side effects due to these drugs are uncommon and transitory. At normal dosage levels decreased accommodation, diplopia, and paralysis of extraocular muscles may be found. Pupillary responses are variable even in drug-induced coma.

Interactions with Other Drugs:

A. Effect of Carisoprodol or Meprobamate on Activity of Other Drugs
   1. Alcohol ↑
   2. Barbiturates ↑
   3. Monoamine oxidase inhibitors ↑
   4. Sedatives and hypnotics ↑
   5. Tricyclic antidepressants ↑
B. Effect of Other Drugs on Activity of Carisoprodol or Meprobamate
   1. Alcohol ↑
   2. Monoamine oxidase inhibitors ↑
   3. Phenothiazines ↑
   4. Tricyclic antidepressants ↑
   5. Barbiturates ↓
   6. Sedatives and hypnotics ↓

References:

American Hospital Formulary Service. Washington, D.C., American Society of Hospital Pharmacists, Vol. I, 12:20, 1978.

Charkes, N. D.: Meprobamate idiosyncrasy. Arch. Intern. Med. *102*:584, 1958.

Friedman, H. T., and Marmelzat, W. L.: Adverse reactions to meprobamate. JAMA *162*:628, 1956.

Hermans, G.: Les psychotropes. Bull. Soc. Belge Ophtalmol. *160*:15, 1972.

Walsh, F. B., and Hoyt, W. F.: Clinical Neuro-Ophthalmology. 3rd Ed., Baltimore, Williams & Wilkins, Vol. III, 1969, pp. 2633–2634.

Generic Name: 1. Chlordiazepoxide; 2. Clonazepam; 3. Clorazepate; 4. Diazepam; 5. Flurazepam; 6. Lorazepam; 7. Nitrazepam; 8. Oxazepam; 9. Prazepam

Proprietary Name: 1. A-Poxide, Brigen-G, Calmoden (G.B.), Chemdipoxide (Canad.), Chlordiazachel, Corax (Canad.), C-Tran (Canad.), Diapax (Canad.), Elenium (Pol.), Libritabs, Librium, Lo Tense, Medilium (Canad.), Menrium, Murcil, Nack (Canad.), Novopoxide (Canad.), Protensin (Canad.), Relaxil (Canad.), Risolid (Swed.), Screen, SK-Lygen, Solium (Canad.), Tenex, Trilium (Canad.), Tropium (G.B.), Via-Quil (Canad.), Zetran; 2. Clonopin, Iktorivil (Swed.), Rivotril (G.B.); 3. Azene, Tranxene, Tranxilene, Tranxilium (Germ.); 4. Apozepam (Swed.), Atensine (G.B.), E-Pam (Canad.), Paxel (Canad.), Relanium (Pol.), Serenack (Canad.), Stesolid (Swed.), Tensium (G.B.), Valium, Vivol (Canad.); 5. Dalmadorm (S. Afr.), Dalmane; 6. Ativan; 7. Apodorm (Swed.), Dumolid (Swed.), Mogadan (Germ.), Mogadon (G.B.), Remnos (G.B.); 8. Adumbran (Austral., Germ., S. Afr.), Oxepam (Scand.), Praxiten (Aust., Germ.), Serax, Serenid (G.B.), Serepax (Austral., Denm., S. Afr., Swed.), Seresta (Belg., Fr., Neth., Switz.), Sobril (Swed.); 9. Centrax, Demetrin (Germ.), Verstran

Primary Use: These benzodiazepine derivatives are effective in the management of psychoneurotic states manifested by anxiety, tension, or agitation. They are also used as adjunctive therapy in the relief of skeletal muscle spasms and as preoperative medications.

Ocular Side Effects:

    A. Systemic Administration
        1. Decreased vision
        2. Eyelids or conjunctiva
            a. Allergic reactions
            b. Erythema
            c. Conjunctivitis — nonspecific
            d. Photosensitivity
            e. Angioneurotic edema

      f. Urticaria

      g. Purpura

      h. Erythema multiforme

3. Decreased corneal reflex (clorazepate, diazepam)
4. Extraocular muscles
    a. Oculogyric crises
    b. Decreased spontaneous movements
    c. Abnormal conjugate deviations
    d. Jerky pursuit movements
    e. Decreased saccadic movements
    f. Nystagmus — horizontal or gaze evoked
    g. Paralysis
5. Decreased accommodation
6. Decreased depth perception (chlordiazepoxide)
7. Diplopia
8. Visual hallucinations (flurazepam)
9. Pupils
    a. Mydriasis — may precipitate narrow-angle glaucoma
    b. Decreased reaction to light
10. Problems with color vision — dyschromatopsia
11. Nonspecific ocular irritation (clorazepate, flurazepam, nitrazepam)
    a. Photophobia
    b. Lacrimation
    c. Burning sensation
12. Abnormal EOG (diazepam)
13. Subconjunctival or retinal hemorrhages secondary to drug-induced anemia
14. Brown lens deposits (?) (diazepam)
15. Loss of eyelashes or eyebrows (?) (clonazepam)

Clinical Significance: In general, significant ocular side effects due to these benzodiazepine derivatives are rare and reversible. At therapeutic dosage levels, these agents may cause decreased corneal reflex, decreased accommodation, decreased depth perception, and abnormal extraocular muscle movements. Recently, it has been well documented that all these drugs can cause an allergic conjunctivitis. Also, it has been suggested that all these drugs can cross-react since they have the common metabolite desmethyldiazepam which is the primary antigen. This may give a type I immune reaction. Typically, the allergic conjunctivitis occurs within 30 minutes after taking these drugs, with the peak reaction occurring within 4 hours and subsiding in 1 to 2 days. Symptoms include blurred vision, burning, tearing, and a foreign body sensation. Contact lens wearers have confused this adverse drug effect

with poorly fitted lenses. To what degree these benzodiazepine derivatives cause pupillary dilatation is uncertain; however, drug manufacturers advise against their use in patients predisposed to narrow-angle
glaucoma. Also, there have been cases reported to the Registry of acute
narrow angle precipitated by diazepam therapy. Flurazepam has only
been reported to have caused decreased vision, decreased accommodation, hallucinations, and nonspecific ocular irritation.

Interactions with Other Drugs:

A. Effect of Benzodiazepine Derivatives on Activity of Other Drugs
   1. Alcohol ↑
   2. Analgesics ↑
   3. Anticholinergics ↑
   4. Antihistamines ↑
   5. Barbiturates ↑
   6. Monoamine oxidase inhibitors ↑
   7. Phenothiazines ↑
   8. Sedatives and hypnotics ↑
   9. Tricyclic antidepressants ↑
  10. Succinylcholine ↓
B. Effect of Other Drugs on Activity of Benzodiazepine Derivatives
   1. Alcohol ↑
   2. Analgesics ↑
   3. Barbiturates ↑
   4. Monoamine oxidase inhibitors ↑
   5. Phenothiazines ↑
   6. Sedatives and hypnotics ↑
   7. Tricyclic antidepressants ↑

References:

Davidson, S. I.: Report of ocular adverse reactions. Trans. Ophthalmol. Soc. U.K.
   93:495, 1973.
Ghosh, J. S.: Allergy to diazepam and other benzodiazepines. Br. Med. J. 1:902,
   1977.
Hyams, S. W., and Keroub, C.: Glaucoma due to diazepam. Am. J. Psychiatry 134:
   447, 1977.
Lutz, E. G.: Allergic conjunctivitis due to diazepam. Am. J. Psychiatry 132:548, 1975.
Majumdar, S. K.: Allergy to diazepam. Br. Med. J. 1:444, 1977.
Miller, J. G.: Objective measurements of the effects of drugs on driver behavior. JAMA
   179:940, 1962.
Mueller, W., and Haase, E.: Fragen zur Beeinflussung des Elektrooculogramms (EOG)
   durch Diazepam (Faustan). Albrecht von Graefes Arch. Klin. Ophthalmol. 197:
   159, 1975.
Murray, N.: Covert effects of chlordiazepoxide therapy. J. Neuropsychiatry 3:168,
   1962.
Orbell, G.: Headaches and migraine associated with eyestrain. Preliminary report of a
   trial of chlordiazepoxide. Br. J. Ophthalmol. 47:246, 1963.

Pau, H.: Braune Einlagerungen in die Linse nach Diazepam (Valium) gaben. Klin. Monatsbl. Augenheilkd. *164*:446, 1974.

Roberts, W.: The use of psychotropic drugs in glaucoma. Dis. Nerv. Syst. (Suppl.) *29*:40, 1968.

Wilkinson, I. M. S.: The influence of drugs and alcohol upon human eye movement. Proc. R. Soc. Med. *69*:479, 1976.

Generic Name: Doxepin. See under *Class: Antidepressants.*

Class: Anticonvulsants

Generic Name: 1. Ethosuximide; 2. Methsuximide; 3. Phensuximide

Proprietary Name: 1. Emeside (G.B.), Epileo Petitmal (Jap.), Petnidan (Germ.), Pyknolepsinum (Germ.), Suxinutin (Germ., Swed.), Zarontin; 2. Celontin, Petinutin (Germ.); 3. Lifene (Fr.), Milontin

Primary Use: These succinimides are effective in the management of petit mal seizures.

Ocular Side Effects:

A. Systemic Administration
1. Decreased vision
2. Diplopia
3. Photophobia
4. Myopia
5. Periorbital edema or hyperemia
6. Subconjunctival or retinal hemorrhages secondary to drug-induced anemia
7. Eyelids or conjunctiva
   a. Allergic reactions
   b. Angioneurotic edema
   c. Lupoid syndrome
   d. Erythema multiforme
   e. Stevens-Johnson syndrome
   f. Exfoliative dermatitis

Clinical Significance: Methsuximide induces ocular side effects more frequently than ethosuximide or phensuximide. All adverse ocular reactions other than those due to anemias or dermatologic conditions are reversible after discontinuation of the drug. This group of drugs can trigger systemic lupus erythematosus by producing antinuclear antibodies.

References:

Alarcón-Segovia, D.: Drug-induced antinuclear antibodies and lupus syndrome. Drugs *12*:69, 1976.
AMA Drug Evaluations. 4th Ed., New York, John Wiley & Sons, 1980, p. 236.
Council on Drugs. New and nonofficial drugs: Methsuximide. JAMA *171*:1506, 1959.
Millichap, J. G.: Anticonvulsant drugs. Clinical and electroencephalographic indications, efficacy and toxicity. Postgrad. Med. *37*:22, 1965.
Walsh, F. B., and Hoyt, W. F.: Clinical Neuro-Ophthalmology. 3rd Ed., Baltimore, Williams & Wilkins, Vol. III, 1969, p. 2645.

Generic Name: 1. Ethotoin; 2. Mephenytoin

Proprietary Name: 1. Peganone; 2. Mesantoin, Mesontoin (G.B.), Methoin (G.B.), Sedantoinal (Fr.)

Primary Use: These hydantoins are effective in the management of psychomotor and grand mal seizures.

Ocular Side Effects:

A. Systemic Administration
   1. Nystagmus
   2. Diplopia
   3. Photophobia
   4. Eyelids or conjunctiva
      a. Allergic reactions
      b. Conjunctivitis — nonspecific
      c. Angioneurotic edema
      d. Lupoid syndrome
      e. Erythema multiforme
      f. Stevens-Johnson syndrome
      g. Exfoliative dermatitis
   5. Subconjunctival or retinal hemorrhages secondary to drug-induced anemia
   6. Corneal or lens opacities (?)
   7. Myasthenic neuromuscular blocking effect (?)
      a. Paresis of extraocular muscles (?)
   8. Loss of eyelashes or eyebrows (?)

Clinical Significance: These hydantoin agents have fewer adverse ocular reactions than phenytoin. Ocular side effects are seen more frequently with mephenytoin than with ethotoin and are reversible either by decreasing the dosage or discontinuing use of the drug. As with phenytoin, nystagmus may persist for some time after use of the drug is stopped. Mephenytoin has been implicated in inducing systemic lupus erythematosus by producing antinuclear antibodies. While in many instances these antibodies are produced, only a small number produce lupus syndromes. Corneal or lens opacities and myasthenic neuromuscular blocking effect have been reported in only one series.

Interactions with Other Drugs:

A. Effect of Hydantoins on Activity of Other Drugs
1. Analgesics ↑
2. Barbiturates ↑
3. Corticosteroids ↓
4. Vitamin D ↓
B. Effect of Other Drugs on Activity of Hydantoins
1. Analgesics ↑
2. Chloramphenicol ↑
3. Oxyphenbutazone ↑
4. Phenothiazines ↑
5. Phenylbutazone ↑
6. Salicylates ↑
7. Sulfonamides ↑
8. Tricyclic antidepressants ↑↓
9. Adrenergic blockers ↓
10. Alcohol ↓
11. Antihistamines ↓
12. Barbiturates ↓
13. Sedatives and hypnotics ↓
C. Cross Sensitivity
1. Barbiturates

References:

Alarcón-Segovia, D.: Drug-induced antinuclear antibodies and lupus syndromes. Drugs *12*:69, 1976.

Gilman, A. G., Goodman, L. S., and Gilman, A. (Eds.): The Pharmacological Basis of Therapeutics. 6th Ed., New York, Macmillan, 1980, pp. 455–456.

Hermans, G.: Les anticonvulsivants. Bull. Soc. Belge Ophtalmol. *160*:89, 1972.

Livingston, S.: Drug Therapy for Epilepsy. Springfield, Charles C Thomas, 1966.

Walsh, F. B., and Hoyt, W. F.: Clinical Neuro-Ophthalmology. 3rd Ed., Baltimore, Williams & Wilkins, Vol. III, 1969, p. 2644.

Generic Name: 1. Paramethadione; 2. Trimethadione

Proprietary Name: 1. Paradione; 2. Epidione (Fr.), Tridione, Trimedone (Canad.), Troxidone (G.B.)

Primary Use: These oxazolidinediones are used primarily in the treatment of refractory petit mal seizures and myoclonic contractions.

Ocular Side Effects:

A. Systemic Administration
1. Glare phenomenon — objects appear covered with white snow
2. Photophobia
3. Night blindness
4. Diplopia
5. Gaze evoked nystagmus
6. Problems with color vision
   a. Dyschromatopsia, red-green or yellow-blue defect
   b. Objects have dazzling white tinge
   c. Colored haloes around lights — mainly white
   d. Colors appear faded
7. Scotomas
8. Eyelids or conjunctiva
   a. Allergic reactions
   b. Photosensitivity
   c. Angioneurotic edema
   d. Lupoid syndrome
   e. Erythema multiforme
   f. Stevens-Johnson syndrome
   g. Exfoliative dermatitis
   h. Lyell's syndrome
9. Subconjunctival or retinal hemorrhages secondary to drug-induced anemia
10. Ocular teratogenic effects (fetal trimethadione syndrome)
    a. "V"-shaped eyebrows
    b. Epicanthus
    c. Strabismus
    d. Hypertelorism
    e. Myopia
11. Myasthenic neuromuscular blocking effect
    a. Paralysis of extraocular muscles
    b. Ptosis
12. Loss of eyelashes or eyebrows (?)

Clinical Significance: The oxazolidinediones have the unusual side effect of causing a prolonged "dazzle" when the eyes are exposed to light. This includes decreased vision, momentary loss of vision, loss of color perception, and illuminated objects appear to be covered by snow. This toxic effect seems to be specific for retinal cones and in all but two instances has been reversible. In general, this phenomenon ceases to occur even if therapy is restarted after a few months. Symptoms often last a few days to a few weeks after use of the drug is discontinued. These drugs can produce antinuclear antibodies; however, lupus erythematosus is rarely precipitated. Paramethadione has significantly fewer and less prolonged ocular side effects than trimethadione. Trimethadione is said to be teratogenic and to cause a typical phenotype with ocular signs as described above.

References:

Alarcón-Segovia, D.: Drug-induced antinuclear antibodies and lupus syndromes. Drugs *12*:69, 1976.

Argov, Z., and Mastaglia, F. L.: Disorders of neuromuscular transmission caused by drugs. N. Engl. J. Med. *301*:409, 1979,

Dekking, H. M.: Visual disturbances due to Tridione. Acta Cong. Ophthalmol. *1*:465, 1950.

Gilman, A. G., Goodman, L. S., and Gilman, A. (Eds.): The Pharmacological Basis of Therapeutics. 6th Ed., New York, Macmillan, 1980, pp. 465–466.

Gordon, N.: Fetal drug syndromes. Postgrad. Med. J. *54*:796, 1978.

Lee, S. L., Rivero, I., and Siegel, M.: Activation of systemic lupus erythematosus by drugs. Arch. Intern. Med. *117*:620, 1966.

Peterson, H. deC.: Association of trimethadione therapy and myasthenia gravis. N. Engl. J. Med. *274*:506, 1966.

Sloan, L. L., and Gilger, A. P.: Visual effects of Tridione. Am. J. Ophthalmol. *30*: 1387, 1947.

Walsh, F. B., and Hoyt, W. F.: Clinical Neuro-Ophthalmology. 3rd Ed., Baltimore, Williams & Wilkins, Vol. III, 1969, pp. 2562, 2639, 2655–2656.

Weisbecker, C. A.: Ophthalmic side effects of systemic medications. Hosp. Form. *12*:709, 1977.

Generic Name: Phenytoin

Proprietary Name: Dantoin (Canad.), Difhydan (Swed.), Dihycon, Di-Hydan (Fr.), Dilabid, Dilantin, Di-Phen, Diphentyn (Canad.), Diphenyl, Diphenylan, Ditoin (Austral.), Divulsan (Canad.), Ekko, Epanutin (G.B.), Fenantoin (Swed.), Kessodanten, Novodiphenyl (Canad.), Phenhydan (Germ.), Phentoin (Austral.), Pyoredol (Fr.), Solantyl (Fr.), Toin, Zentropil (Germ.)

Primary Use: This hydantoin is effective in the prophylaxis and treatment of chronic epilepsy.

Ocular Side Effects:
A. Systemic Administration
    1. Nystagmus—downbeat, horizontal, or vertical
    2. Diplopia
    3. Decreased vision
    4. Pupils
       a. Mydriasis
       b. Decreased reaction to light
    5. Myasthenic neuromuscular blocking effect
       a. Paralysis of extraocular muscles
       b. Ptosis
    6. Decreased accommodation
    7. Decreased convergence
    8. Visual hallucinations
    9. Visual sensations
       a. Glare phenomenon — objects appear covered with white snow
       b. Flashing lights
       c. Oscillopsia
   10. Orbital or periorbital pain
   11. Problems with color vision
       a. Objects have white tinge
       b. Colors appear faded
   12. Eyelids or conjunctiva
       a. Allergic reactions
       b. Ulceration
       c. Purpura
       d. Lupoid syndrome
       e. Erythema multiforme
       f. Stevens-Johnson syndrome
       g. Exfoliative dermatitis
       h. Lyell's syndrome
   13. Ocular teratogenic effects (fetal hydantoin syndrome)
       a. Hypertelorism
       b. Ptosis
       c. Epicanthus
       d. Strabismus
       e. Glaucoma
       f. Optic nerve or iris hypoplasia
       g. Retinal coloboma
       h. Retinoschisis
       i. Trichomegaly
   14. Subconjunctival or retinal hemorrhages secondary to drug-induced anemia

Clinical Significance: Nearly all ocular side effects due to phenytoin are reversible after discontinuation of use of the drug. The first sign of systemic phenytoin toxicity is nystagmus and is directly related to the blood levels of the drug. Instances of nystagmus persisting for 20 months or longer after discontinued use of the drug have been reported. Fine nystagmus may occur even at therapeutic dosages, but coarse nystagmus is indicative of toxic states. Downbeat nystagmus has even been reported due to phenytoin. Paralysis of extraocular muscles is uncommon, reversible, and primarily found in toxic states. Although the fetal hydantoin syndrome is well accepted in the pediatric literature, there is some disagreement in the ophthalmic community as to a true cause-and-effect relationship. However, an increasing number of cases in the literature tends to support the fact that the maternal ingestion of hydantoins can produce congenital abnormalities in their offspring. Ocular abnormalities are quite common in this syndrome.

Interactions with Other Drugs:

A. Effect of Phenytoin on Activity of Other Drugs
   1. Analgesics ↑
   2. Barbiturates ↑
   3. Corticosteroids ↓
   4. Vitamin D ↓
B. Effect of Other Drugs on Activity of Phenytoin
   1. Analgesics ↑
   2. Chloramphenicol ↑
   3. Oxyphenbutazone ↑
   4. Phenothiazines ↑
   5. Phenylbutazone ↑
   6. Salicylates ↑
   7. Sulfonamides ↑
   8. Tricyclic antidepressants ↑↓
   9. Adrenergic blockers ↓
   10. Alcohol ↓
   11. Antihistamines ↓
   12. Barbiturates ↓
   13. Sedatives and hypnotics ↓
C. Cross Sensitivity
   1. Barbiturates

References:

Alpert, J. N.: Downbeat nystagmus due to anticonvulsant toxicity. Ann. Neurol. 4: 471, 1978.

Apt, L., and Gaffney, W. L.: Is there a "fetal hydantoin syndrome?" Am. J. Ophthalmol. 84:439, 1977.

Hanson, J. W., and Smith, D. W.: The fetal hydantoin syndrome. J. Pediatr. 87:285, 1975.
Hoyt, C. S., and Billson, F. A.: Maternal anticonvulsants and optic nerve hypoplasia. Br. J. Ophthalmol. 62:3, 1978.
Majewski, F., et al.: Zur Teratogenität von Antikonvulsiva. Dtsch. Med. Wochenschr. 105:719, 1980.
Manlapaz, J. S.: Abducens nerve palsy in Dilantin intoxication. J. Pediatr. 55:73, 1959.
Morris, J. V., Fischer, E., and Bergin, J. T.: Rare complications of phenytoin sodium treatment. Br. Med. J. 2:1529, 1956.
Spector, R. H., Davidoff, R. A., and Schwartzman, R. J.: Phenytoin-induced ophthalmoplegia. Neurology 26:1031, 1976.
Van Huyssteen, M. P.: Conjunctival ulceration as a complication in the treatment of epilepsy. S. Afr. Med. J. 27:626, 1953.
Wilson, R. S., Smead, W., and Char, F.: Diphenylhydantoin teratogenicity: Ocular manifestations and related deformities. J. Pediatr. Ophthalmol. Strabismus 15:137, 1978.

Generic Name: Sulthiame (Sultiame)

Proprietary Name: Conadil, Elisal (Fr.), Opsolot (G.B.), Trolone

Primary Use: This sulfonamide congener is used in the treatment of psychomotor epilepsy.

Ocular Side Effects:

A. Systemic Administration
  1. Decreased vision
  2. Diplopia
  3. Problems with color vision
    a. Dyschromatopsia
    b. Objects have red tinge
  4. Eyelids or conjunctiva
    a. Edema
    b. Stevens-Johnson syndrome
    c. Ptosis
  5. Papilledema

Clinical Significance: This anticonvulsant has infrequently caused ocular side effects. These adverse ocular reactions are reversible upon discontinuance of the drug. One patient, after ingesting sulthiame for 2 weeks, developed papilledema and transient subjective changes in color vision. Within 2 weeks after the drug was stopped, the papilledema receded. It is possible that these signs and symptoms represented a toxic reaction to sulthiame, but this is unproven.

Interactions with Other Drugs:

A. Effect of Sulthiame on Activity of Other Drugs
  1. Barbiturates ↑

References:

Dukes, M. N. G. (Ed.): Meyler's Side Effects of Drugs. Amsterdam, Excerpta Medica, Vol. IX, 1980, pp. 92, 100.

Garland, H., and Sumner, D.: Sulthiame in treatment of epilepsy. Br. Med. J. *1*:474, 1964.

Grant, W. M.: Toxicology of the Eye. 2nd Ed., Springfield, Charles C Thomas, 1974, pp. 960–961.

Liske, E., and Forster, F. M.: Clinical evaluation of the anticonvulsant effects of sulthiame. J. New Drugs *3*:32, 1963.

Taaffe, A., and O'Brien, C.: A case of Stevens-Johnson syndrome associated with the anti-convulsants sulthiame and ethosuximide. Br. Dent. J. *138*:172, 1975.

Wade, A. (Ed.): Martindale: The Extra Pharmacopoeia. 27th Ed., London, Pharmaceutical Press, 1977, pp. 1245–1246.

Generic Name: 1. Valproate Sodium; 2. Valproic Acid

Proprietary Name: 1. Depakene, Epilim (G.B.); 2. Depakene

Primary Use: Valproic acid is a carboxylic acid derivative, and valproate sodium is the sodium salt of valproic acid. These antiepileptic agents are used in the prophylactic management of petit mal seizures.

Ocular Side Effects:

A. Systemic Administration
  1. Diplopia
  2. Nystagmus
  3. Visual hallucinations
  4. Loss of eyelashes or eyebrows (?)

Clinical Significance: Ocular side effects due to these drugs are rare and seldom of clinical significance. All adverse ocular reactions are reversible with discontinued drug use.

Interactions with Other Drugs:

A. Effect of Valproates on Activity of Other Drugs
  1. Barbiturates ↑

References:

American Hospital Formulary Service. Washington, D.C., American Society of Hospital Pharmacists, Vol. I, 28:12, 1979.

Bellman, M. H., and Ross, E. M.: Side effects of sodium valproate. Br. Med. J. *1*:1662, 1977.

Chadwick, D. W., et al.: Acute intoxication with sodium valproate. Ann. Neurol. *6*: 552, 1979.

Hassan, M. N., Laljee, H. C. K., and Parsonage, M. J.: Sodium valproate in the treatment of resistant epilepsy. Acta Neurol. Scand. *54*:209, 1976.

Physicians' Desk Reference. 35th Ed., Oradell, N.J., Medical Economics Co., 1981, p. 510.

Class: Antidepressants

Generic Name: 1. Amitriptyline; 2. Desipramine; 3. Imipramine; 4. Nortriptyline; 5. Protriptyline

Proprietary Name: 1. Amitid, Amizol (G.B.), Annolytin (Jap.), Deprex (Canad.), Domical (G.B.), Elatrol (Canad.), Elavil, Endep, Larozyl (Swed.), Lentizol (G.B.), Levate (Canad.), Mareline (Canad.), Novotriptyn (Canad.), Saroten (G.B.), SK-Amitriptyline, Tryptanol (Austral., S. Afr.), Tryptizol (G.B.); 2. Depramine (S. Afr.), Norpramin, Pertofran (G.B.), Pertofrane, Pertofrin (Swed.); 3. Berkomine (G.B.), Censtim (Austral.), Chemipramine (Canad.), Co-Caps Imipramine (G.B.), Dimipressin (G.B.), Imavate, Imiprin (Austral.), Impranil (Canad.), Impril (Canad.), Iramil (Austral.), Janimine, Melipramine (Austral.), Norpramine (G.B.), Novopramine (Canad.), Oppanyl (G.B.), Panpramine (S. Afr.), Praminil (G.B.), Presamine, Prodepress (Austral.), SK-Pramine, Somipra (Austral.), Thymopramine (S. Afr.), Tofranil, W.D.D.; 4. Acetexa (Germ.), Allegron (G.B.), Aventyl, Noritren (Swed.), Nortab (Austral.), Nortrilen (Germ.), Nortrilin (S. Afr.), Pamelor, Psychostyl (Fr.), Sensaval (Swed.); 5. Concordin (G.B.), Maximed (Germ.), Triptil, Vivactil

Primary Use: These tricyclic antidepressants are effective in the relief of symptoms of mental depression. Imipramine is also used in the management of enuresis.

Ocular Side Effects:

A. Systemic Administration
   1. Decreased vision
   2. Decrease or paralysis of accommodation
   3. Pupils
      a. Mydriasis — may precipitate narrow-angle glaucoma
      b. Decreased or absent reaction to light

4. Diplopia
5. Photophobia
6. Visual hallucinations
7. Extraocular muscles
    a. Paresis or paralysis — primarily lateral rectus
    b. Oculogyric crises
    c. Decreased spontaneous movements
    d. Abnormal conjugate deviations
    e. Jerky pursuit movements
    f. Blepharospasm
    g. Nystagmus
8. Decreased lacrimation
9. Decreased corneal reflex
10. Retrobulbar or optic neuritis
11. Subconjunctival or retinal hemorrhages secondary to drug-induced anemia
12. Eyelids or conjunctiva
    a. Erythema
    b. Edema
    c. Photosensitivity
    d. Urticaria
    e. Purpura
13. Toxic amblyopia
14. Loss of eyelashes or eyebrows (?)
15. Problems with color vision — dyschromatopsia (?)
B. Local Ophthalmic Use or Exposure — protriptyline
    1. Decreased intraocular pressure — especially if in combination with sympathomimetics
    2. Mydriasis — may precipitate narrow-angle glaucoma
    3. Corneal opacities

Clinical Significance: All adverse ocular reactions due to these tricyclic antidepressants are reversible, transitory, and in most cases, of little clinical significance. The most common ocular side effects are mydriasis and cycloplegia. A number of cases of narrow-angle glaucoma precipitated by amitriptyline have been reported. However, this is indeed a rare finding compared to the number of patients on these drugs. There has also been some question that these agents may cause an increased intraocular pressure in patients with open-angle glaucoma as well. These agents probably cause few ocular sicca problems in normal tear producers. However, in patients with an already compromised tear production, all of these drugs have the potential to aggravate latent or manifested keratoconjunctivitis sicca. This may be due to an initial, probably transitory (a few months) decrease in tear production and an increased frequency of blinking. The clinician needs to be aware always of the interaction between the tricyclic antidepressants and the epinephrine preparations. Deaths have been attributed to the combination use of these drugs. Topical ocular proptriptyline has been used as an antiglaucoma agent, but it has not been marketed since it can cause corneal opacities of unknown composition.

Interactions with Other Drugs:

A. Effect of Tricyclic Antidepressants on Activity of Other Drugs
   1. Alcohol ↑
   2. Analgesics ↑
   3. Anticholinergics ↑
   4. Barbiturates ↑
   5. Monoamine oxidase inhibitors ↑
   6. Phenothiazines ↑
   7. Sedatives and hypnotics ↑
   8. Sympathomimetics ↑
   9. Adrenergic blockers ↓
B. Effect of Other Drugs on Activity of Tricyclic Antidepressants
   1. Adrenergic blockers ↑
   2. Analgesics ↑
   3. Monoamine oxidase inhibitors ↑
   4. Phenothiazines ↑
   5. Sedatives and hypnotics ↑

References:

Azima, H., Silver, A., and Arthurs, D.: Effects of G33040 (Ensidon) and G35020 (Petrofrane) on depressive states. Can. Med. Assoc. J. *87*:1224, 1962.
Blackwell, B., et al.: Anticholinergic activity of two tricyclic antidepressants. Am. J. Psychiatry *135*:722, 1978.
Davidson, S. I.: Reports of ocular adverse reactions. Trans. Ophthalmol. Soc. U.K. *93*:495, 1973.
Edwards, J. G.: Unwanted effects of psychotrophic drugs. Practitioner *218*:862, 1977.
Karson, C. N.: Oculomotor signs in a psychiatric population: A preliminary report. Am. J. Psychiatry *136*:1057, 1979.
Kitazawa, Y., and Langham, M. E.: Influence of an adrenergic potentiator on the ocular response of catecholamines in primates and man. Nature *219*:1376, 1968.
Steel, C. M., O'Duffy, J., and Brown, S. S.: Clinical effects and treatment of imipramine and amitriptyline poisoning in children. Br. Med. J. *3*:663, 1967.

Generic Name: 1. Amoxapine; 2. Clomipramine; 3. Doxepin; 4. Trimipramine

Proprietary Name: 1. Asendin; 2. Anafranil (G.B.); 3. Adapin, Aponal (Germ.), Quitaxon (Austral., Fr., S. Afr.), Sinequan, Sinquan (Germ.); 4. Stangyl (Germ.), Surmontil

Primary Use: These tricyclic antidepressants are used in the treatment of psychoneurotic anxiety or depressive reactions.

Ocular Side Effects:

A. Systemic Administration
  1. Decreased vision
  2. Pupils
    a. Mydriasis — may precipitate narrow-angle glaucoma
    b. Decreased or absent reaction to light — toxic states
  3. Decrease or paralysis of accommodation
  4. Eyelids or conjunctiva
    a. Erythema
    b. Edema
    c. Photosensitivity
    d. Urticaria
    e. Blepharospasm (?)
  5. Nystagmus — horizontal or rotary — toxic states
  6. Visual hallucinations
  7. Keratoconjunctivitis sicca (doxepin)
  8. Lacrimation (amoxapine)
  9. Photophobia (doxepin)
  10. Oculogyric crises (doxepin)
  11. Loss of eyelashes or eyebrows (?) (doxepin)

Clinical Significance: Adverse ocular reactions due to these tricyclic antidepressants are seldom of major clinical importance. Anticholinergic effects are the most frequent and include blurred vision, disturbance of accommodation, and mydriasis. There have been three reports to the Registry of keratoconjunctivitis sicca associated with the use of doxepin. In one case, the onset was dramatic and disappeared when the drug was discontinued. There is a question whether an increase in the blink rate is due to the drug, an associated keratoconjunctivitis sicca, or normally found with mental stress. Since these tricyclic antidepressants may be bound to ocular melanin, there is a potential for retinal damage; however, this side effect has not been reported.

Interactions with Other Drugs:

A. Effect of Tricyclic Antidepressants on Activity of Other Drugs
  1. Alcohol ↑
  2. Analgesics ↑
  3. Anticholinergics ↑
  4. Barbiturates ↑
  5. Monoamine oxidase inhibitors ↑

   6. Phenothiazines ↑
   7. Sedatives and hypnotics ↑
   8. Sympathomimetics ↑
   9. Adrenergic blockers ↓
 B. Effect of Other Drugs on Activity of Tricyclic Antidepressants
   1. Adrenergic blockers ↑
   2. Analgesics ↑
   3. Monoamine oxidase inhibitors ↑
   4. Phenothiazines ↑
   5. Sedatives and hypnotics ↑

References:

Hermans, G.: Les psychotropes. Bull. Soc. Belge Ophtalmol. *160*:15, 1972.
Hobbs, D. C.: Distribution and metabolism of doxepin. Biochem. Pharmacol. *18*:1941, 1969.
Karson, C. N.: Oculomotor signs in a psychiatric population: A preliminary report. Am. J. Psychiatry *136*:1057, 1979.
Penttilä, A., Lehti, H., and Lönnqvist, J.: Psychotropic drugs and impairment of psychomotor functions. Psychopharm. *43*:75, 1975.
Today's drugs. Trimipramine. Br. Med. J. *1*:98, 1967.

Generic Name: Carbamazepine

Proprietary Name: Tegretal (Germ.), Tegretol

Primary Use: This iminostilbene derivative is used in the treatment of pain associated with trigeminal neuralgia.

Ocular Side Effects:

 A. Systemic Administration
   1. Diplopia
   2. Decreased vision
   3. Nystagmus
   4. Decreased spontaneous eye movements
   5. Visual hallucinations
   6. Eyelids or conjunctiva
     a. Allergic reactions
     b. Conjunctivitis — nonspecific
     c. Photosensitivity
     d. Urticaria
     e. Purpura
     f. Lupoid syndrome
     g. Erythema multiforme
     h. Stevens-Johnson syndrome

i. Exfoliative dermatitis
  j. Lyell's syndrome
7. Mydriasis — may precipitate narrow-angle glaucoma — toxic states
8. Decreased accommodation
9. Subconjunctival or retinal hemorrhages secondary to drug-induced anemia
10. Papilledema — toxic states
11. Cataracts (?)
12. Loss of eyelashes or eyebrows (?)
13. Ocular teratogenic effects (?)

Clinical Significance: Probably the most common side effects due to carbamazepine are ocular, with diplopia being the most frequent followed by blurred vision and a "heavy feeling in the eyes." Ocular adverse reactions will occur in most patients when the dosage exceeds 1.2 g and will disappear as the dosage is decreased. Most ocular side effects are reversible and may spontaneously clear even without reduction of the drug dosage. About 25 percent of patients receiving this drug develop neurologic or hematopoietic reactions, some of which are associated with eye abnormalities. The most common drug-related neurologic state is the toxic ataxia syndrome. This may occur as an acute phenomenon with carbamazepine, which may include nystagmus, confusion, drowsiness, and ataxia. Toxic reactions in overdosage situations can cause dilated sluggish or nonreactive pupils and papilledema. This drug can also cause the ocular effects of lupus erythematosus. Carbamazepine can be recovered in the tears, and this method has been advocated to test for blood levels as a noninvasive technique in the pediatric age group.

Interactions with Other Drugs:

A. Effect of Carbamazepine on Activity of Other Drugs
  1. Alcohol ↑
  2. Barbiturates ↑

References:

Alarcón-Segovia, D.: Drug-induced antinuclear antibodies and lupus syndromes. Drugs *12*:69, 1976.
Critchley, E. M. R.: Drug-induced diseases. Drug-induced neurological disease. Br. Med. J. *1*:862, 1979.
Hermans, G.: Les anticonvulsivants. Bull. Soc. Belge Ophtalmol. *160*:89, 1972.
Livingston, S., et al.: Use of carbamazepine in epilepsy. JAMA *200*:204, 1967.
Livingston, S., Pauli, L. L., and Berman, W.: Carbamazepine (Tegretol) in epilepsy. Nine year follow-up study with special emphasis on untoward reactions. Dis. Nerv. Syst. 35:103, 1974.

Lubeck, M. J.: Effects of drugs on ocular muscles. Int. Ophthalmol. Clin. *11*(2):35, 1971.

Monaco, F., et al.: Tears as the best practical indicator of the unbound fraction of an anticonvulsant drug. Epilepsia *20*:705, 1979.

Generic Name: 1. Isocarboxazid; 2. Nialamide; 3. Phenelzine; 4. Tranylcypromine

Proprietary Name: 1. Marplan; 2. Niamid (G.B.); 3. Nardelzine (Fr.), Nardil; 4. Parnate, Tylciprine (Fr.)

Primary Use: These monoamine oxidase inhibitors are used in the symptomatic relief of reactive or endogenous depression.

Ocular Side Effects:

A. Systemic Administration
   1. Decreased vision
   2. Pupils — toxic states
      a. Mydriasis — may precipitate narrow-angle glaucoma
      b. Miosis
      c. Anisocoria
      d. Absence of reaction to light
   3. Extraocular muscles
      a. Diplopia
      b. Ptosis
      c. Nystagmus (phenelzine, tranylcypromine)
      d. Paralysis
      e. Strabismus
   4. Photophobia
   5. Problems with color vision — dyschromatopsia, red-green defect
   6. Photosensitivity
   7. Visual hallucinations (nialamide)
   8. Papilledema (?) (isocarboxazid, tranylcypromine)
   9. Retrobulbar or optic neuritis (?) (isocarboxazid, nialamide, phenelzine)

Clinical Significance: Most ocular side effects due to these monoamine oxidase inhibitors are reversible and insignificant. Pupillary reactions occur primarily in overdose situations. Nystagmus may be induced by phenelzine or tranylcypromine and visual hallucinations by nialamide therapy, but these symptoms have not been reported due to any other monoamine oxidase inhibitors.

Interactions with Other Drugs:

A. Effect of Monoamine Oxidase Inhibitors on Activity of Other Drugs
   1. Analgesics ↑
   2. Anticholinergics ↑
   3. Antihistamines ↑
   4. Barbiturates ↑
   5. Diuretics ↑
   6. General anesthetics ↑
   7. Local anesthetics ↑
   8. Other monoamine oxidase inhibitors ↑
   9. Phenothiazines ↑
   10. Sedatives and hypnotics ↑
   11. Succinylcholine ↑
   12. Sympathomimetics ↑
   13. Tricyclic antidepressants ↑
B. Effect of Other Drugs on Activity of Monoamine Oxidase Inhibitors
   1. Other monoamine oxidase inhibitors ↑
   2. Tricyclic antidepressants ↑
   3. Analgesics ↑↓
   4. Phenothiazines ↓

References:

Grant, W. M.: Toxicology of the Eye. 2nd Ed., Springfield, Charles C Thomas, 1974, pp. 605, 718–719, 744–745, 805–806, 1029–1030.
Hermans, G.: Les psychotropes. Bull. Soc. Belge Ophtalmol. *160*:15, 1972.
Leonard, J. W., Gifford, R. W., Jr., and Williams, G. H., Jr.: Tranylcypromine sulfate therapy. Occurrence of severe paroxysmal headache. JAMA *187*:957, 1964.
Physicians' Desk Reference. 35th Ed., Oradell, N.J., Medical Economics Co., 1981, pp. 1374, 1512, 1684.
Solberg, C. O.: Phenelzine intoxication. JAMA *177*:572, 1961.

Generic Name: Methylphenidate

Proprietary Name: Methidate (Canad.), Ritalin

Primary Use: This piperidine derivative is used in the treatment of mild depression and in the management of children with the hyperkinetic syndrome.

Ocular Side Effects:

A. Systemic Administration — Oral
   1. Eyelids or conjunctiva
      a. Urticaria

        b. Erythema multiforme
        c. Stevens-Johnson syndrome
        d. Exfoliative dermatitis
    2. Visual hallucinations — toxic states
    3. Mydriasis — toxic states
    4. Subconjunctival or retinal hemorrhages secondary to drug-induced anemia
    5. Increased intraocular pressure (?)
  B. Systemic Administration — Intravenous
    1. Talc retinopathy
        a. Small yellow-white emboli
        b. Neovascularization — late
        c. Retinal hemorrhages
    2. Decreased vision
    3. Tractional retinal detachment

Clinical Significance: Ocular side effects due to methylphenidate are rare, reversible, and seldom clinically significant. Mydriasis rarely occurs except in overdose situations. Recently, methylphenidate tablets intended for oral use have become popular among drug addicts who crush the tablets and inject the drug intravenously. The filler in the tablet is insoluble talc, cornstarch, or various binders and lodges in the retina and other tissues as emboli. These glistening refractile particles in the retina which are fairly stationary may cause visual symptoms, and neovascularization may form in time. Severe complications requiring lensectomy, vitrectomy, and retinal surgery have been reported.

Interactions with Other Drugs:

  A. Effect of Methylphenidate on Activity of Other Drugs
    1. Barbiturates ↑
    2. Phenylbutazone ↑
    3. Tricyclic antidepressants ↑
    4. Adrenergic blockers ↓
  B. Contraindications
    1. Monoamine oxidase inhibitors

References:

American Hospital Formulary Service. Washington, D.C., American Society of Hospital Pharmacists, Vol. 1, 28:20, 1973.

Atlee, W. E., Jr.: Talc and cornstarch emboli in eyes of drug abusers. JAMA 219:49, 1972.

Dukes, M. N. G. (Ed.): Meyler's Side Effects of Drugs. Amsterdam, Excerpta Medica, Vol. IX, 1980, pp. 10–11.

Grant, W. M.: Toxicology of the Eye. 2nd Ed., Springfield, Charles C Thomas, 1974, p. 702.

Gunby, P.: Methylphenidate abuse produces retinopathy. JAMA *241*:546, 1979.
Methylphenidate (Ritalin) and other drugs for treatment of hyperactive children. Med. Lett. Drugs Ther. *19*:53, 1977.
Physicians' Desk Reference. 35th Ed., Oradell, N.J., Medical Economics Co., 1981, p. 811.

Class: Antipsychotic Agents

Generic Name: 1. Acetophenazine; 2. Butaperazine; 3. Carphenazine; 4. Chlorpromazine; 5. Diethazine; 6. Ethopropazine (Profenamine); 7. Fluphenazine; 8. Mesoridazine; 9. Methdilazine; 10. Methotrimeprazine (Levomepromazine); 11. Perazine; 12. Periciazine; 13. Perphenazine; 14. Piperacetazine; 15. Prochlorperazine; 16. Promazine; 17. Promethazine; 18. Propiomazine; 19. Thiethylperazine; 20. Thiopropazate; 21. Thioproperazine; 22. Thioridazine; 23. Trifluoperazine; 24. Triflupromazine; 25. Trimeprazine

Proprietary Name: 1. Tindal, Tindala (Swed.); 2. Randolectil (Germ.), Repoise; 3. Proketazine; 4. Chloractil, Chlor-Promanyl (Canad.), Chlorprom-Ez-Ets (Canad.), Chlorzine, Elmarine (Canad.), Hibernal (Swed.), Klorazin (S. Afr.), Klorazine, Klorpromex (Swed.), Komazine, Largactil, Megaphen (Germ.), Onazine (Canad.), Plegomazine (Austral.), Procalm (Austral.), Promachel, Promachlor, Promacid (Austral.), Promapar, Promaz, Promosol (Canad.), Psychozine, Serazone (Austral.), Sonazine, Terpium, Thoradex, Thorazine; 5. Diparcol (Fr.); 6. Lysivane (G.B.), Parkin (Jap.), Parsidol, Parsitan (Canad.); 7. Anatensol (Austral., S. Afr.), Dapotum (Germ.), Lyogen (Germ.), Modecate (G.B.), Moditen (G.B.), Omca (Germ.), Pacinol (Swed.), Permitil, Prolixin, Sevinol (Austral.), Siqualone (Swed.); 8. Inofal (Germ.), Lidanar, Lidanil (Fr.), Serentil; 9. Bristaline (Austral.), Dilosyn (G.B.), Tacaryl; 10. Levoprome, Neurocil (Germ.), Nozinan (Canad., Fr., Swed.), Veractil (G.B.); 11. Taxilan (Germ.); 12. Aolept (Germ.), Neulactil (G.B.), Neuleptil (Canad., Fr.); 13. Decentan (Germ.), Fentazin (G.B.), Trilafon, Trilifan (Fr.); 14. Quide; 15. Anti-Naus (Austral.), Compazine, Stemetil (G.B.), Tementil (Fr.), Vertigon (G.B.); 16. Atarzine (Canad.), Eliranol (Ital.), Hyzine, Intrazine (Canad.), Prazine (Belg., Neth., Switz.), Promanyl (Canad.), Promazettes (Canad.), Promezerine (Canad.), Protactyl (Germ., Norw., Swed.), Sparine; 17. Atosil (Germ.), Avomine (G.B.), Fellozine, Ganphen, Histantil (Canad.), K-Phen, Lemprometh, Lenazine (S. Afr.), Lergigan (Swed.), Methazine, Meth-Zine (Austral.), Pentazine, Phenergan, Phenerhist, Phenerject, Progan (Austral.), Promethapar, Prorex, Prothazine (Austral.), Provigan, Quadnite, Remsed, Rolamethazine, Sigazine, ZiPan; 18. Largon, Popavan (Swed.); 19. Torecan; 20. Dartal (Canad.), Dartalan (G.B.); 21. Majeptil (G.B.), Mayeptil (Germ.); 22. Mallorol (Swed.), Mellaril, Melleretten (Germ.), Melleril (G.B.), Novoridazine (Canad.), Thioril (Canad.); 23. Calmazine (Austral.), Chemflurazine (Canad.), Clinazine (Canad.), Fluazine (Canad.), Jatroneural (Germ.), Novoflurazine (Canad.), Pentazine (Canad.), Solazine (Canad.), Stelazine, Terfluzin (Austral., Swed.), Terfluzine (Canad., Fr.), Trifluoper-Ez-Ets (Canad.), Triflurin (Canad.); 24. Psyquil (Fr., Germ.), Siquil (N.Z.), Vesprin; 25. Penectyl (Canad.), Repeltin (Germ.), Temaril, Theralen (Swed.), Theralene (Fr., Germ.), Vallergan (G.B.)

Primary Use: These phenothiazines are used in the treatment of depressive, involutional, senile, or organic psychoses and various forms of schizophrenia. Some of the phenothiazines are also used as adjuncts to anesthesia, antiemetics, and in the treatment of tetanus.

Ocular Side Effects:

A. Systemic Administration
Not all of the ocular side effects listed have been reported for each phenothiazine.
1. Decreased vision
2. Decrease or paralysis of accommodation
3. Night blindness
4. Problems with color vision
   a. Dyschromatopsia, red-green defect
   b. Objects have yellow or brown tinge
   c. Colored haloes around lights
5. Cornea
   a. Pigmentary deposits
   b. Edema
   c. Punctate keratitis
6. Pupils
   a. Mydriasis — may precipitate narrow-angle glaucoma
   b. Miosis — rare
   c. Decreased reaction to light
7. Retina
   a. Pigmentary changes
   b. Edema
8. Oculogyric crises

9. Visual fields
   a. Scotomas — annular, central, or paracentral
   b. Constriction
10. Nuclear stellate cataracts
11. Visual hallucinations
12. Lacrimation
    a. Increased — rare
    b. Decreased
13. Horner's syndrome
14. Diplopia
15. Nystagmus
16. Jerky pursuit movements
17. Photophobia
18. Optic atrophy
19. Papilledema
20. Myopia
21. Toxic amblyopia
22. Eyelids or conjunctiva
    a. Allergic reactions
    b. Edema
    c. Hyperpigmentation
    d. Photosensitivity
    e. Angioneurotic edema
    f. Lupoid syndrome
    g. Stevens-Johnson syndrome
    h. Exfoliative dermatitis
23. Myasthenic neuromuscular blocking effect
24. Abnormal ERG
25. Subconjunctival or retinal hemorrhages secondary to drug-induced anemia
26. Ocular teratogenic effects (?)

Clinical Significance: The phenothiazines as a class are among the more widely used drugs in the practice of medicine today. The most commonly prescribed drug in this group is chlorpromazine, which has been so thoroughly investigated that over 10,000 publications alone deal with its actions. Even so, these drugs are remarkably safe compared to previously prescribed antipsychotic agents. Their overall rate of all side effects is estimated at only 3 percent. However, if patients are on phenothiazine therapy for a number of years, a 30 percent rate of ocular side effects has been reported. If therapy continues over 10 years, the rate of ocular side effects increases to nearly 100 percent. Side effects are dose- and drug-dependent, with the most significant side effects reported with chlorpromazine and thioridazine therapy, probably since they are most often prescribed. These drugs in high dosages can cause significant adverse effects within a few days, while the same reactions usually would take many years to develop in the normal dosage range. Each phenothiazine has the potential to cause ocular side effects although it is unlikely to cause all of those mentioned. The basic problem is that pinpointing specific toxic effects to a specific phenothiazine is extremely difficult since most patients have been receiving more than one type. The most common adverse ocular effect with this group of drugs is decreased vision, probably due to anticholinergic interference. Chlorpromazine, in chronic therapy, is the most common phenothiazine to cause pigmentary deposits in or on the eye, with multiple reports claiming that other phenothiazines can cause this as well. These deposits are first seen on the lens surface in the pupillary aperture, later near Descemet's membrane, and only in extreme cases in the corneal epithelium. Retinopathy, optic nerve disease, and blindness are exceedingly rare at the recommended dosage levels and then they are almost only found in patients on chronic therapy. Retinal pigmentary changes are most frequently found with thioridazine. This reaction is dose-related and is seldom seen at recommended dosages. A phototoxic process has been postulated to be involved in both the increased ocular pigmentary deposits and the retinal degeneration. The phenothiazines combine with ocular and dermal pigment and are only slowly released. This slow release has in part been given as the reason why adverse ocular reactions may progress even after use of the drug is discontinued.

Interactions with Other Drugs:

    A. Effect of Phenothiazines on Activity of Other Drugs
        1. Alcohol ↑
        2. Analgesics ↑
        3. Antihistamines ↑
        4. Barbiturates ↑
        5. Diuretics ↑
        6. General anesthetics ↑
        7. Other phenothiazines ↑
        8. Salicylates ↑
        9. Sedatives and hypnotics ↑
     10. Adrenergic blockers ↑↓
     11. Anticholinergics ↑↓
     12. Sympathomimetics ↑↓
     13. Miotics ↓
     14. Monoamine oxidase inhibitors ↓

B. Effect of Other Drugs on Activity of Phenothiazines
1. Adrenergic blockers ↑
2. Alcohol ↑
3. Analgesics ↑
4. Anticholinergics ↑
5. Anticholinesterases ↑
6. Diuretics ↑
7. Sedatives and hypnotics ↑
8. Tricyclic antidepressants ↑
9. Antacids ↓
10. Barbiturates ↓
11. Monoamine oxidase inhibitors ↓
12. Sympathomimetics ↓

References:

Delong, S. L., Poley, B. J., and McFarlane, J. R.: Ocular changes associated with long term chlorpromazine therapy. Arch. Ophthalmol. 73:611, 1965.

McClanahan, W. S., et al.: Ocular manifestations of chronic phenothiazine derivative administration. Arch. Ophthalmol. 75:319, 1966.

Meredith, T. A., Aaberg, T. M., and Willerson, W. D.: Progressive chorioretinopathy after receiving thioridazine. Arch. Ophthalmol. 96:1172, 1978.

Potts, A. M.: Drug-induced macular disease. Trans. Am. Acad. Ophthalmol. Otolaryngol. 70:1054, 1966.

Satanove, A., and McIntosh, J. S.: Phototoxic reactions induced by high doses of chlorpromazine and thioridazine. JAMA 200:209, 1967.

Siddall, J. R.: Ocular complications related to phenothiazines. Dis. Nerv. Syst. (Suppl.) 29:10, 1968.

Tamai, A., and Holland, M. G.: Electrophysiological studies on a case of thioridazine pigmentary retinopathy. Acta Soc. Ophthalmol. Jpn. 80:113, 1976.

Vesterhauge, S., and Peitersen, E.: The effects of some drugs on the caloric induced nystagmus. Adv. Otorhinolaryngol. 25:173, 1979.

Weekley, R. D., et al.: Pigmentary retinopathy in patients receiving high doses of a new phenothiazine. Arch. Ophthalmol. 64:65, 1960.

Wetterholm, D. H., Snow, H. L., and Winter, F. C.: A clinical study of pigmentary change in cornea and lens in chronic chlorpromazine therapy. Arch. Ophthalmol. 74:55, 1965.

Generic Name: 1. Chlorprothixene; 2. Thiothixene

Proprietary Name: 1. Taractan, Tarasan (Canad.), Truxal (Austral., Germ., S. Afr., Scand.), Truxaletten (Germ.); 2. Navane, Orbinamon (Germ).

Primary Use: These thioxanthene derivatives are used in the management of schizophrenia. Chlorprothixene is also used in agitation neuroses and as an antiemetic.

Ocular Side Effects:

A. Systemic Administration
    1. Decreased vision
    2. Decrease or paralysis of accommodation
    3. Oculogyric crises
    4. Pupils
       a. Mydriasis — may precipitate narrow-angle glaucoma
       b. Miosis
    5. Diplopia
    6. Cornea
       a. Fine particulate deposits
       b. Keratitis
    7. Lens
       a. Fine particulate deposits
       b. Stellate cataracts
    8. Retinal pigmentary changes
    9. Eyelids or conjunctiva
       a. Allergic reactions
       b. Photosensitivity
       c. Angioneurotic edema
       d. Urticaria
       e. Lupoid syndrome
       f. Exfoliative dermatitis
   10. Subconjunctival or retinal hemorrhages secondary to drug-induced anemia

Clinical Significance: In short-term therapy, ocular side effects due to these thioxanthene derivatives are reversible and usually insignificant. In long-term therapy, however, cases of corneal or lens deposits (chlorprothixene) or lens pigmentation (thiothixene) have been reported. Retinal pigmentary changes are exceedingly rare.

Interactions with Other Drugs:

A. Effect of Thioxanthene Derivatives on Activity of Other Drugs
    1. Alcohol ↑
    2. Analgesics ↑
    3. Anticholinergics ↑
    4. Antihistamines ↑
    5. Barbiturates ↑
    6. Diuretics ↑
    7. General anesthetics ↑
    8. Phenothiazines ↑
    9. Salicylates ↑

      10. Sedatives and hypnotics ↑
      11. Adrenergic blockers ↑↓
      12. Sympathomimetics ↑↓
      13. Monoamine oxidase inhibitors ↓
  B. Effect of Other Drugs on Activity of Thioxanthene Derivatives
      1. Adrenergic blockers ↑
      2. Alcohol ↑
      3. Analgesics ↑
      4. Anticholinergics ↑
      5. Anticholinesterases ↑
      6. Diuretics ↑
      7. Sedatives and hypnotics ↑
      8. Tricyclic antidepressants ↑
      9. Antacids ↓
      10. Barbiturates ↓
      11. Monoamine oxidase inhibitors ↓
      12. Sympathomimetics ↓
  C. Cross Sensitivity
      1. Phenothiazines

References:

AMA Drug Evaluations. 4th Ed., New York, John Wiley & Sons, 1980, pp. 181–182.
Council on Drugs: Evaluation of chlorprothixene (Taractan). JAMA *186*:144, 1963.
Hermans, G.: Les psychotropes. Bull. Soc. Belge Ophtalmol. *160*:15, 1972.
Physicians' Desk Reference. 35th Ed., Oradell, N.J., Medical Economics Co., 1981, pp. 1526, 1542.
Simpson, G. M.: Reactions following the intra-muscular administration of chlorprothixene. Am. J. Psychiatry *120*:1021, 1964.

Generic Name: 1. Droperidol; 2. Haloperidol; 3. Trifluperidol

Proprietary Name: 1. Dridol (Swed.), Droleptan (G.B.), Inapsin (S. Afr.), Inapsine; 2. Haldol, Serenace (G.B.); 3. Psicoperidol (S. Afr., Swed.), Triperidol (G.B.)

Primary Use: These butyrophenone derivatives are used in the management of acute and chronic schizophrenia, and manic depressive, involutional, senile, organic, and toxic psychoses. Droperidol is also used as an adjunct to anesthesia and as an antiemetic.

Ocular Side Effects:

  A. Systemic Administration
      1. Decreased vision

2. Oculogyric crises
3. Decreased intraocular pressure
4. Pupils
   a. Mydriasis — may precipitate narrow-angle glaucoma
   b. Miosis — rare
5. Decreased accommodation
6. Eyelids or conjunctiva
   a. Allergic reactions
   b. Photosensitivity
   c. Angioneurotic edema
   d. Exfoliative dermatitis
7. Visual hallucinations
8. Subconjunctival or retinal hemorrhages secondary to drug-induced anemia
9. Capsular cataracts (?)
10. Loss of eyelashes or eyebrows (?)
11. Myopia (?)

Clinical Significance: Ocular side effects due to these butyrophenone derivatives are often transient and reversible on withdrawal of the medication. There are a number of cases reported to the Registry of bilateral marked pupillary dilatation due to haloperidol. There is one report in the Japanese literature that this group of drugs can cause a rapid onset capsular cataract after long-term therapy. The decreased intraocular pressure due to these drugs is not of a sufficient amount to be of clinical value. There is one case in the Registry of possible increasing myopia associated with haloperidol use.

Interactions with Other Drugs:

A. Effect of Butyrophenones on Activity of Other Drugs
   1. Alcohol ↑
   2. Analgesics ↑
   3. Anticholinergics ↑
   4. Barbiturates ↑
   5. General anesthetics ↑
   6. Phenothiazines ↑
   7. Sedatives and hypnotics ↑
   8. Adrenergic blockers ↓
   9. Sympathomimetics ↓
B. Effect of Other Drugs on Activity of Butyrophenones
   1. Alcohol ↑
   2. Analgesics ↑
   3. Barbiturates ↑

4. Monoamine oxidase inhibitors ↑
5. Phenothiazines ↑
6. Tricyclic antidepressants ↑
7. Sympathomimetics ↓

References:

AMA Drug Evaluations. 4th Ed., New York, John Wiley & Sons, 1980, pp. 182–184, 325, 424.

Barton, D.: Side reactions of drugs in anesthesia. Int. Ophthalmol. Clin. *11*(2):185, 1971.

Clark, M. M.: Droperidol in preoperative anxiety. Anaesthesia *24*:36, 1969.

Ferrari, H. A., and Stephen, C. R.: Neuroleptanalgesia: Pharmacology and clinical experiences with droperidol and fentanyl. South. Med. J. *59*:815, 1966.

Fink, M., et al.: Trifluperidol in the treatment of psychosis. J. New Drugs *6*:174, 1966.

Freeman, J. E., Robertson, A. C., and Ngan, H.: Oculogyric crises due to phenothiazines. (Correspondence). Br. Med. J. *3*:738, 1967.

Hermans, G.: Les psychotropes. Bull. Soc. Belge Ophtalmol. *160*:15, 1972.

Honda, S.: Drug-induced cataract in mentally ill subjects. Rinsho Ganka *28*:521, 1974.

LeVann, L. J.: Haloperidol in the treatment of behavioural disorders in children and adolescents. Can. Psychiatr. Assoc. J. *14*:217, 1969.

Pontinen, P. J., and Miettinen, P.: Neuroleptanalgesia in cataract surgery. Acta Ophthalmol. (Suppl.) *80*:25, 1964.

Generic Name: Lithium Carbonate

Proprietary Name: Camcolit (G.B.), Carbolith (Canad.), Eskalith, Hypnorex (Germ.), Lithane, Lithicarb (Austral.), Lithionit (Swed.), Lithium Duriles (Germ.), Lithium Oligosol (Fr.), Lithobid, Litho-Carb (Canad.), Lithonate, Lithotabs, Maniprex (Belg.), Neurolithium (Fr.), Pfi-Lith, Phasal (G.B.), Priadel (G.B.), Quilonum (Germ., S. Afr.)

Primary Use: This lithium salt is used in the management of the manic phase of manic depressive psychosis.

Ocular Side Effects:

A. Systemic Administration
   1. Decreased vision
   2. Nystagmus — horizontal or vertical
   3. Scotomas
   4. Extraocular muscles
      a. Oculogyric crises
      b. Decreased spontaneous movements
      c. Lateral conjugate deviations
      d. Jerky pursuit movements

    5. Eyelids or conjunctiva — edema
    6. Photophobia
    7. Exophthalmos
    8. Subconjunctival or retinal hemorrhages secondary to drug-induced anemia
    9. Myasthenic neuromuscular blocking effect
    10. Papilledema (?)
    11. Loss of eyelashes or eyebrows (?)

Clinical Significance: Ocular side effects due to lithium are reversible upon withdrawal of the drug. Blurred vision occurs at toxic blood levels (above 2.0 mEq/1). Exophthalmos, either unilateral or bilateral, has occurred at normal dosages of lithium carbonate and may be due to this drug's effect on the thyroid. These changes usually regress on discontinuation of the drug. There has been only one reported case of papilledema due to possible drug-related pseudotumor cerebri. While blindness in toxic states has been reported, it is usually transitory and probably affects vision at the cortical level. Toxic drug responses are closely related to serum lithium blood levels.

Interactions with Other Drugs:
    A. Effect of Other Drugs on Activity of Lithium Carbonate
        1. Carbonic anhydrase inhibitors ↓
        2. Diuretics ↓
        3. Urea ↓

References:

Argov, S., and Mastaglia, F. L.: Disorders of neuromuscular transmission caused by drugs. N. Engl. J. Med. 301:409, 1979.

Baastrup, P. C., and Schou, M.: Lithium as a prophylactic agent. Arch. Gen. Psychiatry 16:162, 1967.

Brown, W. T.: Side effects of lithium therapy and their treatment. Can. Psychiatr. Assoc. J. 21:13, 1976.

Cluff, L. E., Caranasos, G. J., and Stewart, R. B.: Clinical Problems with Drugs. Philadelphia, W. B. Saunders, 1975, pp. 207–212.

Fann, W. E., Asher, H., and Luton, F. H.: Use of lithium in mania. Dis. Nerv. Syst. 30:605, 1969.

Lobo, A., Pilek, E., and Stokes, P. E.: Papilledema following therapeutic dosages of lithium carbonate. J. Nerv. Ment. Dis. 166:526, 1978.

Schlagenhauf, G., Tupin, J., and White, R. B.: Use of lithium carbonate in the treatment of manic psychoses. Am. J. Psychiatry 123:201, 1966.

Generic Name: Loxapine

Proprietary Name: Daxolin, Loxitane

Primary Use: This dibenzoxazepine derivative represents a new subclass of tricyclic antipsychotic agents used in the treatment of schizophrenia.

Ocular Side Effects:

A. Systemic Administration
1. Decreased vision
2. Oculogyric crises
3. Mydriasis — may precipitate narrow-angle glaucoma
4. Decreased accommodation
5. Eyelids or conjunctiva
   a. Edema
   b. Hyperpigmentation
   c. Photosensitivity
   d. Urticaria
6. Ptosis
7. Subconjunctival or retinal hemorrhages secondary to drug-induced anemia

Clinical Significance: Neuromuscular reactions, including oculogyric crises, are frequently reported, usually during the first few days of treatment with loxapine. These reactions occasionally require reduction or temporary withdrawal of the drug. The anticholinergic effects, blurred vision, mydriasis, and decreased accommodation are more likely to occur with concomitant use of antiparkinsonian agents. The possibility of pigmentary retinopathy and lenticular pigmentation from loxapine cannot be excluded but seems quite rare or unlikely.

References:

American Hospital Formulary Service. Washington, D.C., American Society of Hospital Pharmacists, Vol. I, 28:16.08, 1976.

Moyano, C. Z.: A double-blind comparison of Loxitane, loxapine succinate and trifluoperazine hydrochloride in chronic schizophrenic patients. Dis. Nerv. Syst. 36: 301, 1975.

Physicians' Desk Reference. 35th Ed., Oradell, N.J., Medical Economics Co., 1981, p. 1005.

Selman, F. B., McClure, R. F., and Helwig, H.: Loxapine succinate: A double-blind comparison with haloperidol and placebo in acute schizophrenics. Curr. Ther. Res. 19:645, 1976.

Wade, A. (Ed.): Martindale: The Extra Pharmacopoeia. 27th Ed., London, Pharmaceutical Press, 1977, pp. 1550–1551.

Class: Psychedelic Agents

Generic Name: 1. Hashish; 2. Marihuana; 3. Tetrahydrocannabinol, THC

Street Name: 1. Bhang, Charas, Gram, Hash, Keif, Pot, Black Russian; 2. Ace, Acapulco gold, Baby, Belyando sprue, Bhang, Boo, Brown weed, Bush, Cannabis, Charas, Gage, Ganja, Gold, Grass, Gungeon, Hay, Hemp, Herb, Jay, Joint, Kick sticks, Lid, Locoweed, Mary Jane, Mexican green, MJ, Muggles, OJ (opium joint), Panama red, Pot, Rainy-day woman, Reefer, Roach, Rope, Stick, Tea, Twist, Weed, Wheat; 3. The one

Primary Use: These psychedelic agents are occasionally used as cerebral sedatives or narcotics commonly available on the illicit drug market.

Ocular Side Effects:

A. Systemic Administration
   1. Visual hallucinations
   2. Problems with color vision
       a. Dyschromatopsia
       b. Objects have yellow or violet tinge
       c. Colored flashing lights
       d. Heightened color perception
   3. Nystagmus
   4. Nonspecific ocular irritation
       a. Hyperemia
       b. Conjunctivitis
       c. Photophobia (variable)
       d. Burning sensation
   5. Decreased accommodation
   6. Decreased dark adaptation
   7. Diplopia
   8. Decreased vision
   9. Blepharospasm
   10. Impaired oculomotor coordination
   11. Decreased intraocular pressure
   12. Decreased lacrimation
   13. Pupils
       a. Miosis
       b. Anisocoria
   14. Abnormal conjugate deviations (?)
   15. Ocular teratogenic effects (?)

B. Local Ophthalmic Use or Exposure
  1. Decreased intraocular pressure

Clinical Significance: Ocular side effects due to these drugs are transient and seldom of clinical importance. The current area of greatest clinical interest is with the cannabinols found in marihuana. These agents can decrease intraocular pressure, but this varies with the quality of marihuana based on the quantity of the cannabinols contained in the plant. However, even with purified natural occurring cannabinols, one cannot separate the central nervous system high from its ocular pressure lowering effect so its value clinically is quite limited. There is some evidence that marihuana decreases basal lacrimal secretion, decreases photosensitivity, increases dark adaptation, increases color-match limits, and increases Snellen visual acuity. Possibly within the first 5 to 15 minutes, some persons will get some pupillary constriction; however, most do not and, to date, there is no long-term pupillary effect noted. Conjunctival hyperemia is not uncommon and is more pronounced 15 minutes, rather than 90 minutes, after exposure. The sensory perception of one's external environment is altered on this agent. While these drugs are only occasionally used medically, they are in common social usage in many cultures.

References:

Bromberg, W.: Marihuana intoxication; Clinical study of Cannabis sativa intoxication. Am. J. Psychiatry 91:303, 1934.
Cohen, S.: Psychotomimetic agents. Ann. Rev. Pharmacol. 7:301, 1967.
Dawson, W. W., et al.: Marijuana and vision—after ten years' use in Costa Rica. Invest. Ophthalmol. Vis. Sci. 16:689, 1977.
Gilman, A. G., Goodman, L. S., and Gilman, A. (Eds.): The Pharmacological Basis of Therapeutics. 6th Ed., New York, Macmillan, 1980, pp. 560–563.
Hepler, R. S., Frank, I. M., and Petrus, R.: Ocular effects of marihuana smoking. In Braude, M. C., and Szara, S. (Ed.): The Pharmacology of Marihuana. New York, Raven Press, 1976, pp. 815–828.
Mendleson, G.: Effect of cannabis on driving. Med. J. Aust. 1:391, 1978.
Mohan, H., and Sood, G. C.: Conjugate deviation of the eyes after Cannabis indica intoxication. Br. J. Ophthalmol. 48:160, 1964.
Shapiro, D.: The ocular manifestations of the cannabinols. Ophthalmologica 168:366, 1974.
Stuart, K. L.: Ganja (Cannabis sativa L.). West Indian Med. J. 12:156, 1963.
Weil, A. T., Zinberg, N. E., and Nelsen, J. M.: Clinical and psychological effects of marihuana in man. Science 162:1234, 1968.

Generic Name: 1. LSD, Lysergide; 2. Mescaline; 3. Psilocybin

Street Name: 1. Acid, Barrels, Big D, Blue acid, Brown dots, California sunshine, Crackers, Cubes, Cupcakes, Grape parfait, Green domes,

Hawaiian sunshine, Lucy in the sky with diamonds, Micro dots, Purple barrels, Purple haze, Purple ozolone, Sunshine, The animal, The beast, The chief, The hawk, The ticket, Trips, Twenty-five, Yellow dimples; 2. Buttons, Cactus, Mesc, Peyote, The bad seed, Topi; 3. Magic mushroom

Primary Use: These experimental drugs are used in the treatment of chronic alcoholism, character neuroses, and sexual perversions.

Ocular Side Effects:

A. Systemic Administration
  1. Pupils
     a. Mydriasis
     b. Anisocoria
     c. Decreased or absent reaction to light
  2. Visual hallucinations including micro- and macropsia
  3. Problems with color vision
     a. Dyschromatopsia
     b. Heightened color perception
  4. Prolongation of after image
  5. Decreased accommodation
  6. Decreased dark adaptation
  7. Decreased vision
  8. Ocular teratogenic effects (?)
     a. Cataract
     b. Iris coloboma
     c. Microphthalmos
     d. Corneal opacities
     e. Persistent hyperplastic primary vitreous
     f. Retinal dysplasia

Clinical Significance: Ocular side effects due to these drugs are common, but seldom of significant importance except when bizarre visual hallucinations aggravate an already disturbed sensorium. Some claim true visual hallucinations seldom occur with these drugs, but rather a complicated visual experience results from a perceptual disturbance. Perception changes include alterations in colors and shapes. Lysergide is 100 times more potent than psilocybin, which in turn is 4000 times more potent than mescaline. While these drugs are only occasionally used medically, they are easily obtained through illicit channels. There are a significant number of sun gazing reports with irreversible macular damage in persons on lysergide.

References:

Carlson, V. R.: Individual pupillary reactions to certain centrally acting drugs in man. J. Pharmacol. Exp. Ther. *121*:501, 1957.
Ewald, R. A.: Sun gazing associated with the use of LSD. Ann. Ophthalmol. 3:15, 1971.
Gilman, A. G., Goodman, L. S., and Gilman, A. (Eds.): The Pharmacological Basis of Therapeutics. 6th Ed., New York, Macmillan, 1980, pp. 563–567.
Jacobs, B. L., and Trulson, M. E.: Mechanisms of action of LSD. Am. Sci. 67:396, 1979.
Keeler, M. H.: The effects of psilocybin on a test of after-image perception. Psychopharmacologia 8:131, 1965.
Lyle, W. M.: Drugs and conditions which may affect color vision. Part 1. Drugs and chemicals. J. Am. Optometric Assoc. 45:47, 1974.
Payne, J. W.: LSD-25 and accommodative convergence ratios. Arch. Ophthalmol. 74: 81, 1965.
Wade, A. (Ed.): Martindale: The Extra Pharmacopoeia. 27th Ed., London, Pharmaceutical Press, 1977, pp. 880–884.

Generic Name: Phencyclidine

Street Name: Angel Dust, Angel's Mist, Busy Bee, Crystal, DOA, Goon, Hog, Mist, Monkey Tranquilizer, PCP, Peace Pill, Rocket Fuel, Sheets, Super Weed, Tac, Tic

Primary Use: This nonbarbiturate anesthetic was removed from the market because of postoperative psychiatric disturbances; however, it is still commonly available on the illicit drug market.

Ocular Side Effects:

A. Systemic Administration
1. Extraocular muscles
   a. Nystagmus — horizontal, rotary, or vertical
   b. Diplopia
   c. Jerky pursuit movements
2. Pupils
   a. Miosis
   b. Decreased reaction to light
3. Decreased vision
4. Visual hallucinations
5. Ptosis
6. Decreased corneal reflex
7. Increased intraocular pressure

Clinical Significance: Even with relatively low doses (5 mg), phencyclidine may give a characteristic type of nystagmus in which vertical, horizontal, and rotary eye movements occur in sudden bursts. In addition, this drug may produce hallucinations and visual defects, including distortion of body image, hallucinatory voices, and substitution of fairy-tale characters. Acute toxic reactions can last up to a week after a single dose, although the mental effects can linger for more than a month. These effects may keep recurring in sudden episodes, while the patient is apparently recovering.

References:

Corales, R. L., Maull, K. I., and Becker, D. P.: Phencyclidine abuse mimicking head injury. JAMA *243*:2323, 1980.
Dorand, R. D.: Phencyclidine ingestion: Therapy review. South. Med. J. *70*:117, 1977.
Fauman, B., et al.: Psychiatric sequelae of phencyclidine abuse. Clin. Toxicol. *9*:529, 1976.
Tong, T. G., et al.: Phencyclidine poisoning. JAMA *234*:512, 1975.

Class: Sedatives and Hypnotics

Generic Name: Alcohol (Ethanol)

Proprietary Name: Alcohol

Primary Use: This colorless liquid is used as a solvent, an antiseptic, a beverage, and as a nerve block in the management of certain types of intractable pain.

Ocular Side Effects:

A. Systemic Administration — Acute Intoxication
   1. Extraocular muscles
      a. Diplopia
      b. Nystagmus
      c. Esophoria or exophoria
      d. Convergent strabismus
      e. Decreased convergence
      f. Jerky pursuit movements
      g. Decreased spontaneous movements
   2. Pupils
      a. Mydriasis
      b. Decreased or absent reaction to light

        c. Anisocoria
        d. Miosis (coma)
   3. Decreased vision
   4. Decreased accommodation
   5. Problems with color vision
        a. Dyschromatopsia
        b. Objects have blue tinge
   6. Decreased dark adaptation
   7. Decreased intraocular pressure
   8. Constriction of visual fields
   9. Decreased depth perception
  10. Decreased optokinetic nystagmus
  11. Visual hallucinations
  12. Prolonged glare recovery
  13. Ptosis (unilateral or bilateral)
  14. Impaired oculomotor coordination
  15. Toxic amblyopia

B. Systemic Administration — Chronic Intoxication
   1. Paralysis of extraocular muscles
   2. Nystagmus
   3. Paralysis of accommodation
   4. Pupils
        a. Miosis
        b. Decreased or absent reaction to light
   5. Decreased vision
   6. Scotomas — central
   7. Problems with color vision — dyschromatopsia, red-green defect
   8. Lacrimation
   9. Decreased intraocular pressure
  10. Visual hallucinations
  11. Optic neuritis
  12. Corneal deposits (arcus senilis)
  13. Toxic amblyopia
  14. Ocular teratogenic effects (fetal alcohol syndrome)
        a. Narrow palpebral fissure
        b. Hypertelorism
        c. Microphthalmia
        d. Epicanthus
        e. Ptosis
        f. Strabismus
        g. Retinal vascular tortuosity
        h. Pseudopapilledema (enlarged or pale discs)
  15. Subcapsular cataracts

C. Local Ophthalmic Use or Exposure — Retrobulbar Injection
  1. Irritation
     a. Hyperemia
     b. Ocular pain
     c. Edema
  2. Keratitis
  3. Paralysis of extraocular muscles
  4. Nystagmus
  5. Ptosis
  6. Corneal ulceration
  7. Decreased vision
  8. Loss of eyelashes or eyebrows (?)
D. Inadvertent Ocular Exposure
  1. Irritation
     a. Lacrimation
     b. Hyperemia
     c. Ocular pain
     d. Edema
     e. Burning sensation
  2. Keratitis
  3. Corneal necrosis or opacities

Clinical Significance: The large number of adverse ocular effects reported due to ethyl alcohol is in part due to the fact that this agent is second only to water in the volume man consumes. Transient amblyopia lasting up to 5 days is well documented in both acute and chronic alcoholism; however, permanent blindness directly caused by ethyl alcohol is debatable. So-called toxic alcohol amblyopia is probably secondary to a vitamin B deficiency, and if the alcoholic was taking vitamin supplements, it would probably not occur. Intraocular pressure may be significantly lowered in the glaucomatous patient after 40 to 60 ml. of ethyl alcohol; however, this effect lasts only for a few hours. Ethyl alcohol probably has little significant sensory effect on a person's ability to drive; however, nystagmus, diplopia, and incoordinated ocular movements may cause serious problems. Saccadic eye movements in which the eyes are moved rapidly from one object of interest to another are significantly slowed when the person is under the influence of this agent. There is now evidence that perceptual, cognitive, and ocular motor effects of alcohol and tetrahydrocannabinol are additive. The fetal alcohol syndrome is a well-defined entity seen in offsprings whose mothers had high alcohol consumption during pregnancy. The popularity of retrobulbar injections of alcohol is probably not as great today as it was in the past because of numerous untoward, often permanent, ocular and periocular effects.

Interactions with Other Drugs:

A. Effect of Alcohol on Activity of Other Drugs
   1. Anticholinesterases ↑
   2. Barbiturates ↑
   3. Adrenergic blockers ↑
   4. Phenothiazines ↑

B. Effect of Other Drugs on Activity of Alcohol
   1. Analgesics ↑
   2. Antihistamines ↑
   3. Barbiturates ↑
   4. Monoamine oxidase inhibitors ↑
   5. Phenothiazines ↑
   6. Tricyclic antidepressants ↑

References:

Adams, A. J., and Brown, B.: Alcohol prolongs time course of glare recovery. Nature 257:481, 1975.

Altman, B.: Fetal alcohol syndrome. J. Pediatr. Ophthalmol. 13:255, 1976.

Chesher, G. B., et al.: The interaction of ethanol and Δ⁹-tetrahydrocannabinol in man; effects on perceptual, cognitive and motor functions. Med. J. Aust. 2:159, 1976.

González E. R.: New ophthalmic findings in fetal alcohol syndrome. JAMA 245:108, 1981.

Gramberg-Danielsen, B.: Ophthalmological findings after the use of alcohol. Zentralbl. Verkehrs-med. 11:129, 1965.

Newman, H., and Fletcher, E.: Effects of alcohol on driving skill. JAMA 115:1600, 1940.

Olurin, O., and Osuntokun, O.: Complications of retrobulbar alcohol injections. Ann. Ophthalmol. 10:474, 1978.

Peters, H. B.: Changes in color fields occasioned by experimentally induced alcohol intoxication. J. Appl. Psychol. 26:692, 1942.

Sulkowski, A., and Vachon, L.: Side effects of simultaneous alcohol and marijuana use. Am. J. Psychiatry 134:691, 1977.

Wilkinson, I. M. S., Kime, R., and Purnell, M.: Alcohol and human eye movement. Brain 97:785, 1974.

Generic Name: 1. Allobarbital; 2. Amobarbital; 3. Aprobarbital; 4. Barbital; 5. Butabarbital; 6. Butalbital; 7. Butallylonal; 8. Butethal; 9. Cyclobarbital; 10. Cyclopentobarbital; 11. Heptabarbital; 12. Hexethal; 13. Hexobarbital; 14. Mephobarbital (Methylphenobarbital); 15. Metharbital; 16. Methitural; 17. Methohexital; 18. Pentobarbital; 19. Phenobarbital; 20. Primidone; 21. Probarbital; 22. Secobarbital; 23. Talbutal; 24. Thiamylal; 25. Thiopental; 26. Vinbarbital

Proprietary Name: 1. Allobarbital; 2. Amal (Austral.), Amsal (Austral.), Amylbarb (Austral.), Amylobarbitone (G.B.), Amylobeta (Austral.), Amylosol (Austral.), Amytal, Eunoctal (Fr.), Isomyl (Swed.), Isonal

(Canad.), Mylodorm (Austral.), Mylosed (Austral.), Neur-Amyl (Austral.), Novamobarb (Canad.), Restal (Austral.), Schiwanox (Germ.), Sedal (Austral.), Sednotic (Austral.), Stadadorm (Germ.); 3. Alurate, A.P.B.; 4. Barbitone (G.B.), Neuronidia, Veronal; 5. B.B.S., Buta-Barb (Canad.), Butal, Butalan, Butazem, Buticaps, Butisol, Butte, Day-Barb (Canad.), Expansatol, Intasedol, Interbarb (Canad.), Merisyl (Canad.), Neo-Barb (Canad.), Neravan (Germ.), Quiebar, Renbu, Soduben; 6. Sandoptal; 7. Butallylonal; 8. Butobarbitone (G.B.), Sonabarb (Austral.), Soneryl (G.B.); 9. Amnosed (Austral.), Cyclobarbitone (G.B.), Cyklodorm (Swed.), Fabadorm (Austral.), Phanodorm (G.B.), Phanodorn, Placyl (Austral.), Rapidal (G.B.); 10. Cyclopal (Germ.); 11. Medapan (Swed.), Medomin (G.B.), Medomine (Fr.); 12. Hexethal; 13. Evipal, Evipan (Germ.), Hexobarbitone (G.B.), Noctivane (Fr.), Sombulex, Ultra-Sed; 14. Mebaral, Menta-Bal, Mephoral, Methylphenobarbitone (G.B.), Prominal (G.B.), Promitone (Austral.); 15. Gemonil, Gemonit (Swed.); 16. Methitural; 17. Brevimytal (Germ.), Brevital, Brietal (G.B.), Methohexitone (G.B.); 18. Barbopent (Austral.), Dorsital, Hypnol (Canad.), Ibatal (Canad.), Nebralin, Nembutal, Neodorm (Germ.), Nova-Rectal (Canad.), Palapent, Penbarb (Austral.), Penbon (Austral.), Pental (Canad.), Pentanca (Canad.), Pentobarbitone (G.B.), Pentobeta (Austral.), Pentogen (Canad.), Pentone (Austral.), Petab (Austral.), Repocal (Germ.), Schlafen (Jap.), Sodepent (Austral.), Sopental (S. Afr.); 19. Bar, Barbapil, Barbita, Ensobarb (Austral.), Epilol (Canad.), Epsylone (Canad.), Eskabarb, Gardenal (G.B.), Henomint, Hypnette, Hypnolone (Canad.), Infadorm, Luminal, Luminaletten (Germ.), Nova-Pheno (Canad.), Orprine, Parabal (G.B.), PEBA (Canad.), Phenaemal (Germ.), Phenaemaletten (Germ.), Phenased (Austral.), Phen Bar (Canad.), Phenobarbitone (G.B.), Pheno-Caps (Canad.), Pheno-Square, Sedabar (Canad.), Sedadrops, Seda-Tablinen (Germ.), SK-Phenobarbital, Solfoton, Solu-barb, Stental, Talpheno; 20. Elmidone (Austral.), Liskantin (Germ.), Midone (Austral.), Mysoline; 21. Probarbital; 22. Immenoctal (Fr.), Novosecobarb (Canad.), Panasec (S. Afr.), Proquinal (Austral.), Quinalbarbitone (G.B.), Quinaltone (Austral.), Quinbar (Austral.), SCB (Canad.), Secaps (Canad.), Seco-8, Secocaps (Canad.), Secogen (Canad.), Seconal; 23. Lotusate; 24. Surital; 25. Intraval (G.B.), Nesdonal (Fr.), Pentothal, Thiopentone (G.B.), Trapanal (Germ.); 26. Diminal (Swed.)

Primary Use: These barbituric acid derivatives vary primarily in duration and intensity of action and are used as central nervous system depressants, hypnotics, sedatives, and anticonvulsants.

Ocular Side Effects:

  A. Systemic Administration
    1. Eyelids

   a. Ptosis
   b. Blepharoclonus
2. Pupils
   a. Mydriasis
   b. Miosis (coma)
   c. Decreased reaction to light
   d. Hippus
3. Extraocular muscles
   a. Diplopia
   b. Decreased convergence
   c. Paresis
   d. Jerky pursuit movements
   e. Random ocular movements
   f. Vertical gaze palsy
4. Oscillopsia
5. Nystagmus
   a. Downbeat, gaze-evoked, horizontal, jerk, or vertical
   b. Depressed or abolished optokinetic, latent, positional, voluntary, or congenital nystagmus
6. Decreased vision
7. Visual fields
   a. Scotomas
   b. Constriction
8. Problems with color vision
   a. Dyschromatopsia
   b. Objects have yellow or green tinge
9. Visual hallucinations
10. Eyelids or conjunctiva
    a. Allergic reactions
    b. Conjunctivitis — nonspecific
    c. Edema
    d. Photosensitivity
    e. Angioneurotic edema
    f. Urticaria
    g. Lupoid syndrome
    h. Erythema multiforme
    i. Stevens-Johnson syndrome
    j. Exfoliative dermatitis
    k. Lyell's syndrome
11. Decreased intraocular pressure
12. Toxic amblyopia
13. Retinal vasoconstriction
14. Optic nerve disorders
    a. Retrobulbar or optic neuritis

        b. Papilledema
        c. Optic atrophy
   15. Abnormal ERG
   16. Subconjunctival or retinal hemorrhages secondary to drug-induced anemia
   17. Ocular teratogenic effects (?) (primidone)
        a. Optic atrophy
        b. Ptosis
        c. Hypertelorism
        d. Epicanthus
        e. Strabismus
   18. Cortical blindness (?) (thiopental)

Clinical Significance: Numerous adverse ocular side effects have been attributed to barbiturate usage, yet nearly all significant ocular side effects are found in habitual users or in barbiturate poisoning. Few toxic ocular reactions are found due to barbiturate usage at therapeutic dosages or on short-term therapy. The most common ocular abnormalities are disturbances of ocular movement such as decreased convergence, paresis of extraocular muscles, or nystagmus. The pupillary response to barbiturate intake is quite variable, but usually miosis occurs except in the most toxic states when mydriasis is the most frequent side effect. Transient or permanent visual loss is primarily found in patients who are in barbiturate coma. Barbital and phenobarbital have the most frequently reported ocular side effects; however, all barbiturates may produce adverse ocular effects. Chronic barbiturate users have a "tattle tale" ptosis and blepharoclonus. Normally, a tap on the glabella area of the head produces a few eyelid blinks, but in the barbiturate addict the response will be a rapid fluttering of the eyelids. The barbiturates do not appear to have teratogenic effects, except possibly primidone.

Interactions with Other Drugs:

  A. Effect of Barbiturates on Activity of Other Drugs
     1. Alcohol ↑
     2. Antibiotics ↑
       (Kanamycin, Neomycin, Streptomycin)
     3. General anesthetics ↑
     4. Sedatives and hypnotics ↑↓
     5. Analgesics ↓
     6. Antihistamines ↓
     7. Chloramphenicol ↓
     8. Corticosteroids ↓

     9. Local anesthetics ↓
    10. Phenothiazines ↓
    11. Phenylbutazone ↓
    12. Salicylates ↓
    13. Sulfonamides ↓
    14. Tricyclic antidepressants ↓
 B. Effect of Other Drugs on Activity of Barbiturates
     1. Alcohol ↑
     2. Analgesics ↑
     3. Anticholinesterases ↑
     4. Ascorbic acid ↑
     5. Chloramphenicol ↑
     6. Corticosteroids ↑
     7. Monoamine oxidase inhibitors ↑
     8. Phenothiazines ↑
     9. Sulfonamides ↑
    10. Tricyclic antidepressants ↑
    11. Antihistamines ↑↓
    12. Phenylbutazone ↓

References:

Apt, L., and Gaffney, W. L.: Ocular teratogens: A commentary. J. Pediatr. 87:844, 1975.
Bender, M. B., and Gorman, W. F.: Vertical nystagmus on direct forward gaze with vertical oscillopsia. Am. J. Ophthalmol. 32:967, 1949.
Carlson, V. R.: Individual pupillary reactions to certain centrally acting drugs in man. J. Pharmacol. Exp. Ther. 121:501, 1957.
Committee on Alcoholism and Addiction and Council on Mental Health: Dependence on barbiturates and other sedative drugs. JAMA 193:673, 1965.
Edis, R. H., and Mastaglia, F. L.: Vertical gaze palsy in barbiturate intoxication. Br. Med. J. 1:144, 1977.
Rashbass, C.: Barbiturate nystagmus and the mechanisms of visual fixation. Nature 183:897, 1959.
Roth, J. H.: Luminal poisoning with conjunctival residue. Am. J. Ophthalmol. 9:533, 1926.
Westheimer, G.: Amphetamine, barbiturates, and accommodation-convergence. Arch. Ophthalmol. 70:830, 1963.

Generic Name: Bromide

Proprietary Name: Lanabrom

Primary Use: This nonbarbiturate sedative-hypnotic is primarily effective as an anticonvulsant in recalcitrant epilepsy.

Ocular Side Effects:

A. Systemic Administration
    1. Decreased vision
    2. Pupils
       a. Mydriasis
       b. Miosis
       c. Decreased or absent reaction to light
       d. Anisocoria
    3. Problems with color vision — dyschromatopsia
    4. Visual hallucinations — mainly Lilliputian
    5. Eyelids or conjunctiva
       a. Allergic reactions
       b. Erythema
       c. Blepharoconjunctivitis
       d. Stevens-Johnson syndrome
    6. Decreased accommodation
    7. Decreased convergence
    8. Diplopia
    9. Nystagmus
  10. Extraocular muscles
       a. Decreased spontaneous movements
       b. Jerky pursuit movements
  11. Photophobia
  12. Decreased corneal reflex
  13. Apparent movement of stationary objects
  14. Visual fields
       a. Scotomas
       b. Constriction
  15. Papilledema (?)
  16. Optic atrophy (?)

Clinical Significance: The medical use of bromides has been drastically reduced by newer agents since the therapeutic blood level of bromide is so close to its toxic level. Nearly all ocular side effects are reversible after use of the drug is discontinued; however, in acute toxic states, both central and peripheral visual loss may be permanent.

Interactions with Other Drugs:

A. Effect of Bromide on Activity of Other Drugs
    1. Phenothiazines ↑
    2. Tricyclic antidepressants ↑
    3. Analgesics ↓

4. Antihistamines ↓
5. Corticosteroids ↓
B. Effect of Other Drugs on Activity of Bromide
 1. Antihistamines ↑
 2. Corticosteroids ↑
 3. Monoamine oxidase inhibitors ↑
 4. Tricyclic antidepressants ↑

References:

Barbour, R. F., Pilkington, F., and Sargant, W.: Bromide intoxication. Br. Med. J. 2:957, 1936.
Bucy, P. C., Weaver, T. A., and Camp, E. H.: Bromide intoxication of unusual severity and chronicity resulting from self medication with bromoseltzer. JAMA 117:1256, 1941.
Kunze, U.: Chronic bromide intoxication with a severe neurological deficit. J. Neurol. 213:149, 1976.
Levin, M.: Eye disturbances in bromide intoxication. Am. J. Ophthalmol. 50:478, 1960.
Perkins, H. A.: Bromide intoxication: Analysis of cases from a general hospital. Arch. Intern. Med. 85:783, 1950.
Roy, A.: Bromide intoxication. Br. J. Psychiatry 127:415, 1975.
Walsh, F. B., and Hoyt, W. F.: Clinical Neuro-Ophthalmology. 3rd Ed., Baltimore, Williams & Wilkins, Vol. III, 1969, pp. 2541, 2618, 2641.

Generic Name: 1. Bromisovalum (Bromisoval); 2. Carbromal

Proprietary Name: 1. Bromural, Isoval, Somnurol (Germ.); 2. Adalin, Addisomnol (Germ.), Mirfudorm (Germ.)

Primary Use: These brominated monoureides are effective in the management of mild insomnia.

Ocular Side Effects:

A. Systemic Administration
 1. Decreased vision
 2. Nystagmus — horizontal or vertical
 3. Pupils
  a. Mydriasis
  b. Miosis
  c. Decreased reaction to light
  d. Anisocoria
 4. Visual fields
  a. Scotomas — central
  b. Constriction
 5. Retrobulbar or optic neuritis

6. Eyelids or conjunctiva — Stevens-Johnson syndrome
7. Diplopia
8. Decreased convergence (bromisovalum)
9. Ptosis (carbromal)
10. Cataracts (?) (carbromal)

Clinical Significance: Adverse ocular side effects due to these agents are rare except in overdose situations. Except for signs or symptoms related to optic nerve disease, the effects are reversible. Both drugs can elevate serum bromide levels, and this in part may account for some adverse ocular side effects. It is said that nystagmus and diplopia are seen more frequently with bromide poisoning than with these brominated mono-ureides. Only one case of acute reversible cataracts has been reported.

Interactions with Other Drugs:

A. Effect of Brominated Monoureides on Activity of Other Drugs
  1. Phenothiazines ↑
  2. Tricyclic antidepressants ↑
  3. Analgesics ↓
  4. Antihistamines ↓
  5. Corticosteroids ↓
B. Effect of Other Drugs on Activity of Brominated Monoureides
  1. Analgesics ↑
  2. Antihistamines ↑
  3. Corticosteroids ↑
  4. Monoamine oxidase inhibitors ↑
  5. Phenothiazines ↑
  6. Tricyclic antidepressants ↑

References:

Copas, D. E., Kay, W. W., and Longman, V. H.: Carbromal intoxication. Lancet *1*: 703, 1959.
Crawford, R.: Toxic cataract. Br. Med. J. 2:1231, 1959.
Harenko, A.: Irreversible cerebello-bulbar syndrome as the sequela of bromisovalum poisoning. Ann. Med. Interne. Fenn. *56*:29, 1967.
Harenko, A.: Neurologic findings in chronic bromisovalum poisoning. Ann. Med. Interne Fenn. *56*:181, 1967.
Koch, H. R., and Hockwin, O.: Iatrogenic cataracts. Ther. Ggw. *114*:1450, 1975.
Sattler, C. H.: Bromural und Adalinvergiftung des Auges. Klin. Monatsbl. Augenheilkd. *70*:149, 1923.
Stohr, G.: Adalin-Schadigungen. Arztl. Wchnschr. *6*:1097, 1951.

Generic Name: Chloral Hydrate

Proprietary Name: Aquachoral, Chloradorm (Austral.), Chloralate (Austral.), Chloraldurat (Germ.), Chloralex (Canad.), Chloralix (Austral.), Chloralixir (Canad.), Chloralvan (Canad.), Chloratol (Canad.), Cohidrate, Dormel (Austral.), Eudorm (Austral.), Felsules, H.S. Need, Kessodrate, Lanchloral (Austral.), Maso-Chloral, Nigracap (Canad.), Noctec, Novochlorhydrate (Canad.), Oradrate, Rectules, SK-Chloral Hydrate

Primary Use: This nonbarbiturate sedative-hypnotic is effective in the treatment of insomnia.

Ocular Side Effects:

A. Systemic Administration
    1. Decreased vision
    2. Pupils
        a. Mydriasis — toxic states
        b. Miosis
    3. Visual hallucinations — mainly Lilliputian
    4. Ptosis
    5. Decreased convergence
    6. Eyelids or conjunctiva
        a. Allergic reactions
        b. Hyperemia
        c. Edema
    7. Lacrimation
    8. Nonspecific ocular irritation
    9. Nystagmus
    10. Paralysis of extraocular muscles
    11. Optic neuritis (?)

Clinical Significance: While the more serious ocular side effects due to chloral hydrate occur at excessive dosage levels, decreased convergence, miosis, and occasionally ptosis are seen even at recommended therapeutic dosages. Lilliputian hallucinations (in which objects appear smaller than their actual size) are said to be almost characteristic for chloral hydrate-induced delirium. Mydriasis only occurs in severely toxic states.

Interactions with Other Drugs:

A. Effect of Chloral Hydrate on Activity of Other Drugs
    1. Alcohol ↑

    2. Phenothiazines ↑
    3. Tricyclic antidepressants ↑
    4. Analgesics ↓
    5. Antihistamines ↓
    6. Corticosteroids ↓
    7. Phenylbutazone ↓
    8. Sedatives and hypnotics ↓
  B. Effect of Other Drugs on Activity of Chloral Hydrate
    1. Alcohol ↑
    2. Analgesics ↑
    3. Antihistamines ↑
    4. Corticosteroids ↑
    5. Monoamine oxidase inhibitors ↑
    6. Phenothiazines ↑
    7. Tricyclic antidepressants ↑

References:

de Schweinitz, G. E.: Toxic Amblyopias. Philadelphia, Lea Brothers, 1896.
Goldstein, J. H.: Effects of drugs on cornea, conjunctiva, and lids. Int. Ophthalmol. Clin. *11*(2):13, 1971.
Hermans, G.: Les psychotropes. Bull. Soc. Belge Ophtalmol. *160*:15, 1972.
Lubeck, M. J.: Effects of drugs on ocular muscles. Int. Ophthalmol. Clin. *11*(2):35, 1971.
Margetts, E. L.: Chloral delirium. Psychiatr. Q. *24*:278, 1950.
Walsh, F. B., and Hoyt, W. F.: Clinical Neuro-Ophthalmology. 3rd Ed., Baltimore, Williams & Wilkins, Vol. III, 1969, p. 2619.

Generic Name: Ethchlorvynol

Proprietary Name: Placidyl, Serensil

Primary Use: This nonbarbiturate sedative-hypnotic is effective in the treatment of simple insomnia. It is also used as a daytime sedative.

Ocular Side Effects:

  A. Systemic Administration
    1. Decreased vision
    2. Diplopia
    3. Nystagmus
    4. Visual hallucinations
    5. Problems with color vision — dyschromatopsia
    6. Visual fields
      a. Scotomas — central or centrocecal
      b. Constriction

7. Decreased accommodation
8. Toxic amblyopia
9. Anisocoria
10. Optic neuritis

Clinical Significance: Nearly all ocular side effects due to ethchlorvynol are reversible, after discontinuation of the drug. In rare cases, visual defects may be permanent after prolonged therapy. Upon withdrawal of the drug, visual hallucinations are common in patients who have been receiving high doses. Recently, it has been suggested that this is the first drug implicated as causing positional central "vestibular" nystagmus.

Interactions with Other Drugs:

A. Effect of Ethchlorvynol on Activity of Other Drugs
    1. Phenothiazines ↑
    2. Tricyclic antidepressants ↑
    3. Analgesics ↓
    4. Antihistamines ↓
    5. Corticosteroids ↓
B. Effect of Other Drugs on Activity of Ethchlorvynol
    1. Alcohol ↑
    2. Analgesics ↑
    3. Antihistamines ↑
    4. Barbiturates ↑
    5. Corticosteroids ↑
    6. Monoamine oxidase inhibitors ↑
    7. Phenothiazines ↑
    8. Tricyclic antidepressants ↑

References:

American Hospital Formulary Service. Washington, D.C., American Society of Hospital Pharmacists, Vol. I, 28:24, 1975.
Brown, E., and Meyer, G. G.: Toxic amblyopia and peripheral neuropathy with ethchlorvynol abuse. Am. J. Psychiatry 126:882, 1969.
Haining, W. M., and Beveridge, G. W.: Toxic amblyopia in a patient receiving ethchlorvynol as a hypnotic. Br. J. Ophthalmol. 48:598, 1964.
Hudson, H. S., and Walker, H. I.: Withdrawal symptoms following ethchlorvynol (Placidyl) dependence. Am. J. Psychiatry 118:361, 1961.
Millhouse, J., Davies, D. M., and Wraith, S. R.: Chronic ethchlorvynol intoxication. Lancet 2:1251, 1966.
Ropper, A. H.: Unusual nystgamus after ethchlorvynol use. JAMA 232:907, 1975.

Generic Name: 1. Glutethimide; 2. Methyprylon

Proprietary Name: 1. Doriden, Doridene (Fr.), Dorimide, Glimid (Pol.), Gludorm (Austral.), Rolathimide, Somide (Canad.); 2. Methyprylone (G.B.), Noludar

Primary Use: These piperidinedione derivatives are effective in the treatment of simple insomnia or as a mild daytime sedative.

Ocular Side Effects:

A. Systemic Administration
   1. Decreased vision
   2. Pupils
      a. Mydriasis
      b. Miosis (methyprylon)
      c. Decreased or absent reaction to light
   3. Nystagmus — horizontal or vertical
   4. Diplopia
   5. Decreased accommodation
   6. Visual hallucinations
   7. Eyelids or conjunctiva
      a. Allergic reactions
      b. Urticaria
      c. Purpura
      d. Exfoliative dermatitis
   8. Subconjunctival or retinal hemorrhages secondary to drug-induced anemia
   9. Decreased corneal reflex
   10. Papilledema

Clinical Significance: At the recommended dosage, few ocular side effects due to these agents are seen; however, in overdose situations ocular side effects, especially with glutethimide, are common. Papilledema and dilated fixed pupils have only been found in near terminal patients.

Interactions with Other Drugs:

A. Effect of Piperidinedione Derivatives on Activity of Other Drugs
   1. Phenothiazines ↑
   2. Tricyclic antidepressants ↑
   3. Analgesics ↓
   4. Antihistamines ↓

5. Corticosteroids ↓
6. Sedatives and hypnotics ↓
B. Effect of Other Drugs on Activity of Piperidinedione Derivatives
   1. Alcohol ↑
   2. Antihistamines ↑
   3. Barbiturates ↑
   4. Corticosteroids ↑
   5. Monoamine oxidase inhibitors ↑
   6. Tricyclic antidepressants ↑

References:

American Hospital Formulary Service. Washington, D.C., American Society of Hospital Pharmacists, Vol. I, 28:24, 1976.
DeMyttenaere, M., Schoenfeld, L., and Maher, J. F.: Treatment of glutethimide poisoning. JAMA 203:885, 1968.
Hermans, G.: Les psychotropes, Bull. Soc. Belge Ophtalmol. 160:15, 1972.
Maher, J. F., Schreiner, G. E., and Westervelt, F. B.: Acute glutethimide intoxication. Am. J. Med. 33:70, 1962.
Medgyaszay, A.: Impairment of adaptation in response to Noxyron. Szemeszet 100: 228, 1963 (Am. J. Ophthalmol. 57:1073, 1964).
Walsh, F. B., and Hoyt, W. F.: Clinical Neuro-Ophthalmology. 3rd Ed., Baltimore, Williams & Wilkins, Vol. III, 1969, pp. 2647–2648.

Generic Name: Methaqualone

Proprietary Name: Dormir (Austral.), Hyptor (Canad.), Mequelon (Austral.), Mequin, Methalone (Austral.), Methased (Austral.), Nobedorm (Swed.), Normi-Nox (Germ.), Oblioser (Austral.), Optinoxan (Germ.), Parest, Pexaqualone (Canad.), Quaalude, Revonal (G.B.), Rouqualone (Canad.), Sleepinal (Austral.), Somnafac, Sopor, Thendorm (Austral.), Tiqualoine (Canad.), Triador (Canad.), Tualone (Canad.)

Primary Use: This nonbarbiturate sedative-hypnotic is effective in the treatment of simple insomnia or as a daytime sedative.

Ocular Side Effects:

A. Systemic Administration
   1. Nystagmus
   2. Lacrimation
   3. Pupils
      a. Mydriasis — toxic states
      b. Decreased reaction to light — toxic states
      c. Anisocoria

4. Diplopia
5. Decreased vision
6. Problems with color vision — objects have yellow tinge
7. Subconjunctival or retinal hemorrhages secondary to drug-induced anemia
8. Decreased accommodation (?)

Clinical Significance: All ocular side effects due to methaqualone are transient and reversible. Methaqualone has come to be widely abused, and the abuser may employ doses of 75 mg to 2 g a day. Pupillary abnormalities are seen primarily in acute toxic states.

Interactions with Other Drugs:

A. Effect of Methaqualone on Activity of Other Drugs
1. Phenothiazines ↑
2. Tricyclic antidepressants ↑
3. Analgesics ↓
4. Antihistamines ↓
5. Corticosteroids ↓
B. Effect of Other Drugs on Activity of Methaqualone
1. Alcohol ↑
2. Analgesics ↑
3. Antihistamines ↑
4. Barbiturates ↑
5. Corticosteroids ↑
6. Monoamine oxidase inhibitors ↑
7. Phenothiazines ↑
8. Sedatives and hypnotics ↑
9. Tricyclic antidepressants ↑

References:

American Hospital Formulary Service. Washington, D.C., American Society of Hospital Pharmacists, Vol. 1, 28:24, 1976.
Davidson, S. I.: Reports of ocular adverse reactions. Trans. Ophthalmol. Soc. U.K. 93:495, 1973.
Gitelson, S.: Methaqualone-meprobamate poisoning. JAMA 201:977, 1967.
Grant, W. M.: Toxicology of the Eye. 2nd Ed., Springfield, Charles C Thomas, 1974, pp. 676–677.
MacDonald, H. R. F., and Lakshman, A. D.: Poisoning with Mandrax. Br. Med. J. 1:500, 1967.

Generic Name: Methylpentynol

Proprietary Name: Allotropal (Germ.), Insomnol (G.B.), N-Oblivon (Fr.), Oblivon-C (G.B.)

Primary Use: This nonbarbiturate sedative-hypnotic is effective in the treatment of insomnia and as a premedication for minor surgical procedures.

Ocular Side Effects:

A. Systemic Administration
   1. Nystagmus
   2. Diplopia
   3. Conjunctival edema
   4. Mydriasis — may precipitate narrow-angle glaucoma
   5. Visual hallucinations
   6. Ptosis

Clinical Significance: Ocular side effects are commonly seen with methylpentynol, especially nystagmus. Seldom are adverse ocular symptoms of major clinical importance, since this drug is short-acting and is not used for prolonged periods.

Interactions with Other Drugs:

A. Effect of Methylpentynol on Activity of Other Drugs
   1. Phenothiazines ↑
   2. Tricyclic antidepressants ↑
   3. Analgesics ↓
   4. Antihistamines ↓
   5. Corticosteroids ↓
B. Effect of Other Drugs on Activity of Methylpentynol
   1. Analgesics ↑
   2. Antihistamines ↑
   3. Corticosteroids ↑
   4. Monoamine oxidase inhibitors ↑
   5. Phenothiazines ↑
   6. Tricyclic antidepressants ↑

References:

Bartholomew, A. A., et al.: Methylpentynol carbamate and liver function. Lancet *1*:346, 1958.
Hermans, G.: Les psychotropes. Bull. Soc. Belge Ophtalmol. *160*:15, 1972.
Hitzschke, B., and Herbst, A.: Beobachtungen bei Missbrauch von Methylpentinol. Psychiatr. Neurol. (Basel) *153*:308, 1967.
Wade, A. (Ed.): Martindale: The Extra Pharmacopoeia. 27th Ed., London, Pharmaceutical Press, 1977, p. 763.

Generic Name: Paraldehyde

Proprietary Name: Paral

Primary Use: This nonbarbiturate sedative-hypnotic is also effective as an anticonvulsant in epilepsy and in alcohol withdrawal.

Ocular Side Effects:

A. Systemic Administration
   1. Pupils
      a. Mydriasis — toxic states
      b. Miosis
   2. Decreased vision
   3. Visual hallucinations
   4. Decreased corneal reflex
   5. Hemianopsia (?)

Clinical Significance: Ocular side effects due to paraldehyde are common but seldom significant. At therapeutic dosage levels paraldehyde causes miosis; however, at toxic blood levels mydriasis may occur. Visual hallucinations occur primarily during withdrawal of the drug. In one instance of drug withdrawal, a homonymous hemianopsia with loss of corneal reflex occurred.

Interactions with Other Drugs:

A. Effect of Paraldehyde on Activity of Other Drugs
   1. Phenothiazines ↑
   2. Tricyclic antidepressants ↑
   3. Analgesics ↓
   4. Antihistamines ↓
   5. Corticosteroids ↓
   6. Sulfonamides ↓
B. Effect of Other Drugs on Activity of Paraldehyde
   1. Alcohol ↑
   2. Analgesics ↑
   3. Antihistamines ↑
   4. Corticosteroids ↑
   5. Monoamine oxidase inhibitors ↑
   6. Phenothiazines ↑
   7. Tricyclic antidepressants ↑

References:

Grant, W. M.: Toxicology of the Eye. 2nd Ed., Springfield, Charles C Thomas, 1974, p. 786.

Heiman, M.: Visual hallucination during paraldehyde addiction. J. Nerv. Ment. Dis. *96*:251, 1942.

Hermans, G.: Les psychotropes. Bull. Soc. Belge Ophtalmol. *160*:15, 1972.

Lubeck, M. J.: Effects of drugs on ocular muscles. Int. Ophthalmol. Clin. *11*(2):35, 1971.

Walsh, F. B., and Hoyt, W. F.: Clinical Neuro-Ophthalmology. 3rd Ed., Baltimore, Williams & Wilkins, Vol. III, 1969, pp. 2627–2628.

III

Analgesics, Narcotic Antagonists, and Agents Used to Treat Arthritis

Class: Agents Used to Treat Gout

Generic Name: Allopurinol

Proprietary Name: Bloxanth (Canad.), Epidropal (Germ.), Foligan (Germ.), Lopurin, Urosin (Germ.), Zyloprim, Zyloric (G.B.)

Primary Use: This potent xanthine oxidase inhibitor is primarily used in the treatment of chronic hyperuricemia.

Ocular Side Effects:

A. Systemic Administration
   1. Decreased vision
   2. Eyelids or conjunctiva
      a. Allergic reactions
      b. Erythema
      c. Urticaria
      d. Purpura
      e. Stevens-Johnson syndrome
      f. Exfoliative dermatitis
      g. Lyell's syndrome
   3. Subconjunctival or retinal hemorrhages secondary to drug-induced anemia
   4. Cataracts (?)
   5. Macular exudates (?)
   6. Macular hemorrhages (?)
   7. Macular degeneration (?)
   8. Loss of eyelashes or eyebrows (?)
   9. Diplopia (?)

Clinical Significance: Equatorial and posterior subcapsular cataracts are the most significant adverse ocular effects suspected as an allopurinol-related event. To date, 30 cases of cataracts secondary to this agent have been reported either in the literature or to the Registry. These cataracts have been primarily observed in the age groups prior to normal lens aging changes. As commonly as this drug is used, the development of cataracts may only represent the chance occurrence of this type of lens change or may be gout-related, not drug-related. To date, no drug-induced cataract in humans has not already been seen in animals. Thus far, allopurinol has not been known to cause lens changes in animals. However, one investigator has isolated this drug from a human cataract by use of sophisticated analyses; this would appear to indicate a probable cause-and-effect relationship. Since allopurinol is a strong photosensitizer, lenses which decrease light to the eye are possibly indicated for patients using this drug. One case report of Lyell's syndrome has been attributed to allopurinol. In this case, pseudomembranous conjunctivitis, lid and corneal ulcers, corneal abrasions, plus a superficial punctate keratitis were found which persisted for over 14 months. Two reports of maculopathy due to this drug have been published, but a cause-and-effect relationship is difficult to establish. A case of allopurinol hepatotoxicity with diplopia resolved shortly after the drug was discontinued.

Interactions with Other Drugs:

A. Effect of Other Drugs on Activity of Allopurinol
   1. Diuretics ↓

References:

Bennett, T. O., Sugar, J., and Sahgal, S.: Ocular manifestations of toxic epidermal necrolysis associated with allopurinol use. Arch. Ophthalmol. *95*:1362, 1977.

Chawla, S. K., et al.: Allopurinol hepatotoxicity. Case report and literature review. Arthritis Rheum. *20*:1546, 1977.

Davidson, S. I.: Reports of ocular adverse reactions. Trans. Ophthalmol. Soc. U.K. *93*:495, 1973.

Fraunfelder, F. T., et al.: Cataracts associated with allopurinol therapy. Am. J. Ophthalmol. Submitted.

Gilman, A. G., Goodman, L. S., and Gilman, A. (Eds.): The Pharmacological Basis of Therapeutics. 6th Ed., New York, Macmillan, 1980, pp. 720–722.

Laval, J.: Allopurinol and macular lesions. Arch. Ophthalmol. *80*:415, 1968.

Lerman, S., Megaw, J. M., and Gardner, K.: Allopurinol therapy and human cataractogenesis. Am. J. Ophthalmol. Submitted.

Lyell, A.: A review of toxic epidermal necrolysis in Britain. Br. J. Dermatol. *79*:662, 1967.

March, W. F., Goren, S., and Shoch, D.: Action of allopurinol on the lens. In Leopold, I. H. (Ed.): Symposium on Ocular Therapy. St. Louis, C. V. Mosby, Vol. VII, 1974, pp. 83–95.

Pinnas, G.: Possible association between macular lesions and allopurinol. Arch. Ophthalmol. *79*:786, 1968.

Generic Name: Colchicine

Proprietary Name: Aqua-Colchin (Austral.), Colcin (Austral.), Colchineos (Fr., S. Afr.), Colgout (Austral.), Coluric (Austral.)

Primary Use: This alkaloid is used in the prophylaxis and treatment of acute gout.

Ocular Side Effects:

A. Systemic Administration
   1. Cornea
       a. Delayed wound healing
       b. Dellen or erosion
       c. Keratitis
   2. Paresis or paralysis of extraocular muscles
   3. Diplopia
   4. Subconjunctival or retinal hemorrhages secondary to drug-induced anemia
   5. Papilledema — toxic states
   6. Loss of eyelashes or eyebrows (?)
   7. Hypopyon (?)
   8. Cataracts (?)
B. Inadvertent Ocular Exposure
   1. Decreased vision
   2. Conjunctival hyperemia
   3. Corneal clouding

Clinical Significance: Colchicine rarely causes adverse side effects; however, when they do occur, they are usually insignificant and transitory. This antimitotic agent arrests cell division in metaphase, and it is well documented that corneal epithelial replication can be so arrested. With the recent interest in the limbal approach to rectus muscle surgery, there is an increase in limbal edema and perilimbal epithelial disturbances. There are reports that some patients on colchicine have had difficulty in healing of dellen or peripheral corneal erosions. Major ocular side effects have occurred after overdose and have included paresis of extraocular muscles, keratitis, hypopyon, papilledema, and cataracts. The lens changes may have been due to severe dehydration.

Interactions with Other Drugs:

A. Effect of Colchicine on Activity of Other Drugs
   1. Sympathomimetics ↑

References:

American Hospital Formulary Service. Washington, D.C., American Society of Hospital Pharmacists, Vol. II, 92:00, 1977.

Biedner, B. Z., et al.: Colchicine suppression of corneal healing after strabismus surgery. Br. J. Ophthalmol. *61*:496, 1977.

Estable, J. J.: The ocular effect of several irritant drugs applied directly to the conjunctiva. Am. J. Ophthalmol. *31*:837, 1948.

Gilman, A. G., Goodman, L. S., and Gilman, A. (Eds.): The Pharmacological Basis of Therapeutics. 6th Ed., New York, Macmillan, 1980, pp. 718–720.

Grant, W. M.: Toxicology of the Eye. 2nd Ed., Springfield, Charles C Thomas, 1974, pp. 304–305.

Heaney, D., et al.: Massive colchicine overdose: A report on the toxicity. Am. J. Med. Sci. *271*:233, 1976.

Naidus, R. M., Rodvien, R., and Mielke, C. H., Jr.: Colchicine toxicity. A multisystem disease. Arch. Intern. Med. *137*:394, 1977.

Walsh, F. B., and Hoyt, W. F.: Clinical Neuro-Ophthalmology. 3rd Ed., Baltimore, Williams & Wilkins, Vol. III, 1969, p. 2659.

Class: Antirheumatic Agents

Generic Name: 1. Aurothioglucose; 2. Aurothioglycanide; 3. Gold Au^{198}; 4. Gold Sodium Thiomalate (Sodium Aurothiomalate); 5. Gold Sodium Thiosulfate (Sodium Aurothiosulfate)

Proprietary Name: 1. Aureotan (Germ.), Solganal; 2. Aurothioglycanide; 3. Aureotope, Radio Gold (Au 198), Aurocoloid 198; 4. Myochrysine, Myocrisin (G.B.), Tauredon (Germ.); 5. Sodium Aurothiosulphate (G.B.)

Primary Use: These heavy metals are used in the treatment of active rheumatoid arthritis and nondisseminated lupus erythematosus. Radioactive gold (Au^{198}) is also employed for its radiation effects in treating neoplastic growths.

Ocular Side Effects:

   A. Systemic Administration
      1. Red, violet, purple, or brown gold deposits
         a. Eyelids
         b. Conjunctiva
         c. Superficial and deep cornea
         d. Surface of lens

    2. Eyelids or conjunctiva
      a. Allergic reactions
      b. Hyperemia — including ciliary body
      c. Erythema
      d. Blepharoconjunctivitis
      e. Edema
      f. Photosensitivity
      g. Symblepharon
      h. Urticaria
      i. Purpura
      j. Lupoid syndrome
      k. Erythema multiforme
      l. Stevens-Johnson syndrome
      m. Exfoliative dermatitis
      n. Lyell's syndrome
    3. Photophobia
    4. Cornea
      a. Keratitis
      b. Ulceration
      c. Stromal melting
    5. Iritis
    6. Paralysis of extraocular muscles
    7. Ptosis
    8. Diplopia
    9. Nystagmus
   10. Subconjunctival or retinal hemorrhages secondary to drug-induced anemia
   11. Papilledema (?)
   12. Phlyctenular keratoconjunctivitis (?)
   13. Loss of eyelashes or eyebrows (?)
 B. Inadvertent Ocular Exposure
    1. Irritation
    2. Corneal clouding
    3. Iritis

Clinical Significance: Although gold deposition in the conjunctiva and superficial cornea is not uncommon, deposition of gold in the lens or deep cornea is uncommon. Corneal deposition occurs within the epithelium or deep to the epithelium, possibly in the region of the basal lamina. It is usually diffuse, but in some patients, the visual axis is spared and the paralimbal corneal area is more involved. Gold deposition in the cornea may only be in the Hudson-Stähli line region, or it may take a vortex distribution as in Fabry's disease; the gold deposits tend to be increased in areas of corneal scarring. Deep stromal involvement is unusual and possibly only associated with large dosages. Lens deposits of gold are much less frequent than corneal deposits and of little to no clinical importance. They are totally reversible after stopping gold therapy. However, visual acuity is unaffected, and deposition of gold in the cornea or lens is not an indication for cessation of therapy. In general, 1 g of this drug is needed before corneal changes are seen. In total dosages of 1.5 g, from 40 to 75 percent of patients will have gold deposition in the cornea. Corneal deposits may be seen as early as one month after starting therapy; once therapy is ceased, clearing is usually complete within 3 to 5 months. However, cases have been reported requiring 1 year for complete clearing. Corneal ulceration is a rarely encountered manifestation of gold therapy and is theorized to be an allergic reaction due to gold hypersensitivity. Ptosis, diplopia, and nystagmus due to gold therapy are rare.

Interactions with Other Drugs:

A. Contraindications
   1. Oxyphenbutazone
   2. Phenylbutazone

References:

AMA Drug Evaluations. 4th Ed., New York, John Wiley & Sons, 1980, pp. 104–106, 1192.

Austin, P., et al.: Peripheral corneal degeneration and occlusive vasculitis in Wegener's granulomatosis. Am. J. Ophthalmol. 85:311, 1978.

Bron, A. J., McLendon, B. F., and Camp, A. V.: Epithelial deposition of gold in the cornea in patients receiving systemic therapy. Am. J. Ophthalmol. 88:354, 1979.

Gibbons, R. B.: Complications of chrysotherapy. A review of recent studies. Arch. Intern. Med. 139:343, 1979.

Gilman, A. G., Goodman, L. S., and Gilman, A. (Eds.): The Pharmacological Basis of Therapeutics. 6th Ed., New York, Macmillan, 1980, pp. 713–717, 1305.

Gottlieb, N. L., and Gray, R. G.: Diagnosis and management of adverse reactions from gold compounds. J. Anal. Toxicol. 2:173, 1978.

Roberts, W. H., and Wolter, J. R.: Ocular chrysiasis. Arch. Ophthalmol. 56:48, 1956.

Sundelin, F.: Die Goldbehandlung der chronischen Arthritis unter besonderer Berucksichtigung der Komplikationen. Acta Med. Scand. (Suppl.) 117:1, 1941.

Walsh, F. B., and Hoyt, W. F.: Clinical Neuro-Ophthalmology. 3rd Ed., Baltimore, Williams & Wilkins, Vol. III, 1969, pp. 2651–2652, 2686–2687.

Generic Name: Ibuprofen

Proprietary Name: Brufen (G.B.), Motrin

Primary Use: This antipyretic analgesic is used in the treatment of rheumatoid arthritis and osteoarthritis.

Ocular Side Effects:

A. Systemic Administration
    1. Decreased vision
    2. Diplopia
    3. Problems with color vision — dyschromatopsia
    4. Eyelids or conjunctiva
       a. Erythema
       b. Edema
       c. Urticaria
       d. Purpura
       e. Lupoid syndrome
       f. Erythema multiforme
       g. Stevens-Johnson syndrome
       h. Loss of eyelashes or eyebrows (?)
    5. Optic neuritis
    6. Visual fields
       a. Scotomas — centrocecal or paracentral
       b. Constriction
       c. Hemianopsia
       d. Enlarged blind spot
    7. Toxic amblyopia
    8. Cornea
       a. Opacities (?)
       b. Vascularization
    9. Subconjunctival or retinal hemorrhages secondary to drug-induced anemia
    10. Abnormal ERG
    11. Papilledema (?)
    12. Cataracts (?)
    13. Macular degeneration (?)

Clinical Significance: Ibuprofen is one of the largest selling antiarthritic agents in the world. Although over 60 reports of adverse ocular events possibly associated with this drug have been reported to the Registry, most are of little consequence and primarily consist of transient blurred vision. Even so, this is a small number over a 4-year period for such a common drug used for diseases which not infrequently affect the eye. There are enough occasional cases where the drug has been rechallenged that changes in refractive error, diplopia, and decrease in color vision appear to be well documented. Other changes, however, attributed to this drug are debatable. One of these is either a nonrelated chance event occurring or a rare idiosyncratic optic nerve response associated with the use of this drug. The typical sequence is that after 1 to 3 weeks of therapy a unilateral marked decrease in visual acuity occurs, with vision receding to 20/80 to 20/200 range. Visual fields may show various types of central scotomas. If the medication is stopped, visual acuity returns to normal in 1 to 3 months. In one case, it took 8 months for color vision to return to normal. For a drug so commonly used in combination with other agents, it is not possible to implicate specifically this agent. However, many of the cases are outside the usual optic or retrobulbar neuritis age group and occur shortly after starting this medication. Therefore, patients on this drug should be told to stop this medication if a sudden decrease in vision occurs. Although corneal opacities, papilledema, cataracts, and macular degeneration have been suggested as being due to ibuprofen exposure, this is suspective and, to date, must be considered as only coincidental.

References:

Collum, L. M. T., and Bowen, D. I.: Ocular side-effects of ibuprofen. Br. J. Ophthalmol. 55:472, 1971.
Davidson, S. I.: Report of ocular adverse reactions. Trans. Ophthalmol. Soc. U.K. 93:495, 1973.
Dukes, M. N. G. (Ed.): Meyler's Side Effects of Drugs. Amsterdam, Excerpta Medica, Vol. IX, 1980, pp. 150–151.
Filipowicz, M.: Visual disturbances after the use of Brufen. Klin. Oczna 46:339, 1976.
Fraunfelder, F. T.: Interim report: National Registry of Possible Drug-Induced Ocular Side Effects. Ophthalmology 87:87, 1980.
Melluish, J. W., et al.: Ibuprofen and visual function. Arch. Ophthalmol. 93:781, 1975.
Palmer, C. A. L.: Toxic amblyopia from ibuprofen. Br. Med. J. 3:765, 1972.

Generic Name: Indomethacin (Indometacin)

Proprietary Name: Amuno (Germ.), Confortid (Swed.), Imbrilon (G.B.), Inacid (Span.), Indacin (Jap.), Indocid (G.B.), Indocin, Indomee (Swed.), Infrocin (Canad.), Metindol (Pol.), Mezolin (Jap.)

Primary Use: This indole compound is effective as an antipyretic, analgesic, and anti-inflammatory agent in the treatment of rheumatoid arthritis, rheumatoid spondylitis, and degenerative joint disease.

Ocular Side Effects:

A. Systemic Administration
   1. Decreased vision
   2. Diplopia
   3. Problems with color vision — dyschromatopsia
   4. Visual hallucinations

   5. Eyelids or conjunctiva
      a. Angioneurotic edema
      b. Urticaria
   6. Subconjunctival or retinal hemorrhages secondary to drug-induced anemia
   7. Corneal deposits
      a. Superficial whorl pattern
      b. Superficial punctate keratitis
      c. Epithelial erosion
      d. Crystalline deposits
   8. Abnormal scotopic ERG and EOG
   9. Retina (?)
      a. Pigmentary changes
      b. Cystoid degeneration
      c. Edema
      d. Papilledema
      e. Vascular occlusion
  10. Macula (?)
      a. Edema
      b. Degeneration — paramacular
      c. Central serous retinopathy
  11. Decreased dark adaptation (?)
  12. Visual fields (?)
      a. Scotomas
      b. Constriction
      c. Enlarged blind spot
  13. Orbital or periorbital pain (?)
  14. Lacrimation (?)
  15. Mydriasis (?)
  16. Toxic amblyopia (?)
  17. Loss of eyelashes or eyebrows (?)

Clinical Significance: Systemic complications from indomethacin have been reported by some to occur in 35 to 50 percent of patients taking accepted therapeutic doses. The true role of indomethacin-induced ocular adverse effects is clouded by an almost equal number of contradictory reports. Unfortunately, much of the data implicating indomethacin is in retrospective studies. The clinician confronted with a possible adverse ocular effect must judge each case individually, fully aware that the possibility of drug-induced ocular toxic effects may exist. At our current stage of knowledge, however, many investigators feel that indomethacin causes a number of ocular side effects. Increasing data support that superficial corneal crystalline deposits are seen secondary to this drug and resolve on its discontinuation. However, its role in drug-related macular or retinal disease is less clear cut, although there are a number of reports of papilledema secondary to pseudo-tumor cerebri.

Interaction with Other Drugs:

A. Effect of Indomethacin on Activity of Other Drugs
    1. Corticosteroids ↑
    2. Sulfonamides ↑
B. Effect of Other Drugs on Activity of Indomethacin
    1. Salicylates ↓

References:

Burns, C. A.: Indomethacin, reduced retinal sensitivity, and corneal deposits. Am. J. Ophthalmol. *66*:825, 1968.

Carr, R. E., and Siegel, I. M.: Retinal function in patients treated with indomethacin. Am. J. Ophthalmol. *75*:302, 1973.

Davidson, S. I.: Report of ocular adverse reactions. Trans. Ophthalmol. Soc. U.K. *93*:495, 1973.

Henkes, H. E., van Lith, G. H. M., and Canta, L. R.: Indomethacin retinopathy. Am. J. Ophthalmol. *73*:846, 1972.

Kelly, M.: Treatment of 193 rheumatic patients with indomethacin: A new antirheumatic drug. J. Am. Geriat. Soc. *14*:48, 1966.

Palimeris, G., Koliopoulos, J., and Velissaropoulos, P.: Ocular side effects of indomethacin. Ophthalmologica *164*:339, 1972.

Physicians' Desk Reference. 35th Ed., Oradell, N.J., Medical Economics Co., 1981, p. 1210.

Generic Name: Ketoprofen

Proprietary Name: Alrheumat (G.B.), Orudis (G.B.), Profenid (Fr.)

Primary Use: This antipyretic analgesic is used in the treatment of rheumatoid arthritis, osteoarthritis, ankylosing spondylitis, and gout.

Ocular Side Effects:

A. Systemic Administration
    1. Decreased vision
    2. Eyelids or conjunctiva
       a. Conjunctivitis — nonspecific
       b. Angioneurotic edema
    3. Decreased accommodation
    4. Paralysis of extraocular muscles (?)
    5. Papilledema (?)
    6. Visual field defects (?)

6

Clinical Significance: Ketoprofen is not commercially available in the United States but can be obtained in Europe. The only serious side effect thus far reported is pseudotumor cerebri. The usual severe ocular sequelae of papilledema may be found: extraocular muscle paralysis, primarily sixth nerve, and visual field defects. A nonspecific conjunctivitis has been reported which resolved when the medication was discontinued, but this is still an unproven side effect.

References:

Larizza, D., et al.: Ketoprofen causing pseudotumor cerebri in Bartter's syndrome. N. Engl. J. Med. *300:*796, 1979.
Prescott, L. F.: Anti-inflammatory analgesics and drugs used in rheumatism and gout. In Dukes, M. N. G. (Ed.): Side Effects of Drugs Annual 4, Amsterdam, Excerpta Medica, 1980, p. 67.
Umez-Eronini, E. M.: Conjunctivitis due to ketoprofen. Lancet 2:737, 1978.

Generic Name: Naproxen

Proprietary Name: Anaprox, Naprosyn, Naxen (Mex.), Proxen (Aust., Germ., Switz.)

Primary Use: This antipyretic analgesic is used in the treatment of rheumatoid arthritis, osteoarthritis, and ankylosing spondylitis.

Ocular Side Effects:

A. Systemic Administration
   1. Decreased vision
   2. Eyelids or conjunctiva
       a. Conjunctivitis — nonspecific
       b. Edema
       c. Angioneurotic edema
       d. Urticaria
       e. Purpura
   3. Decreased accommodation
   4. Problems with color vision — dyschromatopsia
   5. Subconjunctival or retinal hemorrhages secondary to drug-induced anemia
   6. Cataracts (?)
   7. Optic neuritis (?)

Clinical Significance: With increased use of this nonsteroidal anti-inflammatory agent, probably more adverse ocular effects will be seen. While some patients complain of decreased vision, this is seldom a significant finding and occurs in less than 5 percent of patients. Although three cases of optic neuritis have been reported to the Registry, this may still be only a chance event when starting this drug. Possibly of more concern is the question whether this agent causes anterior or posterior subcapsular cataracts. While there are four such reports in the Registry, there is no proof to date of a cause-and-effect relationship. Because there are a number of adverse ocular effects seen with other anti-inflammatory drugs, the manufacturer recommends periodic ocular examinations. To date, as far as the Registry is concerned, the drug appears to cause few significant adverse ocular effects. A recent report warns of necrotizing vasculitis in the skin; possibly, this should be watched for in the retina.

Interactions with Other Drugs:

A. Effect of Other Drugs on Activity of Naproxen
    1. Antacids ↓
    2. Salicylates ↓

References:

American Hospital Formulary Service. Washington, D.C., American Society of Hospital Pharmacists, Vol. I, 28:08, 1977.

Fraunfelder, F. T.: Interim report: National Registry of Possible Drug-Induced Ocular Side Effects. Ophthalmology 86:126, 1979.

Mordes, J. P., Johnson, M. W., and Soter, N. A.: Possible naproxen-associated vasculitis: Arch. Intern. Med. *140*:985, 1980.

Physicians' Desk Reference. 35th Ed., Oradell, N. J., Medical Economics Co., 1981, p. 1779.

Svihovec, J.: Anti-inflammatory analgesics and drugs used in gout. In Dukes, M. N. G. (Ed.): Meyler's Side Effects of Drugs. Amsterdam, Excerpta Medica, Vol. IX, 1980, p. 152.

Generic Name: 1. Oxyphenbutazone; 2. Phenylbutazone

Proprietary Name: 1. Butapirone (Ital.), Iridil (Ital.), Oxalid, Phlogase (Germ.), Rheumapax (Swed.), Tandacote (G.B.), Tandearil, Tanderil (G.B.); 2. Algoverine (Canad.), Artrizin (Denm.), Artropan (Ital.), Azolid, Butacal (Austral.), Butacote (G.B.), Butagesic (Canad.), Butalan (Austral.), Butalgin (Austral.), Butaphen (Austral.), Butapirazol (Pol.), Butarex (Austral.), Butazolidin, Butazone (G.B.), Butina (S. Afr.), Butoroid (Austral.), Butoz (Austral.), Butozone (S. Afr.), Butrex (S. Afr.), Buzon (Austral.), Chembutazone (Canad.), Diossidone (Ital.), Ecobutazone (Canad.), Elmedal (Germ.), Eributazone (Canad.), Ethibute (G.B.), Flexazone (G.B.), Intrabutazone (Canad.), Kadol (Ital.), Malgesic (Canad.), Merizone (Canad.), Nadozone

(Canad.), Neo-Zoline (Canad.), Novophenyl (Canad.), Oppazone (G.B.), Panazone (S. Afr.), Phenbutazol (Canad.), Phenybute (Austral.), Phenylbetazone (Canad.), Praecirheumin (Germ.), Tazone (Canad.), Tetnor (G.B.), Ticinil (Ital.), Wescozone (Canad.)

Primary Use: These pyrazolone derivatives are effective in the management of acute gout, ankylosing spondylitis, osteoarthritis, and musculo-skeletal disorders.

Ocular Side Effects:

A. Systemic Administration
  1. Decreased vision
  2. Eyelids or conjunctiva
    a. Allergic reactions
    b. Hyperemia
    c. Conjunctivitis — nonspecific
    d. Edema
    e. Urticaria
    f. Symblepharon
    g. Lupoid syndrome
    h. Stevens-Johnson syndrome
    i. Exfoliative dermatitis
    j. Lyell's syndrome
  3. Retinal hemorrhages
  4. Paralysis of extraocular muscles
  5. Diplopia
  6. Problems with color vision — dyschromatopsia
  7. Cornea
    a. Peripheral stromal vascularization
    b. Opacities
    c. Keratitis
    d. Scarring
    e. Ulceration
  8. Toxic amblyopia
  9. Optic neuritis
  10. Optic atrophy
  11. Visual hallucinations
  12. Subconjunctival or retinal hemorrhages secondary to drug-induced anemia

Clinical Significance: Ocular side effects due to these drugs are not uncommon and can be severe. At least 10 to 15 percent of patients taking these agents must discontinue their use due to systemic toxic reactions.

This is due in part to the high dosages necessary in some patients to control their disease. Unlike most drugs, these act so that the older the patient the more likely an untoward side effect. Side effects are so common in patients above the age of 60 that the manufacturers recommend treatment only at weekly intervals. The most common ocular side effect is decreased vision. It has been suggested that this is due to increased lens hydration. However, phenylbutazone-induced hypermetropia up to 3 to 4 diopters has been reported to the Registry. Eyelid or conjunctival changes followed by retinal hemorrhages, not necessarily associated with a drug-induced anemia, are the next most frequent adverse ocular reactions. This group of drugs can elicit an allergic reaction which brings about a lupus syndrome with its associated ocular side effects. Many of the conjunctival or corneal adverse effects may be due to lupoid effects rather than a direct drug effect.

Interactions with Other Drugs:

A. Effect of Pyrazolone Derivatives on Activity of Other Drugs
   1. Penicillins ↑
   2. Sulfonamides ↑
   3. Barbiturates ↓
   4. Corticosteroids ↓
B. Effect of Other Drugs on Activity of Pyrazolone Derivatives
   1. Antacids ↓
   2. Barbiturates ↓
   3. Salicylates ↓
   4. Tricyclic antidepressants ↓

References:

Alarcón-Segovia, D.: Drug-induced antinuclear antibodies and lupus syndromes. Drugs *12*:69, 1976.
Dukes, M. N. G. (Ed.): Meyler's Side Effects of Drugs. Amsterdam, Excerpta Medica, Vol. IX, 1980, pp. 142–145.
Gilman, A. G., Goodman, L. S., and Gilman, A. (Eds.): The Pharmacological Basis of Therapeutics. 6th Ed., New York, Macmillan, 1980, pp. 698–700.
Physicians' Desk Reference. 35th Ed., Oradell, N.J., Medical Economics Co., 1981, pp. 912, 1789.
Raymond, L. F.: Neovascularization of the cornea due to Butazolidin toxicity. Am. J. Ophthalmol. *43*:287, 1957.
Tostevin, A. L.: Retinal haemorrhages associated with the administration of Butazolidin. Med. J. Aust. *1*:69, 1961.
Walsh, F. B., and Hoyt, W. F.: Clinical Neuro-Ophthalmology. 3rd Ed., Baltimore, Williams & Wilkins, Vol. III, 1969, p. 2591.

Generic Name: Sulindac

Proprietary Name: Clinoril

Primary Use: This nonsteroidal anti-inflammatory indene derivative is used in the relief of osteoarthritis, rheumatoid arthritis, and ankylosing spondylitis.

Ocular Side Effects:

A. Systemic Administration
   1. Decreased vision
   2. Diplopia
   3. Eyelids or conjunctiva
      a. Erythema
      b. Angioneurotic edema
      c. Stevens-Johnson syndrome
      d. Lyell's syndrome
   4. Subconjunctival or retinal hemorrhages
   5. Corneal ulceration (?)
   6. Macular pigmentary changes (?)

Clinical Significance: Adverse ocular effects due to sulindac occur rarely and are usually transient visual disturbances. Although the Registry has received several case reports of possible macular pigmentation or perforated corneal ulcers, these reports are only suspected.

Interactions with Other Drugs:

A. Effect of Other Drugs on Activity of Sulindac
   1. Salicylates ↓

References:

American Hospital Formulary Service. Washington, D.C., American Society of Hospital Pharmacists, Vol. I, 28:08, 1979.
Clinoril adverse reactions. FDA Drug Bull. November, 1979, p. 29.
Clinoril-sulindac. Stevens-Johnson syndrome. ADR Highlights. January 29, 1980.
Physicians' Desk Reference. 35th Ed., Oradell, N.J., Medical Economics Co., 1981, p. 1170.
Sanz, M. A., et al.: Sulindac-induced bone marrow toxicity. Lancet 2:802, 1980.

Class: Mild Analgesics

Generic Name: 1. Acetaminophen; 2. Acetanilid; 3. Phenacetin

Proprietary Name: 1. Aceta, Alba-Temp, Alvedon (Swed.), Anapap, Anelix, Anuphen, Apamide, Apap, Atasol (Canad.), Ben-u-ron (Germ.),

Calpol (G.B.), Campain (Canad.), Capital, Ceetamol (Austral.), Cen-Apap, Cetamol (Ire.), Chemcetaphen (Canad.), Datril, Dapa, Dimindol, Dolamin (Austral.), Dolanex, Doliprane (Fr.), Dymadon (Austral.), Febridol, Febrigesic, Febrogesic, G-1, Janupap, Korum, Lestemp, Liquiprin, Lyteca, Med-Apap, Napamol (S. Afr.), Nebs, Neopap, Nevrol (Austral.), Nilprin, Pacemol (N.Z.), Pamol (G.B.), Panado (S. Afr.), Panadol (G.B.), Panodil (Swed.), Paracet (Austral.), Paracetamol (G.B.), Parasin (Austral.), Parmol (Austral.), Parten, Pediaphen (Canad.), Phenaphen, Phendex, Placemol (Austral.), Pirin, Proval, Pyrapap, Restin (S. Afr.), Rounox (Canad.), Salzone (G.B.), SK-Apap, Sub-Due, Tapar, Temetan, Temlo, Tempra, Tenlap, Termidor (Swed.), Ticelgesic (G.B.), Tylenol, Valadol, Valorin; 2. Acetanilide (G.B.); 3. Phenacetin

Primary Use: These para-aminophenol derivatives are used in the control of fever and mild pain.

Ocular Side Effects:

A. Systemic Administration
   1. Decreased vision
   2. Eyelids or conjunctiva
      a. Allergic reactions
      b. Conjunctivitis — nonspecific
      c. Angioneurotic edema
      d. Urticaria
      e. Erythema multiforme
      f. Stevens-Johnson syndrome
   3. Problems with color vision — objects have yellow tinge (phenacetin) — toxic states
   4. Green or chocolate discoloration of subconjunctival or retinal blood vessels
   5. Pupils
      a. Mydriasis
      b. Decreased reaction to light — toxic states
   6. Subconjunctival or retinal hemorrhages secondary to drug-induced anemia

Clinical Significance: Ocular side effects due to these analgesics are quite rare; however, some adverse ocular reactions have occurred at quite low doses, implying a drug idiosyncrasy or a peculiar sensitivity. The most frequent toxic responses have been reported due to acetanilid, followed by phenacetin, and the fewest are due to acetaminophen. In chronic therapy, all of these drugs can produce sulfhemoglobinemia, which accounts for the greenish or chocolate color change in the subconjunctival or retinal blood vessels.

Interactions with Other Drugs:

A. Effect of Para-Aminophenol Derivatives on Activity of Other Drugs
  1. Penicillins ↑ (acetaminophen)
  2. Salicylates ↑ (acetaminophen)
  3. Sulfonamides ↑ (acetaminophen)
  4. Sympathomimetics ↑ (acetaminophen)
  5. Barbiturates ↓ (acetaminophen)
B. Effect of Other Drugs on Activity of Para-Aminophenol Derivatives
  1. Alcohol ↑ (acetaminophen)
  2. Chloramphenicol ↑ (acetanilid)
  3. Phenothiazines ↑ (acetaminophen)
  4. Barbiturates ↓ (acetaminophen, phenacetin)

References:

AMA Drug Evaluations. 4th Ed., New York, John Wiley & Sons, 1980, pp. 77–78.
American Hospital Formulary Service. Washington, D. C., American Society of Hospital Pharmacists, Vol. 1, 28:08, 1973.
Kneezel, L. D., and Kitchens, C. S.: Phenacetin-induced sulfhemoglobinemia: Report of a case and review of the literature. Johns Hopkins Med. J, 139:175, 1976.
Krenzelok, E. P., Best, L., and Manoguerra, A. S.: Acetaminophen toxicity. Am. J. Hosp. Pharm. 34:391, 1977.
Walsh, F. B., and Hoyt, W. F.: Clinical Neuro-Ophthalmology. 3rd Ed., Baltimore, Williams & Wilkins, Vol. III, 1969, pp. 2540–2541.

Generic Name: Antipyrine (Phenazone)

Proprietary Name: Aurone (S. Afr.), Phenazone (G.B.)

Primary Use: This pyrazolone derivative is used as a mild analgesic and antipyretic.

Ocular Side Effects:

A. Systemic Administration
  1. Eyelids or conjunctiva
    a. Allergic reactions
    b. Conjunctivitis — nonspecific
    c. Edema
    d. Discoloration
    e. Urticaria
    f. Stevens-Johnson syndrome
    g. Lyell's syndrome

2. Decreased vision
3. Keratitis
4. Toxic amblyopia
5. Optic atrophy
6. Subconjunctival or retinal hemorrhages secondary to drug-induced anemia

Clinical Significance: Adverse ocular reactions due to antipyrine are not uncommon, with allergic reactions being the most frequent. Fixed eruptions (those occurring at the same site on re-exposure) have also been reported. A transitory decrease in vision or even blindness may occur and last for a few minutes or a few days. Optic atrophy has been reported in two instances.

Interactions with Other Drugs:

A. Effect of Antipyrine on Activity of Other Drugs
   1. General anesthetics ↑
   2. Penicillins ↑
   3. Sulfonamides ↑
B. Effect of Other Drugs on Activity of Antipyrine
   1. Alcohol ↑
   2. General anesthetics ↑
   3. Phenothiazines ↑
   4. Barbiturates ↓
   5. Sedatives and hypnotics ↓

References:

Goldstein, J. H.: Effects of drugs on cornea, conjunctiva, and lids. Int. Ophthalmol. Clin. *11*(2):13, 1971.
Hotz, F. C.: A case of antipyrin amaurosis induced by 130 grains taken in 48 hours. Arch. Ophthalmol. *35*:160, 1906.
Lucas, D. R., and Newhouse, J. P.: Action of metabolic poisons on the isolated retina. Br. J. Ophthalmol. *43*:147, 1959.
Wade, A. (Ed.): Martindale: The Extra Pharmacopoeia. 27th Ed., London, Pharmaceutical Press, 1977, pp. 206–207.
Walsh, F. B., and Hoyt, W. F.: Clinical Neuro-Ophthalmology. 3rd Ed., Baltimore, Williams & Wilkins, Vol. III, 1969, p. 2593.

Generic Name: 1. Aspirin (Acetylsalicylic Acid); 2. Sodium Salicylate

Proprietary Name: 1. Acetophen (Canad.), Acetylin (Germ.), Acetyl-Sal (Canad.), Albyl-Selters (Swed.), Ancasal (Canad.), Apernyl (Swed.), Aquaprin (S. Afr.), A.S.A., Asadrine (Canad.), Asagran (G.B.), Aspasol (S. Afr.), Aspegic (Fr.), Aspergum, Aspirisucre (Fr.), Aspirjen, Aspisol (Austral.), Babiprin (Ire.), Bamyl (Swed.), Bayer Aspirin, Bi-prin (Austral.), Breoprin (G.B.), Buffinol, Caprin (G.B.), Cetasal (Canad.), Chu-Pax (G.B.), Claragine (Fr.), Clariprin (Austral.), Codral Junior (Austral.), Colfarit (Germ.), Dispril (Swed.), Ecotrin, Elsprin (Austral.), Entericin, Entrophen (Canad.), Extren, Godamed (Germ.), Infatabs A (Austral.), Instantine (Swed.), Ivepirine (Fr.), Juvepirine (Fr.), Levius (G.B.), Measurin, Monasalyl (Canad.), Neo-pirine-25 (Canad.), Nova-Phase (Canad.), Novasen (Canad.), Novo-sprin (Austral.), Nu-seals Aspirin (G.B.), Premaspin (Swed.), Prodol (Austral.), Provoprin-500 (Austral.), Rhonal (Canad., Fr.), Sal-Adult/Infant (Canad.), Seclopyrine (Fr.), Solcetas (Austral.), Solusal (Austral.), St. Joseph Aspirin, Supasa (Canad.), Tasprin-Sol (G.B.), Triaphen-10 (Canad.), Zorprin; 2. Alysine, Ancosal (Austral.), Ensalate (Austral.), Enterosalicyl (Fr., Swed.), Enterosalyl (G.B.), Idocyl (Swed.), Klev (Canad.), Rhumax (Austral.), Uracel

Primary Use: These salicylates are used as antipyretics, analgesics, and in the management of gout, acute rheumatic fever, rheumatoid arthritis, subacute thyroiditis, and renal calculi.

Ocular Side Effects:

A. Systemic Administration
1. Eyelids or conjunctiva
   a. Allergic reactions
   b. Conjunctivitis — nonspecific
   c. Edema
   d. Angioneurotic edema
   e. Urticaria
   f. Stevens-Johnson syndrome
2. Decreased vision
3. Problems with color vision
   a. Dyschromatopsia, red-green defect
   b. Objects have yellow tinge
4. Paralysis of extraocular muscles
5. Diplopia
6. Visual hallucinations
7. Myopia
8. Decreased intraocular pressure
9. Nystagmus
10. Pupils
    a. Mydriasis
    b. Decreased or absent reaction to light

11. Visual fields
    a. Scotomas
    b. Constriction
    c. Hemianopsia
12. Scintillating scotomas
13. Papilledema
14. Retinal edema
15. Subconjunctival or retinal hemorrhages — increased rebleeds
16. Toxic amblyopia
17. Keratitis
18. Hyphema (traumatic) — increased rebleeds
19. Optic atrophy
20. Ocular teratogenic effects (?)
    a. Anophthalmos
    b. Microphthalmos
    c. Exophthalmos
21. Loss of eyelashes or eyebrows (?)

B. Inadvertent Ocular Exposure
    1. Conjunctival edema or scarring
    2. Keratitis with or without ulceration

Clinical Significance: While ocular side effects due to salicylates are quite rare, significant adverse effects may occur at therapeutic dosage levels. This is probably due to a drug idiosyncrasy or hypersensitivity. Adverse drug-induced ocular reactions are primarily due to acid-base imbalances, metabolic disturbances, toxic encephalopathy, hemorrhagic phenomena, or hypersensitivity reactions. Sodium salicylate appears to have more toxic ocular reactions than aspirin; however, aspirin has a much higher percentage of hypersensitivity reactions. Toxic responses are more frequent and more severe in infants and children. Neuroophthalmologic defects have been primarily seen with sodium salicylate and are much less frequent with aspirin. A transitory blindness which lasts hours, days, or even weeks may occur. Optic atrophy with permanent blindness has, however, also been reported. In a retrospective study of traumatic hyphemas, the incidence of rebleeding was significantly increased with aspirin administration. Recent data suggest that therapeutic doses of aspirin do not cause fetal damage in humans. Topical ocular aspirin powder has been used for self-mutilation and has caused various degrees of conjunctival and corneal damage. In patients taking high doses of aspirin for rheumatoid or osteoarthritis, acetazolamide may increase the nonionized salicylates in the blood stream. The nonionized salicylates penetrate the central nervous system more easily than the ionized form. Therefore, some carbonic anhydrase inhibitors may increase the risk of salicylate intoxication with its resultant adverse drug effects.

Interactions with Other Drugs:

A. Effect of Salicylates on Activity of Other Drugs
1. Analgesics ↑
2. Penicillins ↑
3. Phenothiazines ↑
4. Phenylbutazone ↓

B. Effect of Other Drugs on Activity of Salicylates
1. Analgesics ↑
2. Carbonic anhydrase inhibitors ↑
3. Penicillins ↑
4. Barbiturates ↓

References:

Copenhaver, R. M.: A report of an unusual self-inflicted eye injury. Arch. Ophthalmol. 63:266, 1960.

Crawford, J. S., Lewandowski, R. L., and Chan, W.: The effect of aspirin on rebleeding in traumatic hyphema. Am. J. Ophthalmol. 80:543, 1975.

Dukes, M. N. G. (Ed.): Meyler's Side Effects of Drugs. Amsterdam, Excerpta Medica, Vol. IX, 1980, pp. 126–133.

Gilman, A. G., Goodman, L. S., and Gilman, A. (Eds.): The Pharmacological Basis of Therapeutics. 6th Ed., New York, Macmillan, 1980, pp. 688–698.

Goldstein, J. H.: Effects of drugs on cornea, conjunctiva, and lids. Int. Ophthalmol. Clin. 11(2):13, 1971.

Gorn, R. A.: The detrimental effect of aspirin on hyphema rebleed. Ann. Ophthalmol. 11:351, 1979.

Kageler, W. V., Moake, J. L., and Garcia, C. A.: Spontaneous hyphema associated with ingestion of aspirin and ethanol. Am. J. Ophthalmol. 82:631, 1976.

Ros, A. M., Juhlin, L. and Michaëlsson, G.: A follow-up study of patients with recurrent urticaria and hypersensitivity to aspirin, benzoates and azo dyes. Br. J. Dermatol. 95:19, 1976.

Slone, D., et al.: Aspirin and congenital malformations. Lancet 1:1373, 1976.

Watson, P. G., and Hazleman, B. L.: The Sclera and Systemic Disorders. Philadelphia, W. B. Saunders, 1976, pp. 384–386.

Generic Name: 1. Codeine; 2. Propoxyphene

Proprietary Name: 1. Codicept (Germ.), Codlin (Austral.), Paveral (Canad.), Tricodein (Germ.); 2. Algaphan (Austral.), Antalvic (Fr.), Darvon, Depronal SA (G.B.), Develin (Germ.), Dextropropoxyphene (G.B.), Dolene, Dolocap, Dolotard (Swed.), Doloxene, Erantin (Germ.), Harmar, Mardon, Pro-65 (Canad.), Propox 65, Propoxychel, Proxagesic, Ropoxy, Scrip-Dyne, SK-65, S-Pain-65

Primary Use: These mild analgesics are used for the relief of mild to moderate pain. Codeine is also used as an antitussive agent.

Ocular Side Effects:

A. Systemic Administration
   1. Miosis
   2. Decreased vision
   3. Myopia (codeine)
   4. Eyelids — exfoliative dermatitis

Clinical Significance: Neither codeine nor propoxyphene causes significant ocular side effects. While codeine frequently may produce miosis, proproxyphene does so only in overdose situations. Visual disturbances are usually insignificant. Codeine has been reported to cause transient myopia.

Interactions with Other Drugs:

A. Effect of Codeine or Propoxyphene on Activity of Other Drugs
   1. Alcohol ↑
   2. Barbiturates ↑
   3. Monoamine oxidase inhibitors ↑
   4. Phenothiazines ↑
   5. Sedatives and hypnotics ↑
   6. Tricyclic antidepressants ↑
B. Effect of Other Drugs on Activity of Codeine or Propoxyphene
   1. Alcohol ↑
   2. Anticholinesterases ↑
   3. Chloramphenicol ↑ (codeine)
   4. Monoamine oxidase inhibitors ↑
   5. Phenothiazines ↑
   6. Tricyclic antidepressants ↑

References:

AMA Drug Evaluations. 4th Ed., New York, John Wiley & Sons, 1980, pp. 61–62, 69–70.
Baron, A., et al.: Myopie spasmodique. Bull. Soc. Ophtalmol. Fr. 67:716, 1967.
Grant, W. M.: Toxicology of the Eye. 2nd Ed., Springfield, Charles C Thomas, 1974, p. 304.
Hermans, G.: Analgesiques majeurs. Bull. Soc. Belge Ophtalmol. 160:116, 1972.
Physicians' Desk Reference. 35th Ed., Oradell, N.J., Medical Economics Co., 1981, p. 1050.

Generic Name: Mefenamic Acid

Proprietary Name: Coslan (Span.), Parkemed (Germ.), Ponstan, Ponstel, Ponstyl (Fr.)

Primary Use: This anthranilic acid derivative is used for the relief of mild to moderate pain.

Ocular Side Effects:

A. Systemic Administration
 1. Decreased vision
 2. Problems with color vision — dyschromatopsia
 3. Nonspecific ocular irritation
 4. Subconjunctival or retinal hemorrhages secondary to drug-induced anemia

Clinical Significance: Ocular side effects due to mefenamic acid are rare, transitory, and seldom require discontinuation of the use of the drug.

Interactions with Other Drugs:

A. Effect of Mefenamic Acid on Activity of Other Drugs
 1. Corticosteroids ↑
 2. Phenylbutazone ↑
 3. Salicylates ↑

References:

AMA Drug Evaluations. 4th Ed., New York, John Wiley & Sons, 1980, pp. 78–79.
American Hospital Formulary Service. Washington, D. C., American Society of Hospital Pharmacists, Vol. 1, 28:08, 1967.
Physicians' Desk Reference. 35th Ed., Oradell, N. J., Medical Economics Co., 1981, p. 1382.

Class: Narcotic Antagonists

Generic Name: 1. Levallorphan; 2. Nalorphine; 3. Naloxone

Proprietary Name: 1. Lorfan; 2. Lethidrone (G.B.), Nalline; 3. Narcan

Primary Use: These narcotic antagonists are used primarily in the management of narcotic-induced respiratory depression.

Ocular Side Effects:

A. Systemic Administration
 1. Pupils
  a. Mydriasis — if a prior narcotic has been given
  b. Miosis

2. Decreased vision
3. Visual hallucinations
4. Pseudoptosis
5. Lacrimation — withdrawal states
B. Local Ophthalmic Use or Exposure — nalorphine
   1. Miosis

Clinical Significance: Although ocular side effects due to these narcotic antagonists are common, they have little clinical significance other than as a screening test to discover narcotic users. These narcotic antagonists produce either a miosis or no effect on the pupils when administered to nonaddicts; however, in addicts, they cause mydriasis. Vivid visual hallucinations are seen both as an adverse ocular reaction and as a withdrawal symptom. Naloxone has only been reported to cause pupillary changes.

Interactions with Other Drugs:

A. Effect of Narcotic Antagonists on Activity of Other Drugs
   1. Alcohol ↑
   2. Barbiturates ↑
   3. Sedatives and hypnotics ↑
   4. Analgesics ↓

References:

AMA Drug Evaluations. 4th Ed., New York, John Wiley & Sons, 1980, pp. 1441–1443.
Gilman, A. G., Goodman, L. S., and Gilman, A. (Eds.): The Pharmacological Basis of Therapeutics. 6th Ed., New York, Macmillan, 1980, pp. 521–525.
Grant, W. M.: Toxicology of the Eye. 2nd Ed., Springfield, Charles C Thomas, 1974, pp. 629, 732–733.
Jasinski, D. R., Martin, W. R., and Haertzen, C.: The human pharmacology and abuse potential of N-Allylnoroxymorphone. (Naloxone). J. Pharmacol. Exp. Ther. *157:* 420, 1967.
Martin, W. R.: Opioid antagonists. Pharmacol. Rev. *19:*463, 1967.

Class: Strong Analgesics

Generic Name: Diacetylmorphine

Proprietary Name: Diamorphine, Heroin

Street Name: Boy, Brother, Caballo, Ca-ca, Crap, H, Harry, Horse, Junk, Poison, Scag, Schmeck, Shit, Smack, Stuff, Tecata

Primary Use: This potent narcotic analgesic is administered pre- and post-operatively and in the terminal stages of cancer for the relief of severe pain.

Ocular Side Effects:

A. Systemic Administration
   1. Pupils
      a. Miosis
      b. Absence of reaction to light
      c. Mydriasis — withdrawal states
      d. Anisocoria — withdrawal states
   2. Decreased accommodation
   3. Nonspecific ocular irritation
      a. Lacrimation
      b. Photophobia
   4. Eyelids or conjunctiva
      a. Hyperemia
      b. Erythema
      c. Edema
      d. Urticaria
   5. Horner's syndrome
      a. Ptosis
      b. Increased sensitivity to sympathetic agents
   6. Endophthalmitis (?)

Clinical Significance: This potent narcotic seldom causes significant ocular side effects. However, heroin addiction has been associated with bacterial and fungal endophthalmitis, probably due to the method of administration and impurities on an embolus basis. If undiagnosed and incompletely treated, these indirect drug-related entities can result in permanent loss of vision. Horner's syndrome has been reported in chronic addicts. Withdrawal of diacetylmorphine in the addict may cause excessive tearing, irregular pupils, and decreased accommodation.

Interactions with Other Drugs:

A. Effect of Other Drugs on Activity of Diacetylmorphine
   1. Analgesics ↓
B. Synergistic Activity
   1. Barbiturates
   2. Local anesthetics

References:

Cosgriff, T. M.: Anisocoria in heroin withdrawal. Arch. Neurol. 29:200, 1973.
Crandall, D. C., and Leopold, I. H.: The influence of systemic drugs on tear constituents. Ophthalmology 86:115, 1979.

Hawkins, K. A., Bruckstein, A. H., and Guthrie, T. C.: Percutaneous heroin injection causing heroin syndrome. JAMA 237:1963, 1977.

Rathod, N. H., De Alarcón, R., and Thomson, I. G.: Signs of heroin usage detected by drug users and their parents. Lancet 2:1411, 1967.

Vastine, D. W., et al.: Endogenous *Candida* endophthalmitis associated with heroin use. Arch. Ophthalmol. 94:1805, 1976.

Generic Name: 1. Hydromorphone; 2. Oxymorphone

Proprietary Name: 1. Dilaudid; 2. Numorphan

Primary Use: These hydrogenated ketones of morphine are used for the relief of moderate to severe pain.

Ocular Side Effects:

  A. Systemic Administration
    1. Decreased vision
    2. Decreased accommodation
    3. Pupils
      a. Miosis
      b. Pinpoint pupils — toxic states
      c. Mydriasis — hypoxic states
    4. Eyelids or conjunctiva
      a. Allergic reactions
      b. Urticaria

Clinical Significance: Adverse ocular effects due to these drugs, although not uncommon, are rarely significant. All ocular side effects are reversible and transitory. Difficulty in focusing is probably the most frequent complaint.

Interactions with Other Drugs:

  A. Effect of Morphine Derivatives on Activity of Other Drugs
    1. Alcohol ↑
    2. Monoamine oxidase inhibitors ↑
    3. Phenothiazines ↑
    4. Sedatives and hypnotics ↑
    5. Tricyclic antidepressants ↑
  B. Effect of Other Drugs on Activity of Morphine Derivatives
    1. Monoamine oxidase inhibitors ↑
    2. Phenothiazines ↑
    3. Tricyclic antidepressants ↑

References:

AMA Drug Evaluations. 4th Ed., New York, John Wiley & Sons, 1980, pp. 62–64.
Gilman, A. G., Goodman, L. S., and Gilman, A. (Eds.): The Pharmacological Basis of Therapeutics. 6th Ed., New York, Macmillan, 1980, pp. 495–511.
Physicians' Desk Reference. 35th Ed., Oradell, N. J., Medical Economics Co., 1981, pp. 882, 966.
Wade, A. (Ed.): Martindale: The Extra Pharmacopoeia. 27th Ed., London, Pharmaceutical Press, 1977, pp. 966, 976.

Generic Name: Meperidine (Pethidine)

Proprietary Name: Demerol, Dolantin (Germ.), Dolosal (Fr.), Pethoid (Austral.), Phytadon (Canad.), Suppolosal (Fr.)

Primary Use: This phenylpiperidine narcotic analgesic is used for the relief of pain, as a preoperative medication, and to supplement surgical anesthesia.

Ocular Side Effects:

A. Systemic Administration
   1. Pupils
      a. Mydriasis
      b. Miosis
      c. Decreased reaction to light
   2. Decreased intraocular pressure
   3. Decreased vision
   4. Corneal deposits (?)
B. Inadvertent Ocular Exposure
   1. Blepharitis
   2. Conjunctivitis — nonspecific

Clinical Significance: None of the ocular side effects due to meperidine are of major importance, and all are transitory. Miosis is uncommon at therapeutic dosages and seldom significant. Mydriasis and decreased pupillary light reflexes are only seen in acute toxicity or in long-term addicts. Ocular side effects, such as blepharitis or conjunctivitis, have been seen secondary to meperidine dust.

Interactions with Other Drugs:

A. Effect of Meperidine on Activity of Other Drugs
   1. Anticholinergics ↑
   2. Anticholinesterases ↓

B. Effect of Other Drugs on Activity of Meperidine
1. Alcohol ↑
2. Analgesics ↑
3. Antacids ↑
4. Anticholinesterases ↑
5. General anesthetics ↑
6. Monoamine oxidase inhibitors ↑
7. Phenothiazines ↑
8. Sedatives and hypnotics ↑
9. Tricyclic antidepressants ↑
10. Barbiturates ↓

References:

Bron, A. J.: Vortex patterns of the corneal epithelium. Trans. Ophthalmol. Soc. U.K. 93:455, 1973.

Grant, W. M.: Toxicology of the Eye. 2nd Ed., Springfield, Charles C Thomas, 1974, pp. 800–801.

Hovland, K. R.: Effects of drugs on aqueous humor dynamics. Int. Ophthalmol. Clin. 11(2):99, 1971.

Lubeck, M. J.: Effects of drugs on ocular muscles. Int. Ophthalmol. Clin. 11(2):35, 1971.

Minton, J.: Occupational Eye Diseases and Injuries. New York, Grune, 1949.

Walsh, F. B., and Hoyt, W. F.: Clinical Neuro-Ophthalmology. 3rd Ed., Baltimore, Williams & Wilkins, Vol. III, 1969, pp. 2664–2665.

Generic Name: Methadone

Proprietary Name: Adanon, Dolophine, Physeptone (G.B.), Polamidon (Germ.), Westadone

Primary Use: This synthetic analgesic is useful in the treatment of chronic painful conditions and in the detoxification treatment of patients dependent on heroin or other morphine-like agents.

Ocular Side Effects:

A. Systemic Administration
1. Decreased vision
2. Pupils
   a. Miosis — toxic states
   b. Mydriasis — withdrawal states
3. Eyelids — urticaria
4. Talc retinopathy
5. Cortical blindness (?) — hypoxic states

Clinical Significance: Methadone seldom causes significant ocular side effects. Although miosis is uncommon, but may occur at therapeutic dosages, it may be so severe in toxic states as to give "pinpoint" pupils. Talc emboli, appearing as small white glistening dots in the macular area, have been reported in addicts who intravenously inject oral medications which contain talc as a filler. A case of cortical blindness, apparently secondary to anoxia, has been reported in a child who experienced severe respiratory depression.

References:

Murphy, S. B., Jackson, W. B., and Pare, J.A.P.: Talc retinopathy. Can. J. Ophthalmol. *13*:152, 1978.

Physicians' Desk Reference. 35th Ed., Oradell, N.J., Medical Economics Co., 1980, p. 1081.

Ratcliffe, S. C.: Methadone poisoning in a child. Br. Med. J. *1*:1069, 1963.

Wade, A. (Ed.): Martindale: The Extra Pharmacopoeia. 27th Ed., London, Pharmaceutical Press, 1977, pp. 967–969.

Generic Name: 1. Morphine; 2. Opium

Proprietary Name: 1. Duna-Phorine (Fr.), Duromorph (G.B.); 2. Pantopon

Primary Use: These opioids are used for the relief of severe pain. Morphine is the alkaloid that gives opium its analgesic action.

Ocular Side Effects:

A. Systemic Administration
   1. Pupils
      a. Miosis
      b. Pinpoint pupils — toxic states
      c. Mydriasis — withdrawal or extreme toxic states
      d. Irregularity — withdrawal states
   2. Decreased vision
   3. Decreased accommodation
   4. Decreased convergence
   5. Decreased intraocular pressure
   6. Myopia
   7. Lacrimation
      a. Increased — withdrawal states
      b. Decreased
   8. Accommodative spasm
   9. Diplopia

      10. Eyelids or conjunctiva
          a. Allergic reactions
          b. Conjunctivitis — nonspecific
          c. Urticaria
      11. Ptosis (opium)
      12. Keratoconjunctivitis
      13. Problems with color vision — dsychromatopsia, red-green defect (?)
      14. Visual fields (?)
          a. Scotomas
          b. Constriction
          c. Hemianopsia
   B. Local Ophthalmic Use or Exposure — Morphine
      1. Miosis
      2. Increased intraocular pressure (?)

Clinical Significance: These narcotics seldom cause significant ocular side effects, and all proven drug-induced toxic effects are transitory. Miosis is the most frequent ocular side effect and is seen routinely even at usual dosage levels. Ocular side effects reported in long-term addicts (#13–14 in the preceding list) are probably due to vitamin deficiency rather than to the drug itself. Withdrawal of morphine or opium in the addict may cause excessive tearing, irregular pupils, decreased accommodation, and diplopia.

Interactions with Other Drugs:

   A. Effect of Opioids on Activity of Other Drugs
      1. Alcohol ↑
      2. Analgesics ↑
      3. Antihistamines ↑
      4. Barbiturates ↑
      5. General anesthetics ↑
      6. Phenothiazines ↑
      7. Sedatives and hypnotics ↑
      8. Tricyclic antidepressants ↑
   B. Effect of Other Drugs on Activity of Opioids
      1. Anticholinesterases ↑ (morphine)
      2. Monoamine oxidase inhibitors ↑
      3. Phenothiazines ↑ (morphine)
      4. Tricyclic antidepressants ↑ (opium)
      5. Anticholinergics ↓ (morphine)
   C. Synergistic Activity
      1. Adrenergic blockers
      2. Alcohol
      3. Anticholinergics

References:

Crandall, D. C., and Leopold, I. H.: The influence of systemic drugs on tear con-
  stituents. Ophthalmology 86:115, 1979.
Cross, D. A., and Krupin, T.: Implications of the effects of general anesthesia on
  basal tear production. Anesth. Analg. 56:35, 1977.
Duncalf, D.: Anesthesia and intraocular pressure. Bull. N.Y. Acad. Med. 51:374, 1975.
Goldstein, J. H.: Effects of drugs on cornea, conjunctiva, and lids. Int. Ophthalmol.
  Clin. 11(2):13, 1971.
Grant, W. M.: Toxicology of the Eye. 2nd Ed., Springfield, Charles C Thomas, 1974,
  pp. 720–722, 767–768.
Hovland, K. R.: Effects of drugs on aqueous humor dynamics. Int. Ophthalmol. Clin.
  11(2):99, 1971.
Walsh, F. B., and Hoyt, W. F.: Clinical Neuro-Ophthalmology. 3rd Ed., Baltimore,
  Williams & Wilkins, Vol. III, 1969, pp. 2707–2709.

Generic Name: Pentazocine

Proprietary Name: Fortal (Belg., Fr.), Fortalgesic (Swed., Switz.), For-
tral (G.B.), Fortralin (Scand.), Talwin

Primary Use: This benzomorphan narcotic analgesic is used for the relief
of pain, as a preoperative medication, and to supplement surgical anesthesia.

Ocular Side Effects:

  A. Systemic Administration
     1. Miosis
     2. Decreased vision
     3. Visual hallucinations
     4. Nystagmus
     5. Diplopia
     6. Lacrimation — abrupt withdrawal states
     7. Decreased accommodation

Clinical Significance: Ocular side effects due to pentazocine are usually
insignificant and reversible. Miosis is the most frequent and is seen
routinely even at suggested dosage levels. Although visual complaints
are seldom of major consequence, diplopia may be incapacitating. Vivid
visual hallucinations, some of which are threatening, have been reported with this drug; once pentazocine is discontinued, the hallucinations cease. All other ocular side effects are rare.

Interactions with Other Drugs:

  A. Effect of Pentazocine on Activity of Other Drugs
     1. Analgesics ↓

References:

AMA Drug Evaluations. 4th Ed., New York, John Wiley & Sons, 1980, pp. 70–72.

American Hospital Formulary Service. Washington, D.C., American Society of Hospital Pharmacists, Vol. 1, *28*:08, 1969.

Jones, K. D.: A novel side-effect of pentazocine. Br. J. Clin. Pract. *29*:218, 1975.

Martin, W. R.: Opioid antagonists. Pharmacol. Rev. *19*:463, 1967.

Physicians' Desk Reference. 35th Ed., Oradell, N.J., Medical Economics Co., 1981, p. 1908.

IV

Agents Used in Anesthesia

Class: Adjuncts to Anesthesia

Generic Name: Hyaluronidase

Proprietary Name: Alidase, Hyalas (Swed.), Hyalase (G.B.), Hyason (Belg.), Jalovis (Ital.), Jaluran (Ital.), Kinetin (Germ.), Permease (Aust.), Seravase (S. Afr.), Wydase

Primary Use: This enzyme is added to local anesthetic solutions to enhance the effect of infiltrative anesthesia. It has also been used in paraphimosis, lepromatous nerve reactions, and in the management of carpal tunnel syndrome.

Ocular Side Effects:

A. Local Ophthalmic Use or Exposure — Subconjunctival or Retrobulbar Injection
  1. Eyelids or conjunctiva
     a. Allergic reactions
     b. Conjunctivitis — follicular
  2. Irritation
  3. Myopia
  4. Astigmatism
  5. Decreases the duration of local anesthetic
  6. Increases the frequency of local anesthetic reactions
  7. Increases cystoid macular edema

Clinical Significance: Adverse ocular reactions due to periocular injection of hyaluronidase are either quite rare or masked by the postoperative surgical reactions. Subconjunctival injection of this drug causes myopia and astigmatism secondary to changes in the corneal curvature. This is a transitory phenomenon with recovery occurring within a few weeks. Irritative or allergic reactions are often stated to be due to impurities in the preparation since pure hyaluronidase is felt to be nontoxic. Hyaluronidase decreases the duration of action of local anesthetic drugs by allowing them to diffuse out of the tissue more rapidly. Side effects of the local anesthetic are probably more frequent when it is used with hyaluronidase, since its absorption rate is increased. Of marked clinical importance is a prospective double blind study which suggests cystoid macular edema is possibly caused by the use of hyaluronidase. To date, these data are not completely accepted, and the mechanism of this drug causing cystoid macular edema is unknown. If the patient is on heparin or if there is associated bleeding in the area of injection, the effect of hyaluronidase may be decreased since both human serum and heparin inhibit this agent.

Interactions with Other Drugs:

A. Effect of Hyaluronidase on Activity of Other Drugs
  1. Parenteral medications ↑
  2. Salicylates ↓
B. Effect of Other Drugs on Activity of Hyaluronidase
  1. Heparin ↓

References:

Barton, D.: Side reactions to drugs in anesthesia. Int. Ophthalmol. Clin. *11*(2):185, 1971.

Havener, W. H.: Ocular Pharmacology. 4th Ed., St. Louis, C. V. Mosby, 1978, pp. 81–85.

Roper, D. L., and Nisbet, R. M.: Effect of hyaluronidase on the incidence of cystoid macular edema. Ann. Ophthalmol. *10*:1673, 1978.

Salkie, M. L.: Inhibition of Wydase by human serum. Can. Med. Assoc. J. *121*:845, 1979.

Stanworth, A.: The ocular effects of local corticosteroids and hyaluronidase. In Paterson, G., Miller, S. J. H., and Paterson, G. D. (Eds.): Drug Mechanisms in Glaucoma. Boston, Little, Brown and Co., 1966, pp. 231–248.

Treister, G., Romano, A., and Stein, R.: The effect of subconjunctivally injected hyaluronidase on corneal refraction. Arch. Ophthalmol. *81*:645, 1969.

Wade, A. (Ed.): Martindale: The Extra Pharmacopoeia. 27th Ed., London, Pharmaceutical Press, 1977, pp. 578–579.

Generic Name: 1. Methscopolamine; 2. Scopolamine (Hyoscine)

Proprietary Name: *Systemic:* 1. Holopane (S. Afr.), Holopon (Germ.), Pamine, Scoline, Scordin (Jap.); 2. Scopolamina Lux (Ital.), Scopos (Fr.) *Ophthalmic:* 2. Isopto Hyoscine

Primary Use: *Systemic:* These quaternary ammonium derivatives are used as preanesthetic medications to decrease bronchial secretions, as sedatives and antispasmodics, and in the prophylaxis of motion sickness. *Ophthalmic:* Scopolamine, a topical parasympatholytic mydriatic and cycloplegic agent, is used in refractions, in accommodative spasm, and in the management of uveitis.

Ocular Side Effects:

A. Systemic Administration
1. Mydriasis — may precipitate narrow-angle glaucoma
2. Decrease or paralysis of accommodation
3. Decreased vision
4. Decreased lacrimation
5. Visual hallucinations
B. Local Ophthalmic Use or Exposure
1. Decreased vision
2. Mydriasis — may precipitate narrow-angle glaucoma
3. Decrease or paralysis of accommodation
4. Eyelids or conjunctiva
   a. Allergic reactions
   b. Conjunctivitis — follicular
5. Irritation
   a. Hyperemia
   b. Photophobia
   c. Edema
6. Increased intraocular pressure
7. Decreased lacrimation
8. Visual hallucinations

Clinical Significance: Although ocular side effects from systemic administration of these drugs are common, they are reversible and seldom serious. Occasionally, patients on scopolamine have aggravated keratoconjunctivitis sicca problems due to decreased tear production. This is the only autonomic drug which has been reported to cause decreased tear lysozymes, of which the importance to the clinician is unknown to date. Mydriasis and paralysis of accommodation are intended ocular effects resulting from topical application of scopolamine. This drug may elevate the intraocular pressure in open-angle glaucoma and can precipitate narrow-angle glaucoma. Allergic reactions are not uncommon after topical ocular application.

Interactions with Other Drugs:

A. Effect of Quaternary Ammonium Derivatives on Activity of Other Drugs
1. Phenothiazines ↑

B. Effect of Other Drugs on Activity of Quaternary Ammonium Derivatives
   1. Antihistamines ↑
   2. Monoamine oxidase inhibitors ↑
   3. Phenothiazines ↑
   4. Tricyclic antidepressants ↑
   5. Adrenergic blockers ↓
C. Synergistic Activity
   1. Analgesics

References:

Crandall, D. C., and Leopold, I. H.: The influence of systemic drugs on tear constituents. Ophthalmology 86:115, 1979.

Erickson, O. F.: Drug influences on lacrimal lysozyme production. Stanford Med. Bull. *18*:34, 1960.

Freund, M., and Merin, S.: Toxic effects of scopolamine eye drops, Am. J. Ophthalmol. 70:637, 1970.

Harris, L. S.: Cycloplegic-induced intraocular pressure elevations. Arch. Ophthalmol. 79:242, 1968.

Leopold, I. H., and Comroe, J. H., Jr.: Effect of intramuscular administration of morphine, atropine, scopolamine and neostigmine on the human eye. Arch. Ophthalmol. *40*:285, 1948.

Young, S. E., Ruiz, R. S., and Falletta, J.: Reversal of systemic toxic effects of scopolamine with physostigmine. Am. J. Ophthalmol. 72:1136, 1971.

Generic Name: 1. Metocurine Iodide; 2. Tubocurarine

Proprietary Name: 1. Auxoperan (Fr.), Diamethine, Metubine Iodide; 2. Tubarine

Primary Use: These neuromuscular blocking agents are used as adjuncts to anesthesia, primarily as skeletal muscle relaxants.

Ocular Side Effects:

A. Systemic Administration
   1. Decreased convergence
   2. Diplopia
   3. Nystagmus
   4. Paresis or paralysis of extraocular muscles
   5. Ptosis
   6. Decreased intraocular pressure — minimal

Clinical Significance: The extraocular muscles, especially the abductors, are selectively affected as the first signs of toxicity due to these curare agents. These drugs, unlike succinylcholine, do not cause a transitory elevation of intraocular pressure, so they are safe to use if the globe is perforated.

Interactions with Other Drugs:

A. Effect of Other Drugs on Activity of Neuromuscular Blocking Agents
  1. Antibiotics (apnea) ↑
     (Bacitracin, Colistin, Kanamycin, Neomycin, Polymyxin B, Streptomycin)
  2. Diuretics ↑
  3. Local anesthetics ↑
  4. Monoamine oxidase inhibitors ↑
  5. Anticholinesterases ↑↓
  6. Adrenergic blockers ↓
  7. Sympathomimetics ↓
B. Synergistic Activity
  1. General anesthetics

References:

Duke-Elder, S.: Systems of Ophthalmology. St. Louis, C. V. Mosby, Vol. XIV, Part 2, 1972, p. 1339.
Duncalf, D.: Anesthesia and intraocular pressure. Trans. Am. Acad. Ophthalmol. Otolaryngol. 79:562, 1975.
Gilman, A. G., Goodman, L. S., and Gilman, A. (Eds.): The Pharmacological Basis of Therapeutics. 6th Ed., New York, Macmillan, 1980, pp. 220–232.
Grant, W. M.: Toxicology of the Eye. 2nd Ed., Springfield, Charles C Thomas, 1974, p. 332.
Kornblueth, W., et al.: Influence of general anesthesia on intraocular pressure in man. Arch. Ophthalmol. 61:84, 1959.
Walsh, F. B., and Hoyt, W. F.: Clinical Neuro-Ophthalmology. 3rd Ed., Baltimore, Williams & Wilkins, Vol. III, 1969, pp. 2656–2657.

Generic Name: Succinylcholine (Suxamethonium)

Proprietary Name: Anectine, Brevidil E/M (G.B.), Celocurin-Klorid (Swed.), Lysthenon (Germ.), Pantolax (Germ.), Quelicin, Scoline (Austral., Canad., S. Afr.), Succinyl (Germ.), Sucostrin, Sux-Cert

Primary Use: This neuromuscular blocking agent is used as an adjunct to general anesthesia to obtain relaxation of skeletal muscles.

Ocular Side Effects:

A. Systemic Administration
  1. Extraocular muscles

        a. Eyelid retraction
        b. Enophthalmos
        c. Globe rotates inferiorly
        d. Paralysis
        e. Adduction of abducted eyes
        f. Alters forced duction tests
    2. Intraocular pressure
        a. Increased — initial
        b. Decreased
    3. Ptosis
    4. Diplopia
    5. Eyelids or conjunctiva
        a. Allergic reactions
        b. Erythema
        c. Edema

Clinical Significance: All ocular side effects due to succinylcholine are transitory; however, some have major clinical importance. A transient contraction of extraocular muscles may cause intraocular pressure elevations within 1 minute after succinylcholine is given from 5 to 15 mm Hg for as long as 1 to 4 minutes. While this short-term elevation of intraocular pressure has little or no effect in the normal or glaucomatous eye, it has the potential to cause expulsion of the intraocular contents in a surgically opened or perforated globe. A slight decrease in intraocular pressure occurs in normal or glaucomatous eyes after this initial increase. Extraocular muscle contraction induced by succinylcholine may cause lid retraction or an enophthalmos, which may cause the surgeon to misjudge the amount of resection needed in ptosis procedures. Eyelid retraction may be due to a direct action on Müller's muscle. Both eyelid retraction and enophthalmos seldom last for over 5 minutes after drug administration. Succinylcholine may cause abnormal forced duction tests up to 20 minutes after the drug is administered. In anesthetized patients, succinylcholine may cause abduction-deviated eyes to return to their normal conscious position. Also, prior suggestions that small subparalytic doses of the drug given before the standard dose would lessen the increase in intraocular pressure were not found to be true.

Interactions with Other Drugs:

A. Effect of Other Drugs on Activity of Succinylcholine
    1. Antibiotics ↑
       (Bacitracin, Colistin, Kanamycin, Neomycin, Polymyxin B, Streptomycin)

2. Anticholinesterases ↑
3. EDTA ↑
4. General anesthetics ↑
5. Local anesthetics ↑
6. Phenothiazines ↑

References:

France, N. K., et al.: Succinylcholine alteration of the forced duction test. Ophthalmology 87:1282, 1980.
Hovland, K. R.: Effects of drugs on aqueous humor dynamics. Int. Ophthalmol. Clin. 11(2):99, 1971.
Katz, R. L., Eakins, K. E., and Lord, C. O.: The effects of hexafluorenium in preventing the increase in intraocular pressure produced by succinylcholine. Anesthesiology 29:70, 1968.
Lubeck, M. J.: Effects of drugs on ocular muscles. Int. Ophthalmol. Clin. 11(2):35, 1971.
Macri, F. J., and Grimes, P. A.: The effects of succinylcholine on the extraocular striate muscles and on the intraocular pressure. Am. J. Ophthalmol. 44:221, 1957.
Meyers, E. F., Singer, P., and Otto, A.: A controlled study of the effect of succinylcholine self-taming on intraocular pressure. Anesthesiology 53:72, 1980.
Mindel, J. S., et al.: Succinylcholine-induced return of the eyes to the basic deviation. Ophthalmology 87:1288, 1980.
Taylor, T. H., Mulcahy, M., and Nightingale, D. A.: Suxamethonium chloride in intraocular surgery. Br. J. Anaesthesiol. 40:113, 1968.

Class: General Anesthetics

Generic Name: Chloroform (Anesthetic Chloroform)

Proprietary Name: Chloroform

Primary Use: This potent inhalation anesthetic, analgesic, and muscle relaxant is used in obstetrical anesthesia. It is also used as a solvent.

Ocular Side Effects:

A. Systemic Administration
    1. Pupils — dependent on plane of anesthesia
        a. Mydriasis — reactive to light (initial)
        b. Miosis — reactive to light (deep level of anesthesia)
        c. Mydriasis — nonreactive to light (coma)
    2. Strabismus — convergent or divergent
    3. Nystagmus
    4. Decreased intraocular pressure

5. Decreased vision
6. Cortical blindness (?)
B. Inadvertent Ocular Exposure
   1. Irritation
      a. Hyperemia
      b. Ocular pain
      c. Edema
      d. Burning sensation
   2. Keratitis
   3. Corneal opacities
   4. Corneal ulceration

Clinical Significance: Ocular side effects due to chloroform are common, transitory, and seldom of clinical significance other than as an aid in judging the level of anesthesia. During early levels of anesthesia induction, the eyes are convergent; however, with deeper levels they become divergent. Nystagmus most often occurs during the recovery phase of anesthesia. Blindness has been reported secondary to central anoxic episodes.

Interactions with Other Drugs:

A. Effect of Chloroform on Activity of Other Drugs
   1. Adrenergic blockers ↑
   2. Analgesics ↑
   3. Antihistamines ↑
   4. Local anesthetics ↑
   5. Phenothiazines ↑
   6. Sympathomimetics ↑
B. Effect of Other Drugs on Activity of Chloroform
   1. Adrenergic blockers ↑
   2. Antihistamines ↑
   3. Monoamine oxidase inhibitors ↑
   4. Phenothiazines ↑

References:

Duke-Elder, S.: Systems of Ophthalmology. St. Louis, C. V. Mosby, Vol. XIV, Part 2, 1972, pp. 1040, 1164, 1337, 1340.
Gilman, A. G., Goodman, L. S., and Gilman, A. (Eds.): The Pharmacological Basis of Therapeutics. 6th Ed., New York, Macmillan, 1980, pp. 291–292.
Grant, W. M.: Toxicology of the Eye. 2nd Ed., Springfield, Charles C Thomas, 1974, pp. 135–136, 267–268.
Hovland, K. R.: Effects of drugs on aqueous humor dynamics. Int. Ophthalmol. Clin. 11(2):99, 1971.
Howie, T. O.: Eye signs of anaesthesia. Br. Med. J. 1:540, 1944.

Generic Name: Ether (Anesthetic Ether)

Proprietary Name: Ether

Primary Use: This potent inhalation anesthetic, analgesic, and muscle relaxant is used during induction of general anesthesia.

Ocular Side Effects:

A. Systemic Administration
    1. Pupils — dependent on plane of anesthesia
        a. Mydriasis — reactive to light (initial)
        b. Miosis — reactive to light (deep level of anesthesia)
        c. Mydriasis — nonreactive to light (coma)
    2. Extraocular muscles — dependent on plane of anesthesia
        a. Slow oscillations (initial)
        b. Eccentric placement of globes (initial)
        c. Concentric placement of globes (coma)
    3. Nonspecific ocular irritation
    4. Conjunctival hyperemia
    5. Lacrimal secretion — dependent on plane of anesthesia
        a. Increased (initial)
        b. Decreased (coma)
        c. Abolished (coma)
    6. Decreased intraocular pressure
    7. Decreased vision
    8. Cortical blindness (?)
B. Inadvertent Ocular Exposure
    1. Irritation
    2. Punctate keratitis
    3. Corneal opacities

Clinical Significance: Adverse ocular reactions due to ether are common, reversible, and seldom of clinical importance other than in the determination of the plane of anesthesia. Ether decreases intraocular pressure probably on the basis of increasing the facility of outflow. Ether vapor is an irritant to all mucous membranes, including the conjunctiva. Regardless of this irritant effect, ether vapor has, in addition, a vasodilator property. Permanent corneal opacities have been reported due to direct contact of liquid ether with the cornea. Blindness after induction of general anesthesia is probably due to asphyxic cerebral cortical damage.

Interactions with Other Drugs:

A. Effect of Ether on Activity of Other Drugs
   1. Adrenergic blockers ↑
   2. Analgesics ↑
   3. Local anesthetics ↑
   4. Phenothiazines ↑
   5. Sympathomimetics ↑
B. Effect of Other Drugs on Activity of Ether
   1. Adrenergic blockers ↑
   2. Antihistamines ↑
   3. Monoamine oxidase inhibitors ↑
   4. Phenothiazines ↑
   5. Anticholinergics ↓

References:

Gilman, A. G., Goodman, L. S., and Gilman, A. (Eds.): The Pharmacological Basis of Therapeutics. 6th Ed., New York, Macmillan, 1980, p. 291.
Grant, W. M.: Toxicology of the Eye. 2nd Ed., Springfield, Charles C Thomas, 1974, pp. 135–136, 464–465.
Kornblueth, W., et al.: Influence of general anesthesia on intraocular pressure in man. Arch. Ophthalmol. *61*:84, 1959.
Wade, A. (Ed.): Martindale: The Extra Pharmacopoeia. 27th Ed., London, Pharmaceutical Press, 1977, pp. 696–697.
Walsh, F. B., and Hoyt, W. F.: Clinical Neuro-Ophthalmology. 3rd Ed., Baltimore, Williams & Wilkins, Vol. III, 1969, pp. 2675–2676.

Generic Name: Ketamine

Proprietary Name: Ketaject, Ketalar, Ketanest (Germ.), Ketaset, Vetalar

Primary Use: This intravenous nonbarbiturate anesthetic is used for short-term diagnostic or surgical procedures. It may also be used as an adjunct to anesthesia.

Ocular Side Effects:

A. Systemic Administration
   1. Decreased vision
   2. Diplopia
   3. Horizontal nystagmus
   4. Postsurgical visually induced "emergence reactions"
   5. Extraocular muscles
      a. Abnormal conjugate deviations
      b. Random ocular movements
   6. Lacrimation

7

7. Visual hallucinations
8. Increased intraocular pressure — minimal (deep level of anesthesia)

Clinical Significance: All ocular side effects due to ketamine are transient and reversible. After ketamine anesthesia, diplopia may persist up to 30 minutes during the recovery phase and may be particularly bothersome to some patients. "Emergence reactions" occur in 12 percent of patients and may consist of various psychological manifestations varying from pleasant dream-like states to irrational behavior. The incidence of these reactions is increased by visual stimulation as the effect of the drug is wearing off. Three cases of transient blindness following ketamine anesthesia have recently been reported. The blindness lasts about half an hour with complete restoration of sight and no apparent sequelae. This is thought to be a toxic cerebral-induced phenomenon. The effect of ketamine on intraocular pressure is somewhat confusing with various authors obtaining different results. Probably, if intraocular pressure is taken before this drug increases muscle tone (just prior to anesthesia), there is an 8- to 10-minute period when intraocular pressure is not elevated. Ketamine is also being used by lay people for its psychedelic effect, and abusers may develop visual hallucinations, coarse horizontal nystagmus, abnormal conjugate eye deviations, and diplopia.

Interactions with Other Drugs:

A. Effect of Ketamine on Activity of Other Drugs
    1. Adrenergic blockers ↑
B. Effect of Other Drugs on Activity of Ketamine
    1. Monoamine oxidase inhibitors ↑
    2. Phenothiazines ↑

References:

Barton, D.: Side reactions of drugs in anesthesia. Int. Ophthalmol. Clin. *11*(2):185, 1971.
Corssen, G., and Hoy, J. E.: A new parenteral anesthetic. Cl–581: Its effect on intraocular pressure. J. Pediatr. Ophthalmol. *4*:20, 1967.
Fine, J., Weissman, J., and Finestone, S. C.: Side effects after ketamine anesthesia: Transient blindness. Anesth. Analg. *53*:72, 1974.
Harris, J. E., Letson, R. D., and Buckley, J. J.: The use of Cl–581. A new parenteral anesthetic in ophthalmic practice. Trans. Am. Ophthalmol. Soc. *66*:206, 1968.
Hovland, K. R.: Effects of drugs on aqueous humor dynamics. Int. Ophthalmol. Clin. *11*(2):99, 1971.
Ketamine. Med. Lett. Drugs Ther. *19*:58, 1977.
Marynen, L., and Libert: Ocular tonometry in the child under general anesthesia with IM ketamine. Acta Anaesthesiol. Belg. (Suppl.) *27*:29, 1976.
Shaffer, L. L.: Ketamine. JAMA *229*:763, 1974.

Generic Name: Methoxyflurane

Proprietary Name: Penthrane

Primary Use: This methyl ether is used as an inhalation anesthetic with good analgesic and muscle relaxant properties.

Ocular Side Effects:

A. Systemic Administration
1. Decreased intraocular pressure
2. "Flecked retinal syndrome"
3. Myasthenic neuromuscular blocking effect
    a. Paralysis of extraocular muscles
    b. Ptosis

Clinical Significance: Ocular side effects due to methoxyflurane are rare, but recently a unique adverse ocular reaction has been reported. If this drug is used for an extended period of time, especially in a patient with renal insufficiency, irreversible renal failure may occur. Oxalosis occurs for unknown reasons, with calcium oxalate crystal deposits throughout the body including the retinal pigmentary epithelium. The deposition of these crystals in the retina gives the clinical picture of an apparent "flecked retinal syndrome." This drug can also aggravate or unmask myasthenia gravis.

Interactions with Other Drugs:

A. Effect of Methoxyflurane on Activity of Other Drugs
1. Adrenergic blockers ↑
2. Analgesics ↑
3. Local anesthetics ↑
4. Phenothiazines ↑
5. Sympathomimetics ↑
B. Effect of Other Drugs on Activity of Methoxyflurane
1. Adrenergic blockers ↑
2. Antihistamines ↑
3. Barbiturates ↑
4. Monoamine oxidase inhibitors ↑
5. Phenothiazines ↑
6. Tetracyclines ↑
7. Anticholinergics ↓

References:

Argov, Z., and Mastaglia, F. L.: Disorders of neuromuscular transmission caused by drugs. N. Engl. J. Med. *301*:409, 1979.
Bullock, J. D., and Albert, D. M.: Flecked retina. Arch. Ophthalmol. *93*:26, 1975.
Gilman, A. G., Goodman, L. S., and Gilman, A. (Eds.): The Pharmacological Basis of Therapeutics. 6th Ed., New York, Macmillan, 1980, pp. 286–288.
Grant, W. M.: Toxicology of the Eye. 2nd Ed., Springfield, Charles C Thomas, 1974, pp. 678–679.
Schettini, A., Owre, E. S., and Fink, A. I.: Effect of methoxyflurane anaesthesia on intraocular pressure. Can. Anaesth. Soc. J. *15*:172, 1968.
Wade, A. (Ed.): Martindale: The Extra Pharmacopoeia. 27th Ed., London, Pharmaceutical Press, 1977, pp. 703–706.

———————

Generic Name: Nitrous Oxide

Proprietary Name: Entonox (G.B.)

Primary Use: This inhalation anesthetic and analgesic is used in dentistry, in the second stage of labor in pregnancy, and during induction of general anesthesia.

Ocular Side Effects:

A. Systemic Administration
   1. Pupils — dependent on plane of anesthesia
      a. Mydriasis — reactive to light (initial)
      b. Miosis — reactive to light (deep level of anesthesia)
      c. Mydriasis — nonreactive to light (coma)
   2. Intraocular pressure
      a. Increased
      b. Decreased
   3. Decreased vision
   4. Decreased lacrimation
   5. Cortical blindness (?)

Clinical Significance: Pupillary changes due to nitrous oxide are common; however, other than aiding in determination of the anesthetic plane, they are seldom of importance. Nitrous oxide as well as other anesthetics produce the transitory effect of decreased basal tear production during general anesthesia. While decreased vision or blindness after induction of general anesthesia is quite rare, this phenomenon is more frequent with nitrous oxide than with most other general anesthetics. Visual loss is probably secondary to asphyxic cerebral cortical damage.

Interactions with Other Drugs:

  A. Effect of Nitrous Oxide on Activity of Other Drugs
      1. Adrenergic blockers ↑
      2. Sympathomimetics ↑
  B. Effect of Other Drugs on Activity of Nitrous Oxide
      1. Monoamine oxidase inhibitors ↑
      2. Phenothiazines ↑

References:

Hart, S. M., and Fitzgerald, P. G.: Unexplained jaundice following non-halothane anaesthesia. Br. J. Anaesth. 47:1321, 1975.
Hovland, K. R.: Effects of drugs on aqueous humor dynamics. Int. Ophthalmol. Clin. 11(2):99, 1971.
Kornblueth, W., et al.: Influence of general anesthesia on intraocular pressure in man. Arch. Ophthalmol. 61:84, 1959.
Krupin, T., Cross, D. A., and Becker, B.: Decreased basal tear production associated with general anesthesia. Arch. Ophthalmol. 95:107, 1977.
Walsh, F. B., and Hoyt, W. F.: Clinical Neuro-Ophthalmology. 3rd Ed., Baltimore, Williams & Wilkins, Vol. III, 1969, p. 2676.

Generic Name: Trichloroethylene

Proprietary Name: Anamenth (Germ.), Trilene (G.B.)

Primary Use: This potent inhalation anesthetic is used primarily for short-term diagnostic or surgical procedures and in obstetrics. It may also be used as an adjunct to anesthesia.

Ocular Side Effects:

  A. Systemic Administration
      1. Paresis or paralysis of extraocular muscles
      2. Diplopia
      3. Ptosis
      4. Decreased vision
      5. Visual fields
         a. Scotomas — central or paracentral
         b. Constriction
         c. Enlarged blind spot
      6. Photophobia
      7. Extraocular muscles
         a. Pain on ocular movements
         b. Limitation of ocular movements
      8. Paralysis of accommodation

9. Pupils
    a. Decreased or absent reaction to light
    b. Anisocoria
10. Problems with color vision — dyschromatopsia
11. Horizontal nystagmus
12. Decreased lacrimation
13. Retrobulbar or optic neuritis
14. Optic atrophy
15. Toxic amblyopia
16. Decreased intraocular pressure
17. Peripapillary hemorrhages
18. Decreased corneal reflex
19. Retinal edema
20. Retinal vasoconstriction
21. Visual hallucinations
22. Corneal ulceration
B. Inadvertent Ocular Exposure
    1. Irritation
        a. Lacrimation
        b. Hyperemia
        c. Edema
        d. Burning sensation
    2. Punctate keratitis
    3. Corneal opacities

Clinical Significance: Ocular side effects due to trichloroethylene are uncommon since the discovery that most of the adverse reactions were
due to toxic decomposition products of the drug. With adjustments in
anesthetic equipment and technique such as using this drug for only
short procedures, adverse ocular reactions are seldom seen. The most
severe toxic response occurs in the central nervous system, and the
cranial nerves are the most susceptible. Trichloroethylene may cause
toxic ocular side effects from industrial exposure.

Interactions with Other Drugs:

A. Effect of Trichloroethylene on Activity of Other Drugs
    1. Adrenergic blockers ↑
B. Effect of Other Drugs on Activity of Trichloroethylene
    1. Monoamine oxidase inhibitors ↑
    2. Phenothiazines ↑

References:

Duke-Elder, S.: Systems of Ophthalmology. St. Louis, C. V. Mosby, Vol. XIV, Part 2,
    1972, pp. 1165, 1315, 1337, 1344.

Hovland, K. R.: Effects of drugs on aqueous humor dynamics. Int. Ophthalmol. Clin. *11*(2):99, 1971.
Humphrey, J. H., and McClelland, M.: Cranial nerve palsies with herpes following general anesthesia. Br. Med. J. *1*:315, 1944.
Maloof, C. C.: Burns of the skin produced by trichloroethylene vapors at room temperature. J. Ind. Hyg. *31*:295, 1949.
Smith, G. F.: Trichloroethylene: A review. Br. J. Ind. Med. *23*:249, 1966.
Vernon, R. J., and Ferguson, R. K.: Effects of trichloroethylene on visual motor performance. Arch. Environ. Health *18*:894, 1969.

Class: Local Anesthetics

Generic Name: 1. Bupivacaine; 2. Chloroprocaine; 3. Etidocaine; 4. Lidocaine; 5. Mepivacaine; 6. Prilocaine; 7. Procaine; 8. Propoxycaine

Proprietary Name: 1. Carbostesin (Germ.), Marcain (G.B.), Marcaine; 2. Nesacaine; 3. Duranest; 4. Anaesthol (Germ.), Anestacon, Ardecaine, Canocaine, Dolicaine, Indolor (S. Afr.), L-Caine, Leostesin (S. Afr.), Lida-Mantle, Lidocaton (G.B.), Lidothesin (G.B.), Lignane (S. Afr.), Lignocaine (G.B.), Lignostab (G.B.), Nervocaine, Norocaine, Nurocain (Austral.), Rocaine, Sarnacaine (Austral.), Stanacaine, Ultracaine, Xylestesin (Germ.), Xylocaine, Xylocard (G.B.), Xylotox (G.B.); 5. Carbocaine, Cavacaine, Scandicain (Germ.); 6. Citanest, Xylonest (Germ.); 7. Anucaine, Durathesia, Neocaine, Novocain, P45 (Austral.), Planocaine (S. Afr.), Rectocaine, Unicaine, Westocaine (Canad.); 8. Blockain, Ravocaine

Primary Use: These amides or esters of para-aminobenzoic acid are used in infiltrative, epidural block, and peripheral or sympathetic nerve block anesthesia or analgesia.

Ocular Side Effects:

A. Systemic Administration
　1. Decreased vision
　2. Horner's syndrome (transitory — lumbar extradural blockade)
　　a. Miosis
　　b. Ptosis
　3. Extraocular muscles
　　a. Paresis or paralysis
　　b. Diplopia
　　c. Nystagmus
　　d. Jerky pursuit movements

    4. Eyelids or conjunctiva
       a. Allergic reactions
       b. Hyperemia
       c. Edema
       d. Urticaria
       e. Exfoliative dermatitis
       f. Blepharoclonus
    5. Problems with color vision — dyschromatopsia (lidocaine)
    6. Retrobulbar neuritis (?)
    7. Papilledema (?)
    8. Optic atrophy (?)
B. Local Ophthalmic Use or Exposure — (Bupivacaine, Lidocaine, Procaine)
    1. Decreased vision
    2. Paresis or paralysis of extraocular muscles
    3. Decreased intraocular pressure
    4. Optic atrophy (?)
    5. Retinal vasoconstriction (?)

Clinical Significance: Ocular side effects due to these drugs are directly dependent on their method of administration. Significant ocular side effects due to intravenous or spinal injections have been reported; however, nearly all are transitory. Cranial nerve paralyses of various kinds including extraocular muscle paralysis have been reported. The sixth cranial nerve has been the one most frequently affected, although the third and fourth nerves have occasionally also been involved. The paralysis may develop almost immediately, although it usually occurs a number of days later. Recovery usually occurs within a few days; however, in some instances it may take from 1 to 2 years. Exceptional cases of permanent optic nerve damage have also been seen and are probably due to impurities or other chemicals inadvertently administered. Transient loss of vision is practically routine from retrobulbar injections of lidocaine or procaine. Adverse ocular reactions from retrobulbar injections of local anesthetics have been difficult to prove since direct trauma from the needle pressure from a subdural injection on the optic nerve or from pressure from a traumatic hematoma may cause optic nerve damage mimicking a drug-induced toxicity.

Interactions with Other Drugs:

A. Effect of Local Anesthetics on Activity of Other Drugs
    1. Sulfonamides ↓
B. Effect of Other Drugs on Activity of Local Anesthetics
    1. Anticholinesterases ↑

References:

American Hospital Formulary Service. Washington, D.C., American Society of Hospital Pharmacists, Vol. II, 72:00, 1974.

de Jong, P. T. V. M., et al.: Ataxia and nystagmus induced by injection of local anesthetics in the neck. Ann. Neurol. *1*:240, 1977.

Faulkner, S. H.: Ocular paralysis following spinal anaesthesia. Trans. Ophthalmol. Soc. U.K. *64*:234, 1944.

Phillips, O. C., et al.: Neurologic complications following spinal anesthesia with lidocaine: A prospective review of 10,440 cases. Anesthesiology *30*:284, 1969.

Class: Therapeutic Gases

Generic Name: Carbon Dioxide

Proprietary Name: Carbon Dioxide

Primary Use: This odorless, colorless gas is used as a respiratory stimulant to increase cerebral blood flow and in the maintenance of acid-base balance.

Ocular Side Effects:

A. Systemic Administration
1. Decreased vision
2. Decreased convergence
3. Paralysis of accommodation
4. Decreased dark adaptation
5. Photophobia
6. Visual fields
   a. Constriction
   b. Enlarged blind spot
7. Problems with color vision
   a. Dyschromatopsia
   b. Objects have yellow tinge
8. Retinal vascular engorgement
9. Pupils
   a. Mydriasis
   b. Absence of reaction to light
10. Visual hallucinations
11. Diplopia
12. Abnormal conjugate deviations

13. Papilledema
14. Increased intraocular pressure
15. Ptosis
16. Decreased corneal reflex
17. Proptosis

Clinical Significance: Ocular side effects due to carbon dioxide are not uncommon. While most of them are reversible, some are permanent and have major clinical significance. Carbon dioxide may have a specific toxicity for the retinal ganglion cells which accounts for severe visual defects due to this agent. Nonreactive dilated pupils only occur in severe toxic states.

References:

Duke-Elder, S.: Systems of Ophthalmology. St. Louis, C. V. Mosby, Vol. XIV, Part 2, 1972, pp. 1350–1351.
Freedman, A., and Sevel, D.: The cerebro-ocular effects of carbon dioxide poisoning. Arch. Ophthalmol. 76:59, 1966.
Sevel, D., and Freedman, A.: Cerebro-retinal degeneration due to carbon dioxide poisoning. Br. J. Ophthalmol. 51:475, 1967.
Sieker, H. O., and Hickam, J. B.: Carbon dioxide intoxication: The clinical syndrome, its etiology and management, with particular reference to the use of mechanical respirators. Medicine 35:389, 1956.
Walsh, F. B., and Hoyt, W. F.: Clinical Neuro-Ophthalmology. 3rd Ed., Baltimore, Williams & Wilkins, Vol. III, 1969, pp. 2601–2602.

———————

Generic Name: Oxygen

Proprietary Name: Oxygen

Primary Use: This colorless, odorless, tasteless gas is used in inhalation anesthesia and in hypoxia.

Ocular Side Effects:

A. Systemic Administration
  1. Retinal vascular changes
     a. Constriction
     b. Spasms
     c. Hemorrhages
  2. Decreased vision
  3. Visual fields
     a. Scotomas — paracentral
     b. Constriction
  4. Retrolental fibroplasia — in newborns or young infants

5. Mydriasis
6. Heightened color perception
7. Retinal detachment
8. Decreased intraocular pressure

Clinical Significance: The toxic ocular effects due to oxygen are most prominent in premature infants but may be found in any age group under hyperbaric conditions. Ocular side effects secondary to oxygen therapy are otherwise uncommon. While the ocular changes due to retrolental fibroplasia are irreversible, nearly all other side effects are transient after use of oxygen is discontinued. A report of permanent bilateral blindness probably due to 80 percent oxygen during general anesthesia has been reported. It has been suggested that in some susceptible people severe retinal vasoconstriction or even direct retinal toxicity may occur from oxygen therapy. Bilateral retinal hemorrhages with permanent partial visual loss were reported secondary to sudden increase in CSF pressure after an excessive volume of oxygen was used to increase a myelogram contrast.

References:

Gallin-Cohen, P. F., Podos, S. M., and Yablonski, M. E.: Oxygen lowers intraocular pressure. Invest. Ophthalmol. Vis. Sci. *19*:43, 1980.

Gilman, A. G., Goodman, L. S., and Gilman, A. (Eds.): The Pharmacological Basis of Therapeutics. 6th Ed., New York, Macmillan, 1980, pp. 321–331.

Havener, W. H.: Ocular Pharmacology. 4th Ed., St. Louis, C. V. Mosby, 1978, pp. 464–467.

Kobayashi, T., and Murakami, S.: Blindness of an adult caused by oxygen. JAMA *219*:741, 1972.

Kushner, B. J., et al.: Retrolental fibroplasia. II. Pathologic correlations. Arch. Ophthalmol. *95*:29, 1977.

Nichols, C. W., Lambertsen, C. J., and Clark, J. M.: Transient unilateral loss of vision associated with oxygen at high pressure. Arch. Ophthalmol. *81*:548, 1969.

Oberman, J., Cohn, H., and Grand, M. G.: Retinal complications of gas myelography. Arch. Ophthalmol. 97:1905, 1979.

Slagsvold, J. E., and Larsen, J. L.: Retinal haemorrhage as a complication of gas encephalography and gas myelography. Prospective study using oxygen gas with a discussion of pathogenic mechanisms. J. Neurol. Neurosurg. Psychiatry *40*:1049, 1977.

V

Gastrointestinal Agents

Class: Agents Used to Treat Acid Peptic Disorders

Generic Name: Cimetidine

Proprietary Name: Tagamet

Primary Use: This histamine H_2 receptor antagonist is used in the treatment of confirmed duodenal ulcers.

Ocular Side Effects:

A. Systemic Administration
   1. Visual hallucinations
   2. Photophobia
   3. Eyelids or conjunctiva
      a. Hyperemia
      b. Stevens-Johnson syndrome
   4. May precipitate narrow-angle glaucoma (?)

Clinical Significance: Cimetidine has been marketed in Great Britain since 1976 and in the United States since 1977. Since that time, only a few adverse ocular effects have been reported. Visual hallucinations have occurred particularly with high doses, with renal impairment, and in elderly patients. All of these adverse ocular reactions are transient and disappear with the withdrawal of the drug therapy. A few cases of angle-closure glaucoma secondary to cimetidine have been reported to the Registry.

References:

Adler, L. E., Sadja, L., and Wilets, G.: Cimetidine toxicity manifested as paranoia and hallucinations. Am. J. Psychiatry 137:1112, 1980.
Agarwal, S. K.: Cimetidine and visual hallucinations. JAMA 240:214, 1978.

Ahmed, A. H., et al.: Stevens-Johnson syndrome during treatment with cimetidine. Lancet 2:433, 1978.

Cimetidine (Tagamet): Update on adverse effects. Med. Lett. Drugs Ther. 20:77, 1978.

Hoskyns, B. L.: Cimetidine withdrawal. Lancet 1:254, 1977.

Class: Antacids

Generic Name: 1. Acid Bismuth Sodium Tartrate; 2. Bismuth Oxychloride; 3. Bismuth Sodium Tartrate; 4. Bismuth Sodium Thioglycollate; 5. Bismuth Sodium Triglycollamate; 6. Bismuth Subcarbonate; 7. Bismuth Subsalicylate

Proprietary Name: 1. Acid Bismuth Solution (G.B.); 2. Bismuth Oxychloride; 3. Bismuth Sodium Tartrate; 4. Bismuth Sodium Thioglycollate; 5. Bistrimate (Canad.); 6. Bismuth Carbonate, Muthanol (Fr.); 7. Bismuth Salicylate

Primary Use: Bismuth salts are primarily used as antacids and in the treatment of syphilis and yaws.

Ocular Side Effects:

A. Systemic Administration
  1. Eyelids or conjunctiva
     a. Blue discoloration (?)
     b. Exfoliative dermatitis
     c. Lyell's syndrome
  2. Subconjunctival hemorrhages
  3. Corneal deposits
  4. Visual hallucinations — toxic states
  5. Decreased vision (?) — toxic states

Clinical Significance: Adverse ocular reactions to bismuth preparations are quite rare and seldom of clinical significance. Bismuth-containing corneal deposits have been documented. Only one case of decreased vision has been reported after an overdose of bismuth.

Interactions with Other Drugs:

A. Effect of Bismuth Salts on Activity of Other Drugs
  1. Tetracyclines ↓

References:

AMA Drug Evaluations. 4th Ed., New York, John Wiley & Sons, 1980, p. 966.
Cohen, E. L.: Conjunctival haemorrhage after bismuth injection. Lancet *1*:627, 1945.
Fischer, F. P.: Bismuthiase secondaire de la cornee. Ann. Oculist (Paris) *183*:615, 1950.
Grant, W. M.: Toxicology of the Eye. 2nd Ed., Springfield, Charles C Thomas, 1974, pp. 191–192.
Supino-Viterbo, V., et al.: Toxic encephalopathy due to ingestion of bismuth salts: Clinical and EEG studies of 45 patients. J. Neurol. Neurosurg. Psychiatry *40*:748, 1977.
Walsh, F. B., and Hoyt, W. F.: Clinical Neuro-Ophthalmology. 3rd Ed., Baltimore, Williams & Wilkins, Vol. III, 1969, p. 2686.

Class: Antiemetics

Generic Name: 1. Chlorcyclizine; 2. Cyclizine; 3. Meclizine (Meclozine)

Proprietary Name: 1. Di-Paralene (Austral., Fr., Swed.), Perazil; 2. Marezine, Marzine (G.B.), Valoid (G.B.); 3. Antivert, Bonamine (Canad., Germ.), Bonine, Calmonal (Germ.), Eldezine, Lamine, Mecazine (Canad.), Navicalm (S. Afr.), Postafen (Germ., Swed.), Roclizine, Veritab, Vertizine, Vertrol, Wehvert

Primary Use: These piperazine antihistaminic derivatives are effective in the management of nausea and vomiting.

Ocular Side Effects:

A. Systemic Administration
   1. Decreased vision
   2. Pupils
      a. Mydriasis – may precipitate narrow-angle glaucoma
      b. Decreased reaction to light
   3. Decreased tolerance to contact lenses
   4. Diplopia
   5. Visual hallucinations
   6. Ocular teratogenic effects (?)
      a. Cataracts
      b. Tapetoretinal degeneration

Clinical Significance: Ocular side effects due to these drugs are rare, reversible, and usually of little clinical significance. Pupillary changes and visual hallucinations primarily occur in overdose situations. A few reports of ocular teratogenic abnormalities have been reported with cyclizine and meclizine therapy; however, these findings may be coincidental.

References:

Gilman, A. G., Goodman, L. S., and Gilman, A. (Eds.): The Pharmacological Basis of Therapeutics. 6th Ed., New York, Macmillan, 1980, pp. 623–629.
Gott, P. H.: Cyclizine toxicity. Intentional drug abuse of a proprietary antihistamine. N. Engl. J. Med. 279:596, 1968.
Grant, W. M.: Toxicology of the Eye. 2nd Ed., Springfield, Charles C Thomas, 1974, pp. 256, 341–342.
McBride, W.: Cyclizine and congenital abnormalities. Br. Med. J. 1:1157, 1963.
Physicians' Desk Reference. 35th Ed., Oradell, N.J., Medical Economics Co., 1981, pp. 759, 1535.

Generic Name: Metoclopramide

Proprietary Name: Donopon-GP (Jap.), Maxeran (Canad.), Maxolon (G.B.), Metoclol (Jap.), Moriperan (Jap.), Paspertin (Germ.), Primperan (G.B.), Reglan

Primary Use: This orthopramide is used as adjunctive therapy in roentgen-ray examination of the stomach and duodenum and for the prevention and treatment of irradiation sickness.

Ocular Side Effects:

A. Systemic Administration
 1. Extraocular muscles
  a. Oculogyric crises
  b. Diplopia
  c. Paralysis
  d. Nystagmus
  e. Strabismus
 2. Decreased vision
 3. Eyelids or conjunctiva
  a. Edema
  b. Urticaria

Clinical Significance: Ocular side effects secondary to metoclopramide are rare; however, the drug can produce acute dystonic reactions, particularly in children. This includes transitory oculogyric crises, inability to close the eyes, nystagmus, and various extraocular muscle abnormalities. These dystonic reactions usually occur within 36 hours of starting treatment and subside within 24 hours after stopping the drug. Long-term use of the drug, especially in high dosage, should be avoided if possible.

Interactions with Other Drugs:

A. Effect of Other Drugs on Activity of Metoclopramide
   1. Anticholinesterases ↑
   2. Anticholinergics ↓

References:

Casteels-Van Daele, M., et al.: Dystonic reactions in children caused by metoclopramide. Arch. Dis. Child. *45*:130, 1975.

Kataria, M., Traub, M., and Marsden, C. D.: Extrapyramidal side-effects of metoclopramide. Lancet *2*:1254, 1978.

Melmed, S., and Bank, H.: Metoclopramide and facial dyskinesia. Br. Med. J. *1*:331, 1975.

Metoclopramide (Reglan), a new promotility agent. Physicians' Drug Alert *1*:35, 1980.

Stewart, I. A., and Maran, A. G. D.: The effects of metoclopramide on nystagmus and vertigo. Postgrad. Med. J. (Suppl.) *4*:19, 1973.

Vesterhauge, S., and Peitersen, E.: The effects of some drugs on the caloric induced nystagmus. Adv. Otorhinolaryngol. *25*:173, 1979.

Class: Antilipidemic Agents

Generic Name: Clofibrate

Proprietary Name: Aterosol (Swed.), Atheromide (Jap.), Atheropront (Germ.), Atromidin (Swed.), Atromid-S, Claresan (Fr.), Lipavlon (Fr.), Liprinal (G.B.), Recolip (Swed.), Regelan (Germ.), Skleromexe (Germ.)

Primary Use: This aryloxyisobutyric acid derivative is effective in the treatment of hypercholesterolemia and/or hypertriglyceridemia.

Ocular Side Effects:

A. Systemic Administration
   1. Decreased vision
   2. Eyelids or conjunctiva
      a. Erythema
      b. Conjunctivitis — nonspecific

    c. Edema
    d. Urticaria
    e. Purpura
    f. Lupoid syndrome
    g. Blepharoclonus
3. Subconjunctival or retinal hemorrhages secondary to drug-induced anemia
4. Myopia
5. Loss of eyelashes or eyebrows (?)
6. Decreased intraocular pressure (?)

Clinical Significance: Ocular side effects due to clofibrate are quite rare and seldom of major clinical significance. All reactions seem to clear on cessation of the drug. Controversy has surrounded this agent, but most feel that its value in glaucoma and reversing diabetic retinopathy is questionable. One case in the Registry seems to document a +2.50 refractive change, lasting for 6 weeks after cessation of the drug.

Interactions with Other Drugs:

A. Effect of Clofibrate on Activity of Other Drugs
    1. Anticholinesterases ↑
B. Effect of Other Drugs on Activity of Clofibrate
    1. Neomycin ↑

References:

Arif, M. A., and Vahrman, J.: Skin eruption due to clofibrate. Lancet 2:1202, 1975.
Clements, D. B., Elsby, J. M., and Smith, W. D.: Retinal vein occlusion. A comparative study of factors affecting the prognosis, including a therapeutic trial of Atromid S in this condition. Br. J. Ophthalmol. 52:111, 1968.
Cullen, J. F.: Clofibrate in glaucoma. Lancet 2:892, 1967.
Orban, T.: Clofibrate in glaucoma. Lancet 1:47, 1968.
Physicians' Desk Reference. 35th Ed., Oradell, N.J., Medical Economics Co., 1981, p. 605.

Class: Antispasmodics

Generic Name: 1. Adiphenine; 2. Ambutonium; 3. Anisotropine (Octatropine); 4. Clidinium; 5. Dicyclomine (Dicycloverine); 6. Diphemanil; 7. Glycopyrrolate; 8. Hexocyclium; 9. Isopropamide; 10. Mepenzolate; 11. Methantheline; 12. Methixene; 13. Methylatropine Nitrate (Atropine Methonitrate); 14. Oxyphencyclimine; 15. Oxyphenonium; 16. Pipenzolate (Pipenzolone); 17. Piperidolate; 18. Poldine; 19. Propantheline; 20. Tridihexethyl

Proprietary Name: *Systemic:* 1. Adiphenine; 2. Ambutonium; 3. Valpin; 4. Quarzan; 5. Antispas, Atumin (Germ.), Benacol, Bentyl, Bentylol (Canad.), Clomin (S. Afr.), Diclomyl (Austral.), Dicycol (Austral.), Incron (Jap.), Mamiesan (Jap.), Merbentyl (G.B.), Nospaz, Pasmin, Procyclomin (Austral.), Rocyclo, Rotyl, Sawamin (Jap.), Stannitol, Wyovin (N.Z.); 6. Demotil (Swed.), Prantal; 7. Asecryl (Fr.), Robinul, Tarodyn (Swed.); 8. Tral, Traline (Fr., Germ.); 9. Darbid, Priamide (Belg., Fr., Germ.), Tyrimide (G.B.); 10. Cantil; 11. Banthine, Vagantin (Germ.); 12. Methyloxan (Jap.), Tremaril (S. Afr., Switz.), Tremarit (Germ.), Tremonil (G.B.), Tremoquil (Swed.), Trest; 13. Metropine; 14. Daricol (Swed.), Daricon, Spazamin (Austral.); 15. Antrenyl, Spastrex (S. Afr.); 16. Piptal (G.B.), Piptil; 17. Dactil; 18. Nactate (Swed.), Nacton (G.B.); 19. Banlin (Canad.), Ercotina (Swed.), Neo-Banex (Canad.), Norpanth, Pantheline (Austral.), Pro-Banthine, Pro-dixamon (Swed.), Robantaline, Ropanth, SK-Propantheline, Spastil; 20. Pathilon *Ophthalmic:* 11. Methantheline; 13. Eumydrin; 15. Oxyphenonium; 19. Propantheline

Primary Use: *Systemic:* These anticholinergic agents are effective in the management of gastrointestinal tract spasticity and peptic ulcers. *Ophthalmic:* These topical anticholinergic mydriatic and cycloplegic agents are used in refractions and fundus examinations.

Ocular Side Effects:

    A. Systemic Administration
        1. Decreased vision
        2. Mydriasis — may precipitate narrow-angle glaucoma
        3. Paralysis of accommodation
        4. Photophobia
        5. Problems with color vision
           a. Dyschromatopsia (piperidolate)
           b. Colored flashing lights (propantheline)
        6. Flashing lights (piperidolate)
        7. Eyelids or conjunctiva
           a. Allergic reactions
           b. Exfoliative dermatitis
        8. Loss of eyelashes or eyebrows (?) (glycopyrrolate)
    B. Local Ophthalmic Use or Exposure
        1. Mydriasis — may precipitate narrow-angle glaucoma
        2. Photophobia

3. Paralysis of accommodation
4. Eyelids or conjunctiva (oxyphenonium)
   a. Allergic reactions
   b. Conjunctivitis — nonspecific
5. Increased intraocular pressure (oxyphenonium)

C. Inadvertent Ocular Exposure
   1. Pupils (propantheline)
      a. Mydriasis
      b. Absence of reaction to light

Clinical Significance: Ocular side effects due to these anticholinergic agents vary, depending on the drug; however, adverse ocular reactions are seldom significant and are reversible. None of the preceding drugs have little more than 10 to 15 percent of the anticholinergic activity of atropine. The most frequent ocular side effects are decreased vision, mydriasis, decreased accommodation, and photophobia. While these effects are not uncommon with some of these agents, rarely are they severe enough to cause a change in the medication. The weak anticholinergic effect of these agents seldom aggravates open-angle glaucoma; however, it has the potential to precipitate narrow-angle glaucoma attacks. Recently, two cases of unilateral pupillary dilatation were seen in patients who inadvertently got antiperspirants containing propantheline on their fingers and transferred it to their eyes.

Interactions with Other Drugs:

A. Effect of Anticholinergics on Activity of Other Drugs
   1. Barbiturates ↑ (adiphenine)
B. Effect of Other Drugs on Activity of Anticholinergics
   1. Antihistamines ↑
   2. Monoamine oxidase inhibitors ↑
   3. Phenothiazines ↑
   4. Tricyclic antidepressants ↑

References:

AMA Drug Evaluations. 4th Ed., New York, John Wiley & Sons, 1980, pp. 989–1000.
Dukes, M. N. G. (Ed.): Meyler's Side Effects of Drugs. Amsterdam, Excerpta Medica, Vol. IX, 1980, pp. 230–231.
Gilman, A. G., Goodman, L. S., and Gilman, A. (Eds.): The Pharmacological Basis of Therapeutics. 6th Ed., New York, Macmillan, 1980, pp. 128–132.
Havener, W. H.: Ocular Pharmacology. 4th Ed., St. Louis, C. V. Mosby, 1978, p. 261.
Leopold, I. H. (Ed.): Glaucoma Drug Therapy: Monograph I Parasympathetic Agents. Irvine, Calif., Allergan Pharmaceuticals, 1975, pp. 19–21.
Nissen, S. H., and Nielsen, P. G.: Unilateral mydriasis after use of propantheline bromide in an antiperspirant. Lancet 2:1134, 1977.

Generic Name: 1. Atropine; 2. Belladonna; 3. Homatropine

Proprietary Name: *Systemic:* 1. Atropinol (Germ.), Atropt (Austral.), Atroptol (Austral.), Spersatropine (S. Afr.); 2. Belladonna Extract, Leaf, or Tincture, Bellafolin (Germ.), Bellafoline (Fr.); 3. Homapin, Novatrin, Omatropina Lux (Ital.), Sed-Tens SE *Ophthalmic:* 1. Atropisol, BufOpto Atropine, Isopto Atropine; 3. Homatrocel, Isopto Homatropine, SMP Homatropine (G.B.)

Primary Use: *Systemic:* These anticholinergic agents are used in the management of gastrointestinal tract spasticity and peptic ulcers, and to decrease secretions of the respiratory tract. Atropine is also used in the treatment of hyperactive carotid sinus reflex and Parkinson's disease. Homatropine is also used in the treatment of dysmenorrhea. *Ophthalmic:* These topical anticholinergic mydriatic and cycloplegic agents are used in refractions, semiocclusive therapy, accommodative spasms, and uveitis.

Ocular Side Effects:

A. Systemic Administration
 1. Decreased vision
 2. Mydriasis — may precipitate narrow-angle glaucoma
 3. Decrease or paralysis of accommodation
 4. Photophobia
 5. Micropsia
 6. Decreased lacrimation
 7. Visual hallucinations
 8. Problems with color vision
   a. Dyschromatopsia
   b. Objects have red tinge
 9. Eyelids or conjunctiva — Stevens-Johnson syndrome (belladonna)
B. Local Ophthalmic Use or Exposure — Topical Application
 1. Decreased vision
 2. Decrease or paralysis of accommodation
 3. Mydriasis — may precipitate narrow-angle glaucoma
 4. Irritation
   a. Hyperemia
   b. Photophobia
   c. Edema
 5. Increased intraocular pressure
 6. Eyelids or conjunctiva
   a. Allergic reactions
   b. Blepharoconjunctivitis—follicular

7. Micropsia
8. Decreased lacrimation
9. Visual hallucinations
C. Local Ophthalmic Use or Exposure — Subconjunctival Injection
    1. Brawny scleritis

Clinical Significance: Atropine and homatropine have essentially the same ocular side effects whether they are administered systemically or by topical ocular application. Systemic administration causes fewer and less severe ocular side effects, since significantly smaller amounts of the drugs reach the eye. However, transient loss of vision following an intravenous injection of atropine has been reported. Topical ocular atropine and homatropine may elevate the intraocular pressure in eyes with open-angle glaucoma, but seldom in normal eyes. Probably the most common side effect which requires the discontinuation of these agents is contact dermatitis. Conjunctival papillary hypertrophy usually suggests a hypersensitivity reaction, while a follicular response suggests a toxic or irritative reaction. These drugs are said to produce a greater pupillary response in patients with Down's syndrome. Systemic reactions may occur after ocular instillation of these anticholinergic drugs, particularly in children and elderly patients. Symptoms of systemic toxicity include dryness of the mouth and skin, flushing, fever, rash, thirst, tachycardia, irritability, hyperactivity, ataxia, confusion, somnolence, hallucinations, and delirium. These reactions have been observed most frequently after the use of atropine. Rarely, convulsions, coma, and death occurred after ocular instillation of this drug in young children. In the primate, topical ocular atropine appears to decrease or slow echothiophate-induced lens changes.

Interactions with Other Drugs:

A. Effect of Anticholinergics on Activity of Other Drugs
    1. Phenothiazines ↑
    2. Analgesics ↑↓
    3. Anticholinesterases ↓
B. Effect of Other Drugs on Activity of Anticholinergics
    1. Analgesics ↑
    2. Antihistamines ↑
    3. Monoamine oxidase inhibitors ↑
    4. Phenothiazines ↑
    5. Tricyclic antidepressants ↑

References:

Crandall, D. C., and Leopold, I. H.: The influence of systemic drugs on tear constituents. Ophthalmology 86:115, 1979.

Fraunfelder, F. T., Hanna, C., and Meyer, M.: Drug-induced ocular side effects. In Leopold, I. H., and Burns, R. P. (Eds.): Symposium on Ocular Therapy. New York, John Wiley & Sons, Vol. XI, 1979, p. 116.

Garin, P.: Les medicaments en rapport avec le systeme digestif. Bull. Soc. Belge Ophtalmol. *160*:267, 1972.

German, E., and Siddiqui, N.: Atropine toxicity from eyedrops. N. Engl. J. Med. *282*:689, 1970.

Gilman, A. G., Goodman, L. S., and Gilman, A. (Eds.): The Pharmacological Basis of Therapeutics. 6th Ed., New York, Macmillan, 1980, pp. 120–128, 133–137.

Gleason, M. N., et al.: Clinical Toxicology of Commercial Products. 3rd Ed., Baltimore, Williams & Wilkins, 1969.

Gooding, J. M., and Holcomb, M. C.: Transient blindness following intravenous administration of atropine. Anesth. Analg. *56*:872, 1977.

Havener, W. H.: Ocular Pharmacology. 4th Ed., St. Louis, C. V. Mosby, 1978, pp. 244–252.

Kaufman, P. L., Axelsson, U., and Bárány, E. H.: Atropine inhibition of echothiophate cataractogenesis in monkeys. Arch. Ophthalmol. *95*:1262, 1977.

Lazenby, G. W., Reed, J. W., and Grant, W. M.: Anticholinergic medication in open-angle glaucoma. Long-term tests. Arch. Ophthalmol. *84*:719, 1970.

Lazenby, G. W., Reed, J. W., and Grant, W. M.: Short-term tests of anticholinergic medication in open-angle glaucoma. Arch. Ophthalmol. *80*:443, 1968.

Leopold, I. H., and Comroe, J. H., Jr.: Effect of intramuscular administration of morphine, atropine, scopolamine and neostigmine on the human eye. Arch. Ophthalmol. *40*:285, 1948.

Stokes, H. R.: Drug reactions reported in a survey of South Carolina. Ophthalmology *86*:161, 1979.

Class: Stimulants of the Gastrointestinal and Urinary Tracts

Generic Name: Bethanechol

Proprietary Name: Besacolin (Jap.), Duvoid, Iricoline (Fr.), Mechothane (G.B.), Mictrol, Myotonachol, Myotonine (G.B.), Urecholine, Uro-Carb (Austral.), Urolax, Vesicholine

Primary Use: This quaternary ammonium parasympathomimetic agent is effective in the management of postoperative abdominal distention and nonobstructive urinary retention.

Ocular Side Effects:

  A. Systemic Administration
   1. Nonspecific ocular irritation
     a. Lacrimation

     b. Hyperemia
     c. Burning sensation
  2. Decreased accommodation

Clinical Significance: Adverse ocular reactions due to bethanechol are unusual, but they may continue long after use of the drug is discontinued. Some advocate use of this agent in the treatment of Riley Day syndrome and ocular pemphigoid because of the possible increase in lacrimal secretion.

Interactions with Other Drugs:

  A. Effect of Other Drugs on Activity of Bethanechol
     1. Anticholinergics ↓
     2. Sympathomimetics ↓

References:

Gilman, A. G., Goodman, L. S., and Gilman, A. (Eds.): The Pharmacological Basis of Therapeutics. 6th Ed., New York, Macmillan, 1980, pp. 91–96.

Grant, W. M.: Toxicology of the Eye. 2nd Ed., Springfield, Charles C Thomas, 1974, p. 188.

Perritt, R. A.: Eye complications resulting from systemic medications. Ill. Med. J. *117*:423, 1960.

Wade, A. (Ed.): Martindale: The Extra Pharmacopoeia. 27th Ed., London, Pharmaceutical Press, 1977, p. 992.

Generic Name: Carbachol

Proprietary Name: *Systemic:* Carbyl (Ital.), Doryl (Germ.) *Ophthalmic:* Carbacel, Isopto Carbachol, Isopto-Karbakolin (Swed.), Miostat, Mistura, PV Carbachol (Canad.)

Primary Use: *Systemic:* This quaternary ammonium parasympathomimetic agent is effective in the management of postoperative intestinal atony and urinary retention. *Ophthalmic:* This topical or intraocular agent is used in open-angle glaucoma.

Ocular Side Effects:

  A. Systemic Administration
     1. Decreased accommodation
  B. Local Ophthalmic Use or Exposure — Topical Application
     1. Miosis
     2. Decreased vision
     3. Decreased intraocular pressure

    4. Accommodative spasm
    5. Eyelids or conjunctiva
       a. Allergic reactions
       b. Hyperemia
       c. Conjunctivitis — follicular
    6. Ocular pain
    7. Blepharoclonus
    8. Myopia
    9. Retinal detachment
C. Local Ophthalmic Use or Exposure — Intracameral Injection
    1. Miosis
    2. Corneal edema
    3. Decreased vision

Clinical Significance: Probably the most frequent ocular side effect due to carbachol is a decrease in vision secondary to miosis or accommodative spasms. In the younger age groups, transient drug-induced myopia may be quite bothersome. Follicular conjunctivitis is common after long-term therapy, but this in general has minimal clinical significance. Miotics can induce retinal detachments but probably only in eyes with preexisting retinal pathologic condition. If there are significant breaks in the conjunctiva or corneal epithelium, care must be taken not to apply topical ocular carbachol since major systemic side effects may occur. In addition, this topical ocular medication used in glaucoma therapy may be one of the more toxic agents on the corneal epithelium. Case reports in the Registry and experimental data implicated commercially available intraocular carbachol as possibly having an inadequate buffering system, too low a pH, or some other unknown factors which have been associated occasionally with transitory and persistent corneal edema. The manufacturer has now modified the formulation, but this preparation should be carefully watched to make sure the problem has been solved with the new formulation.

Interactions with Other Drugs:

A. Effect of Other Drugs on Activity of Carbachol
    1. Anticholinergics ↓
    2. Sympathomimetics ↓

References:

Beasley, H., and Fraunfelder, F. T.: Retinal detachments and topical ocular miotics. Ophthalmology 86:95, 1979.

Beasley, H., et al.: Carbachol in cataract surgery. Arch. Ophthalmol. 80:39, 1968.

Fraunfelder, F. T.: Corneal edema after use of carbachol. Arch. Ophthalmol. 97:975, 1979.

Krejci, L., and Harrison, R.: Antiglaucoma drug effects on corneal epithelium. A comparative study in tissue culture. Arch. Ophthalmol. *84:*766, 1970.

Pape, L. G., and Forbes, M.: Retinal detachment and miotic therapy. Am. J. Ophthalmol. *85:*558, 1978.

Vaughn, E. D., Hull, D. S., and Green, K.: Effect of intraocular miotics on corneal endothelium. Arch. Ophthalmol. *96:*1897, 1978.

VI

Cardiac, Vascular, and Renal Agents

Class: Agents Used to Treat Migraine

Generic Name: 1. Ergonovine (Ergometrine); 2. Ergotamine; 3. Methylergonovine; 4. Methysergide

Proprietary Name: 1. Ergomine (Austral.), Ergotrate, Ermalate (Austral.); 2. Ergate (S. Afr.), Ergomar, Ergostat, Ergotart (Austral.), Etin (Austral.), Exmigra (Neth.), Exmigrex (Fin.), Femergin (G.B.), Gynergen, Lingraine (G.B.), Lingran (Swed.), Lingrene (Norw.); 3. Levospan (Jap.), Methergin (Austral., Fr., Germ., S. Afr., Swed.), Methergine, Methylergobasine (Canad.), Methylergometrine (G.B.); 4. Deseril (G.B.), Desernil (Fr.), Sansert

Primary Use: These ergot alkaloids and derivatives are effective in the management of migraine or other vascular types of headaches and as oxytocic agents.

Ocular Side Effects:

A. Systemic Administration
   1. Decreased vision
   2. Retinal vascular disorders
      a. Spasms
      b. Constriction
      c. Stasis
      d. Thrombosis
      e. Occlusion
   3. Miosis (ergotamine)
   4. Decreased intraocular pressure — minimal
   5. Visual fields
      a. Scotomas (methysergide)
      b. Hemianopsia (ergonovine)

6. Decreased accommodation (methysergide)
7. Problems with color vision
   a. Dyschromatopsia
   b. Objects have red tinge
8. Eyelids or conjunctiva
   a. Edema
   b. Lupoid syndrome
9. Loss of eyelashes or eyebrows (?)
10. Optic neuritis (?)
11. Cataracts (?)
12. Cortical blindness (?) (methylergonovine)

Clinical Significance: Ocular side effects due to these ergot alkaloids are rare; however, patients on standard therapeutic dosages may develop significant adverse ocular effects. This is probably due to an unusual susceptibility, sensitivity, or a preexisting disease which is exacerbated by the ergot preparations. Increased ocular vascular complications have been seen in patients with a preexisting occlusive peripheral vascular disease. The course of patients with retinal vascular disease should be followed closely if ergot preparations are necessary for the management of their nonophthalmic disease. Even in a healthy 19 year old, a standard therapeutic injection of ergotamine apparently precipitated a central retinal artery occlusion. There are sporadic reports of ischemic optic neuritis, as well as cataracts, in the literature, but these are rare and difficult to prove a cause-and-effect relationship.

Interactions with Other Drugs:

A. Effect of Ergot Alkaloids on Activity of Other Drugs
   1. Analgesics ↓ (methysergide)
B. Synergistic Activity
   1. Sympathomimetics

References:

Alarcón-Segovia, D.: Drug-induced antinuclear antibodies and lupus syndrome. Drugs *12*:69, 1976.

Christensen, L., and Swan, K. C.: Adrenergic blocking agents in the treatment of glaucoma. Trans. Am. Acad. Ophthalmol. Otolaryngol. 53:489, 1949.

Crews, S. J.: Toxic effects on the eye and visual apparatus resulting from the systemic absorption of recently introduced chemical agents. Trans. Ophthalmol. Soc. U.K. 82:387, 1962.

Gilman, A. G., Goodman, L. S., and Gilman, A. (Eds.): The Pharmacological Basis of Therapeutics. 6th Ed., New York, Macmillan, 1980, pp. 939–947.

Peters, G. S., and Horton, B. T.: Headache: With special reference to the excessive use of ergotamine preparations and withdrawal effects. Proc. Staff Meet. Mayo Clin. *26*:153, 1951.

Class: Antianginal Agents

Generic Name: Amiodarone

Proprietary Name: Cordarone (Belg., Fr.)

Primary Use: This benzofuran derivative is effective in the treatment of angina pectoris.

Ocular Side Effects:

A. Systemic Administration
1. Yellow-brown deposits
   a. Cornea
   b. Conjunctiva
   c. Lens
2. Decreased vision
3. Problems with color vision — colored haloes around lights
4. Corneal ulceration
5. Eyelids or conjunctiva
   a. Photosensitivity
   b. Stevens-Johnson syndrome
6. Retinal depigmentation (?)

Clinical Significance: Ocular deposits due to amiodarone probably occur in nearly all patients on long-term usage. The only significant ocular side effect is a whorl-like corneal epithelial pattern indistinguishable from that due to chloroquine. These deposits are dose- and time-related, and in some patients appear to reach a steady state with no progression even with continued drug use. The usual pattern for corneal deposition initially is a horizontal, irregular, branching line near the junction of the mid and outer one third of the cornea (stage 1). In stage 2, this increases, so that 6 to 10 branches increase in length and curve superiorly. Any increase in the number of branches constitutes stage 3. The deposits may be seen as early as 2 weeks after starting the drug and probably occur in most patients by 4 months. They are completely reversible but may take as long as 1 year to clear. In general, patients taking 100 to 200 mg/day have only minimal or even no corneal deposits. At dosages of 400 mg or more, however, most patients will show corneal deposits. Histologically, these deposits appear to be a drug-induced lipid complex or lipofuscin. One author claims that if the drug is withheld for 1 week every 1 to 2 months this side effect will not occur. Visual changes are unusual and most often consist of complaints of hazy vision. Slate-gray periocular skin pigmentation has been seen secondary to photosensitivity reactions. Corneal ulcerations that appear during treatment with amiodarone have been reported to heal without complications. Retinal depigmentation has been suggested as being caused by this drug. Two case reports of retinal depigmentation have been received by the Registry. However, no clearcut documented evidence that this drug causes human retinal damage has been found to date, although the intracytoplasmic granulations have been found in the retinal pigment epithelium of animals.

References:

D'Amico, D. J., Kenyon, K. R., and Ruskin, J. N.: Amiodarone keratopathy: Drug-induced lipid storage disease. Arch. Ophthalmol. *99*:257, 1981.

Dudognon, P., et al.: Neuropathie au chlorhydrate d'amiodarone. Étude clinique et histopathologique d'une nouvelle lipidose médicamenteuse. Rev. Neurol. *135*:527, 1979.

Kaplan, L. J., and Cappaert, W. E.: Amiodarone keratopathy. Correlation to dosage and duration. Arch. Ophthalmol. *100*:601, 1982.

Wilson, F. M., II, Schmitt, T. E., and Grayson, M.: Amiodarone-induced cornea verticillata. Ann. Ophthalmol. *12*:657, 1980.

Generic Name: Amyl Nitrite

Proprietary Name: Aspirols, Vaporole

Primary Use: This short-acting nitrite antianginal agent is effective in the treatment of acute attacks of angina pectoris.

Ocular Side Effects:

A. Inhalation Administration
   1. Mydriasis
   2. Decreased vision
   3. Problems with color vision
      a. Dyschromatopsia
      b. Objects have yellow tinge
      c. Colored haloes around objects — mainly blue or yellow
   4. Decreased intraocular pressure — transient
   5. Color hallucinations
   6. Eyelids or conjunctiva — allergic reactions
   7. Retinal vasodilatation

Clinical Significance: Ocular side effects due to amyl nitrite are transient and reversible. Adverse ocular reactions are not uncommon but seldom of clinical significance. There is no evidence that this drug has precipitated narrow-angle glaucoma. Amyl nitrite ordinarily causes a fall in intraocular pressure for only 10 to 20 minutes. Prior reports of elevation of intraocular pressure with this drug are being questioned.

Interactions with Other Drugs:

A. Effect of Amyl Nitrite on Activity of Other Drugs
1. Analgesics ↑
2. Anticholinergics ↑
3. Antihistamines ↑
4. Sympathomimetics ↑
5. Tricyclic antidepressants ↑
6. Anticholinesterases ↓
B. Effect of Other Drugs on Activity of Amyl Nitrite
1. Adrenergic blockers ↑
2. Anticholinesterases ↓

References:

Cristini, G., and Pagliarani, N.: Amyl nitrite test in primary glaucoma. Br. J. Ophthalmol. 37:741, 1953.
Cristini, G., and Pagliarani, N.: Slitlamp study of the aqueous veins in simple glaucoma during the amyl nitrite test. Br. J. Ophthalmol. 39:685, 1955.
Grant, W. M.: Physiological and pharmacological influences upon intraocular pressure. Pharmacol. Rev. 7:143, 1955.
Grant, W. M.: Toxicology of the Eye. 2nd Ed., Springfield, Charles C Thomas, 1974, pp. 134–135.
Robertson, D., and Stevens, R. M.: Nitrates and glaucoma. JAMA 237:117, 1977.
Variations and patterns of IOP. Ann. Ophthalmol. 8:1027, 1976.

Generic Name: 1. Erythrityl Tetranitrate; 2. Isosorbide Dinitrate; 3. Mannitol Hexanitrate; 4. Pentaerythritol Tetranitrate; 5. Trolnitrate

Proprietary Name: 1. Anginar, Cardilate, Cardiwell (Fr.); 2. Angidil, Carvasin (Austral.), Cedocard (G.B.), Coronex (Canad.), Dilatrate, Directan (Jap.), ISDN, Iso-Bid, Iso-D, Isoket (Germ.), Isordil, Isosorb, Isotrate, Maycor (Germ.), Nitrol (Jap.), Onset, Risordan (Fr.), Sorate, Sorbangil (Swed.), Sorbide, Sorbidilat (Germ.), Sorbitrate, Sorquad, Vascardin (G.B.); 3. Moloid (Germ.), SDM No. 5, Vascunitol; 4. Angijen, Antime, Antora, Arcotrate, Auxinutril (Fr.), Baritrate, Blaintrate, Cardiacap (G.B.), Cordilate (S. Afr.), Corodyl, Desatrate, Dilac 80, Dilanca (Canad.), Dilcoran (Germ.), Dinate, Duotrate, Kortrate, Maso-Trol, Metranil, Mycardol (G.B.), Naptrate, Neo-Corodil (Canad.), Neo-Corovas, Niritol (Canad.), Nitrin, Nitropent (Swed.), Nitropenthrite (Fr.), Pantrate (S. Afr.), Penritol (Austral.), Penta-Cap, PentaE, Penta-Forte-T, Pentanitrine (Fr.), Penta-Tal, Pentathryn (Austral.), Pentestan, Pentetra, Pentral (G.B.), Pentrate, Pentritol, Pentryate,

Pent-T, Pentylan, Pentytrit (Denm.), Perispan, Peritrate, Perynitrate (Canad.), PETN, Petro, P-T (Canad.), P-T-T, Quintrate, Rate, Reithritol, SDM No. 23/35, SK-Petn, Tentrate, Terpate, Tetracap, Tetranite (Canad.), Tetrasule, Tetratab, Tranite, Vasolate; 5. Angitrit (Germ., Norw.), Duronitrin (Austral.), Metamine, Nitroduran (Swed.), Ortin (Switz.), Praenitron (Austral.)

Primary Use: These long-acting vasodilators are used in the treatment of chronic angina pectoris.

Ocular Side Effects:

A. Systemic Administration
   1. Decreased vision
   2. Intraocular pressure
      a. Decreased
      b. Increased (?)
   3. Eyelids — exfoliative dermatitis

Clinical Significance: Ocular side effects due to the nitrate vasodilators are uncommon, transitory, and reversible. The primary adverse ocular reaction is transitory blurred vision. Use of these vasodilators is probably not contraindicated in glaucomatous patients; however, there have been a few reports to the contrary. Clinically, no adverse glaucoma effects have been reported to date of any practical importance.

Interactions with Other Drugs:

A. Effect of Nitrates on Activity of Other Drugs
   1. Analgesics ↑
   2. Anticholinergics ↑
   3. Antihistamines ↑
   4. Sympathomimetics ↑
   5. Tricyclic antidepressants ↑
   6. Anticholinesterases ↓
B. Effect of Other Drugs on Activity of Nitrates
   1. Adrenergic blockers ↑
   2. Anticholinesterases ↓

References:

American Hospital Formulary Service. Washington, D.C., American Society of Hospital Pharmacists, Vol. 1, *24*:12, 1979.
Grant, W. M.: Toxicology of the Eye. 2nd Ed., Springfield, Charles C Thomas, 1974, pp. 611–612, 795–796.

Leydhecker, H. C. W.: Glaukom und gefässerweiternde Medikamente. Dtsch. Med. Wochenschr. *104*:1330, 1979.
Whitworth, C. G., and Grant, W. M.: Use of nitrate and nitrite vasodilators by glaucomatous patients. Arch. Ophthalmol. *71*:492, 1964.

Generic Name: Nitroglycerin

Proprietary Name: Anginine (Austral.), Angised (S. Afr.), Ang-O-Span, Cardabid, Corobid, Gilucor Nitro (Germ.), Glyceryl Trinitrate (G.B.), Glynite (Canad.), Gly-Trate, Klavi Kordal, Lenitral (Fr.), Niglycon, Niong, Nitora, Nitrangin (Germ.), Nitrine, Nitro-Bid, Nitrocap, Nitrocels, Nitrocontin (G.B.), Nitro-Dial, Nitrodyl, Nitroglyn, Nitrol, Nitrolar, Nitrolex TD, Nitrolingual (Germ.), Nitro-Lyn, Nitro Mack Retard (Germ.), Nitronet, Nitrong, Nitroprn, Nitrorectal (Germ.), Nitroretard (Swed.), Nitro-SA, Nitrospan, Nitrostabilin (Canad.), Nitrostat, Nitro-TD, Nitrotym, Nitrozell Retard (Germ.), Sustac (G.B.), Trates, Triagin (Austral.), Vasitrin (Austral.), Vasoglyn

Primary Use: This short-acting trinitrate vasodilator is effective in the treatment of acute attacks of angina pectoris.

Ocular Side Effects:

A. Systemic Administration
   1. Decreased vision
   2. Intraocular pressure
      a. Decreased
      b. Increased (?)
   3. Retinal vasodilatation
   4. Problems with color vision — colored haloes around lights, mainly yellow or blue
   5. Subconjunctival or retinal hemorrhages secondary to drug-induced anemia
   6. Eyelids — exfoliative dermatitis
   7. Visual hallucinations (?)
   8. Optic atrophy (?)

Clinical Significance: Ocular side effects due to nitroglycerin are uncommon, transient, and reversible. No clinically important evidence of significant ocular pressure elevation due to nitroglycerin usage exists in patients with open- or narrow-angle glaucoma. Theoretically, however, the drug does have the potential to precipitate narrow-angle glaucoma, and patients with narrow angles taking this drug should be closely followed. Transitory and reversible blindness due to ingestion of nitro-glycerin has been seen, and in one instance, optic atrophy was reported.

Interactions with Other Drugs:

A. Effect of Nitroglycerin on Activity of Other Drugs
    1. Analgesics ↑
    2. Anticholinergics ↑
    3. Antihistamines ↑
    4. Sympathomimetics ↑
    5. Tricyclic antidepressants ↑
    6. Anticholinesterases ↓
B. Effect of Other Drugs on Activity of Nitroglycerin
    1. Adrenergic blockers ↑
    2. Anticholinesterases ↓

References:

Laws, C. E.: Nitroglycerine head. JAMA 54:793, 1910.
Leydhecker, W.: Glaukom und gefässerweiternde Medikamente. Dtsch. Med. Wo-chenschr. 104:1330, 1979.
Resnick, L.: Eye Hazards in Industry. Extent, Cause and Means of Prevention. New York, Columbia University Press, 1941, p. 266.
Robertson, D., and Stevens, R. M.: Nitrates and glaucoma. JAMA 237:117, 1977.
Stecher, P. G. (Ed.): The Merck Index: An Encyclopedia of Chemicals and Drugs. 8th Ed., Rahway, N.J., Merck and Co., Inc., 1968, pp. 75, 727–728.
Whitworth, C. G., and Grant, W. M.: Use of nitrate and nitrite vasodilators by glau-comatous patients. Arch. Ophthalmol. 71:492, 1964.
Zahn, K. I.: The effect of nitroglycerine on the retinal circulation. Cesk. Oftalmol. 13:146, 1957.

Generic Name: Perhexilene

Proprietary Name: Pexid

Primary Use: This antianginal agent reduces the severity of anginal attacks in patients with coronary artery disease.

Ocular Side Effects:

A. Systemic Administration
    1. Decreased vision
    2. Nystagmus
    3. Papilledema
    4. Problems with color vision — dyschromatopsia

8

Clinical Significance: Neurologic complications are common among adverse effects of perhexilene, and several cases of bilateral papilledema have been reported. Normally, the papilledema improved within 6 weeks of discontinuing the drug. Permanent changes may ensue if the drug-induced increased intracranial pressure remains unrecognized. Decreased vision and nystagmus may occur with or without an increase in intracranial pressure.

References:

Gras, H., et al.: Les troubles de l'equilibre provoques par le malleate de perhexilline. Nouv. Presse Med. 3:2338, 1974.
Laroche, J., and Laroche, C.: Nouvelles recherches sur la modification de la vision des couleurs sous l'action des medicaments a dose therapeutique. Ann. Pharm. Fr. 35:173, 1977.
Murray, W., MacNair, D. R., and Talbot, M. D.: Ataxia during perhexiline maleate therapy. Practitioner 221:757, 1978.
Poisson, M., et al.: Thrombose post-arteriographique des veines ophtalmiques dans 2 cas de neuropathie peripherique au maleate de perhexiline avec signes neurologiques centraux. Nouv. Presse Med. 6:3550, 1977.
Stephens, W. P., et al.: Raised intracranial pressure due to perhexiline maleate. Br. Med. J. 1:21, 1978.

Class: Antiarrhythmic Agents

Generic Name: Disopyramide

Proprietary Name: Norpace, Rythmodan (G.B.)

Primary Use: This anticholinergic agent is indicated for suppression and prevention of recurrence of cardiac arrhythmias.

Ocular Side Effects:

A. Systemic Administration
   1. Decreased vision
   2. Eyelids or conjunctiva
      a. Erythema
      b. Conjunctivitis — nonspecific
      c. Photosensitivity
   3. Mydriasis — may precipitate narrow-angle glaucoma
   4. Diplopia (?)

Clinical Significance: The anticholinergic effects of disopyramide can cause blurred vision and fluctuation of visual acuity. The drug can cause mydriasis and has precipitated narrow-angle glaucoma. In one case report submitted to the Registry, narrow-angle glaucoma did not occur until 7 days after the patient was started on the medication. A few cases of diplopia have also been reported, but these patients were also on digitalis drugs as well.

Interactions with Other Drugs:

A. Synergistic Effect
  1. Anticholinergics

References:

American Hospital Formulary Service. Washington, D.C., American Society of Hospital Pharmacists, Vol. I, 24:04, 1979.
Disopyramide (Norpace) for ventricular arrhythmias. Med. Lett. Drugs Ther. 19: 101, 1977.
Photosensitivity from drugs, perfumes and cosmetics. Med. Lett. Drugs Ther. 22:64, 1980.
Trope, G. E., and Hind, V. M. D.: Closed-angle glaucoma in patient on disopyramide. Lancet 1:329, 1978.
Wayne, K., Manolas, E., and Sloman, G.: Fatal overdose with disopyramide. Med. J. Aust. 1:231, 1980.

Generic Name: Methacholine

Proprietary Name: Methacholine

Primary Use: *Systemic:* This quaternary ammonium parasympathomimetic agent is primarily used in the management of paroxysmal tachycardia, Raynaud's syndrome, and scleroderma. *Ophthalmic:* This topical agent is used in the management of narrow-angle glaucoma and in the diagnosis of Adie's pupil.

Ocular Side Effects:

A. Systemic Administration
  1. Decreased accommodation
B. Local Ophthalmic Use or Exposure
  1. Pupils
    a. No effect — normal pupil
    b. Miosis — Adie's pupil
  2. Decreased intraocular pressure

3. Eyelids or conjunctiva
   a. Allergic reactions
   b. Hyperemia
4. Myopia
5. Bloody tears
6. Blepharoclonus
7. Lacrimation

Clinical Significance: Topical ocular application of methacholine causes a number of ocular side effects; however, all are reversible and of minimal clinical importance. While miosis normally occurs with topical ocular 10 percent methacholine solutions, no effect is seen with 2.5 percent solutions except in patients with Adie's pupil or familial dysautonomia.

Interactions with Other Drugs:

A. Effect of Other Drugs on Activity of Methacholine
   1. Anticholinergics ↓
   2. Sympathomimetics ↓

References:

Ellis, P. P.: Ocular Therapeutics and Pharmacology. 5th Ed., St. Louis, C. V. Mosby, 1977, pp. 16, 47, 50, 187.
Gilman, A. G., Goodman, L. S., and Gilman, A. (Eds.): The Pharmacological Basis of Therapeutics. 6th Ed., New York, Macmillan, 1980, pp. 91–96.
Grant, W. M.: Toxicology of the Eye. 2nd Ed., Springfield, Charles C Thomas, 1974, pp. 706–718.
Havener, W. H.: Ocular Pharmacology. 4th Ed., St. Louis, C. V. Mosby, 1978, pp. 263 264.
Wade, A. (Ed.): Martindale: The Extra Pharmacopoeia. 27th Ed., London, Pharmaceutical Press, 1977, p. 997.

Generic Name: Metoprolol

Proprietary Name: Betaloc (G.B.), Lopressor, Seloken (Swed.)

Primary Use: This beta-adrenergic blocking agent is effective in the management of angina pectoris.

Ocular Side Effects:

A. Systemic Administration
   1. Decreased vision
   2. Eyelids or conjunctiva
      a. Hyperemia

    b. Conjunctivitis — nonspecific
    c. Urticaria
    d. Purpura
  3. Ocular pain
  4. Decreased lacrimation (?)
  5. Keratoconjunctivitis sicca (?)
  6. Visual hallucinations (?)
  7. Loss of eyelashes or eyebrows (?)

Clinical Significance: This beta blocker only rarely has been associated with adverse ocular effects. To date, the oculomucocutaneous syndrome associated with practolol use has not occurred with metoprolol. Some patients, however, have experienced dry eyes, decreased tear production, and minimal injection of conjunctiva and/or eyelids. Therefore, patients receiving metoprolol should be observed for potential ocular sicca problems.

Interactions with Other Drugs:

A. Effect of Metoprolol on Activity of Other Drugs
  1. Adrenergic blockers ↑
  2. Sympathomimetics ↓
B. Effect of Other Drugs on Activity of Metoprolol
  1. Adrenergic blockers ↑
C. Contraindications
  1. Myocardial depressant general anesthetic

References:

American Hospital Formulary Service. Washington, D.C., American Society of Hospital Pharmacists, Vol. I, 24:08, 1979.
Furhoff, A.-K., Nordlander, M., and Peterson, C.: Cross-sensitivity between practolol and other beta-blockers? Br. Med. J. 1:831, 1976.
Scott, D.: Another beta-blocker causing eye symptoms? Br. Med. J. 2:1221, 1977.
Van Joost, Th., Middelkamp Hup, J., and Ros, F. E.: Dermatitis as a side-effect of long-term topical treatment with certain beta-blocking agents. Br. J. Dermatol. 101:171, 1979.

Generic Name: Oxprenolol

Proprietary Name: Trasicor (G.B.)

Primary Use: This beta-adrenergic blocking agent is effective in the management of cardiac arrhythmias, angina pectoris, and hypertension.

Ocular Side Effects:

  A. Systemic Administration
      1. Decreased vision
      2. Eyelids or conjunctiva
          a. Allergic reactions
          b. Hyperemia
          c. Erythema
          d. Conjunctivitis — nonspecific
          e. Edema
          f. Hyperpigmentation
          g. Purpura
          h. Loss of eyelashes or eyebrows (?)
      3. Visual hallucinations
      4. Decreased lacrimation
      5. Myasthenic neuromuscular blocking effect (?)
      6. Oculomucocutaneous syndrome — keratoconjunctivitis sicca (?)
  B. Local Ophthalmic Use or Exposure
      1. Decreased intraocular pressure
      2. Miosis
      3. Punctate keratitis

Clinical Significance: This beta blocker only rarely causes ocular side effects, and they are usually transitory and insignificant. There is a suspicion, but no conclusive data, that oxprenolol has the potential to cause an oculomucocutaneous syndrome similar to that seen with practolol. At present, one can only closely follow the course of patients on this drug for ocular changes, especially signs of irritation and keratoconjunctivitis sicca. However, there have been a number of cases reported to the Registry of sudden onset keratoconjunctivitis sicca with marked conjunctival hyperemia.

Interactions with Other Drugs:

  A. Effect of Oxprenolol on Activity of Other Drugs
      1. Phenothiazines ↑
      2. Sympathomimetics ↑
      3. Tricyclic antidepressants ↑
      4. Antihistamines ↓

References:

Argov, A., and Mastaglia, F. L.: Disorders of neuromuscular transmission caused by drugs. N. Engl. J. Med. *301*:409, 1979.
Bron, A. J.: Mechanisms of ocular toxicity. In Gorrod, J. W. (Ed.): Drug Toxicity. London, Taylor & Frances, 1979, p. 237.

Bucci, M. G.: Topical administration of oxprenolol (beta blocking agent) in the therapy of the glaucoma. Preliminary note. Boll. Oculist. *54*:.235, 1975.

Harrower, A. D. B., and Strong, J. A.: Hyperpigmentation associated with oxprenolol administration. Br. Med. J. 2:296, 1977.

Holt, P. J. A., and Waddington, E.: Oculocutaneous reaction to oxprenolol. Br. Med. J. 2:539, 1975.

Hudson, W. A., and Finnis, W. A.: Oxprenolol and psoriasis-like eruptions. Lancet *1*:932, 1975.

Lewis, B. S., Setzen, M., and Kokoris, N.: Ocular reaction to oxprenolol. A case report. S. Afr. Med. J. *50*:482, 1976.

Wright, P., and Fraunfelder, F. T.: Practolol-induced oculomucocutaneous syndrome. In Leopold, I. H., and Burns, R. P. (Eds.): Symposium on Ocular Therapy. New York, John Wiley & Sons, Vol. IX, 1976, pp. 97–110.

Generic Name: Practolol

Proprietary Name: Eraldin (G.B.)

Primary Use: This beta-adrenergic blocking agent is effective in the management of angina pectoris, certain arrhythmias, and hypertension. It is also used as an adjunct to anesthesia and as a bronchodilator.

Ocular Side Effects:

A. Systemic Administration
1. Oculomucocutaneous syndrome — keratoconjunctivitis sicca
2. Foreign body sensation
3. Photophobia
4. Decreased lacrimation
5. Decreased vision
6. Conjunctiva
   a. Hyperemia
   b. Prominence of papillary tufts
   c. Areas of increased or decreased vascularity
   d. Scarring
   e. Keratinization
   f. Shrinkage — with obliteration of fornix
   g. Edema
7. Cornea
   a. Dense yellow or white stromal opacities
   b. Loss of stroma
   c. Perforation
   d. Ulceration
8. Eyelids
   a. Edema
   b. Erythema

      c. "Cafe au lait" pigmentation
      d. Lupoid syndrome
      e. Urticaria
      f. Exfoliative dermatitis
      g. Eczema
    9. Decreased tear lysozymes
   10. Myasthenic neuromuscular blocking effect (?)
  B. Local Ophthalmic Use or Exposure
    1. Decreased intraocular pressure

Clinical Significance: Ocular side effects due to practolol occur in approximately 0.2 percent of patients. The severity of the practolol-induced ocular changes is directly proportional to the length of time the patient has been taking the drug. If at the first signs of ocular involvement the drug is discontinued, all the ocular changes are reversible. However, if it remains unrecognized, this may lead to severe irreversible ocular changes including blindness. The most frequent adverse ocular reaction includes various degrees of keratoconjunctivitis sicca. This may progress to severe keratinization, scarring, and loss of conjunctival fornices. Sudden onset of corneal opacities with loss of stromal thickness leading to perforation has been seen. Adverse ocular reactions due to practolol may be unique since a serum intercellular antibody has been found in several patients. This antibody has also been found in the epithelium of eyes with practolol-induced disease. Possibly, this syndrome is due to an antibody that is a metabolite of practolol. While many of the signs and symptoms improve on withdrawal of the drug, reduction of tear secretion persists in most patients. The drug has been withdrawn from the market for general use but is still available in an injectable form for hospital use. To date, no clearcut oculomucocutaneous syndrome has been seen with any other beta-blocking drug.

Interactions with Other Drugs:

  A. Effect of Practolol on Activity of Other Drugs
    1. Alcohol ↑
    2. Analgesics ↑
    3. Barbiturates ↑
    4. General anesthetics ↑
    5. Phenothiazines ↑
    6. Sympathomimetics ↑↓
  B. Effect of Other Drugs on Activity of Practolol
    1. Alcohol ↑
    2. Analgesics ↑
    3. Barbiturates ↑

4. General anesthetics ↑
5. Phenothiazines ↑
6. Anticholinergics ↓

References:

Amos, H. E., Brigden, W. D., and McKerron, R. A.: Untoward effects associated with practolol: Demonstration of antibody binding to epithelial tissue. Br. Med. J. *1*:598, 1975.

Amos, H. E., Lake, B. G., and Artis, J.: Possible role of antibody specific for a practolol metabolite in the pathogenesis of oculomucocutaneous syndrome. Br. Med. J. *1*:402, 1978.

Felix, R. H., Ive, F. A., and Dahl, M. G. C.: Cutaneous and ocular reactions to practolol. Br. Med. J. *4*:321, 1974.

Raftery, E. B., and Denman, A. M.: Systemic lupus erythematosus syndrome induced by practolol. Br. Med. J. *2*:452, 1973.

Rahi, A. H. S., et al.: Pathology of practolol-induced ocular toxicity. Br. J. Ophthalmol. *60*:312, 1976.

Wright, P., and Fraunfelder, F. T.: Practolol-induced oculomucocutaneous syndrome. In Leopold, I. H., and Burns, R. P. (Eds.): Symposium on Ocular Therapy. New York, John Wiley & Sons, Vol. IX, 1976, pp. 97–110.

Wright, P.: Untoward effects associated with practolol administration: Oculomucocutaneous syndrome. Br. Med. J. *1*:595, 1975.

Generic Name: Propranolol

Proprietary Name: Dociton (Germ.), Herzul (Jap.), Inderal, Kemi (Jap.)

Primary Use: This beta-adrenergic blocking agent is effective in the management of angina pectoris, certain arrhythmias, hypertrophic subaortic stenosis, pheochromocytoma, and certain hypertensive states.

Ocular Side Effects:

A. Systemic Administration
1. Diplopia
2. Decreased vision
3. Eyelids or conjunctiva
   a. Allergic reactions
   b. Erythema
   c. Conjunctivitis — nonspecific
   d. Purpura
   e. Lupoid syndrome
   f. Erythema multiforme
   g. Stevens-Johnson syndrome
   h. Exfoliative dermatitis
   i. Loss of eyelashes or eyebrows (?)
4. Decreased intraocular pressure

5. Visual hallucinations
6. Decreased lacrimation (?)
7. Exophthalmos — withdrawal states
8. Myasthenic neuromuscular blocking effect
    a. Paralysis of extraocular muscles
    b. Ptosis

B. Local Ophthalmic Use or Exposure
    1. Decreased corneal reflex
    2. Conjunctival hyperemia
    3. Irritation
    4. Decreased intraocular pressure
    5. Miosis
    6. Decreased lacrimation (?)

Clinical Significance: Adverse ocular side effects due to propranolol are usually insignificant and transient. As with all beta-adrenergic blocking agents, one needs to be aware of the possibility of sicca-like syndrome. Although there now seem to be enough cases in the literature and in the Registry to implicate this drug in causing a keratoconjunctivitis sicca-like syndrome, it is not proved; if it does occur, it is a rare event. Topical ocular use has little clinical application, although it has been advocated for thyrotoxic lid retraction and glaucoma therapy. Although the combined use of oral propranolol and topical ophthalmic timolol is contraindicated, it is apparent that a synergistic effect in lowering intraocular pressure may occur in an occasional patient.

Interactions with Other Drugs:

A. Effect of Propranolol on Activity of Other Drugs
    1. Alcohol ↑
    2. Analgesics ↑
    3. Barbiturates ↑
    4. General anesthetics ↑
    5. Phenothiazines ↑
    6. Sympathomimetics ↑↓
B. Effect of Other Drugs on Activity of Propranolol
    1. Alcohol ↑
    2. Analgesics ↑
    3. Barbiturates ↑
    4. General anesthetics ↑
    5. Phenothiazines ↑
    6. Anticholinergics ↓
C. Synergistic Effect
    1. Timolol

References:

Argov, Z., and Mastaglia, F. L.: Disorders of neuromuscular transmission caused by drugs. N. Engl. J. Med. *301*:409, 1979.

Cass, E., Kadar, D., and Stein, H. A.: Hazards of phenylephrine topical medication in persons taking propranolol. Can. Med. Assoc. J. *120*:1261, 1979.

Cote, G., and Drance, S. M.: The effect of propranolol on human intraocular pressure. Can. J. Ophthalmol. 3:207, 1968.

Crombie, A. L., and Lawson, A. A. H.: Adrenergic blocking agents. Br. J. Ophthalmol. *52*:616, 1968.

Davidson, S. I.: Report of ocular adverse reactions. Trans. Ophthalmol. Soc. U.K. *93*:495, 1973.

Shenkman, L., Podrid, P., and Lowenstein, J.: Hyperthyroidism after propranolol withdrawal. JAMA *238*:237, 1977.

Sneddon, J. M., and Turner, P.: Adrenergic blockade and the eye signs of thyrotoxicosis. Lancet 2:525, 1966.

Generic Name: Quinidine

Proprietary Name: Biquin (Canad.), Cardioquin, Cin-Quin, Duraquin, Galactoquin (Germ.), Kinidin (G.B.), Maso-Quin, Prosedyl (Canad.), Quinaglute, Quinate (Canad.), Quinicardine, Quinidex, Quinora, SK-Quinidine

Primary Use: This isomer of quinine is effective in the treatment and prevention of atrial, nodal, and ventricular arrhythmias.

Ocular Side Effects:

A. Systemic Administration
   1. Decreased vision
   2. Problems with color vision — dyschromatopsia
   3. Mydriasis
   4. Visual fields
      a. Scotomas
      b. Constriction
   5. Photophobia
   6. Diplopia
   7. Night blindness
   8. Eyelids or conjunctiva
      a. Allergic reactions
      b. Photosensitivity
      c. Angioneurotic edema
      d. Urticaria
      e. Lupoid syndrome
      f. Exfoliative dermatitis

9. Subconjunctival or retinal hemorrhages secondary to drug-induced anemia
10. Optic neuritis
11. Myasthenic neuromuscular blocking effect
12. Anterior uveitis
13. Toxic amblyopia

Clinical Significance: Ocular side effects due to quinidine are rare, and most are transitory and reversible with discontinued use of the drug. Adverse ocular reactions are primarily dose-dependent and are cumulative. A presumably allergic reaction, including keratitic precipitates, flare and cells, and Koeppe nodules, has been described secondary to quinidine.

Interactions with Other Drugs:
A. Effect of Quinidine on Activity of Other Drugs
   1. Adrenergic blockers ↑
   2. Antibiotics (apnea) ↑
   3. Anticholinergics ↑
   4. Phenothiazines ↑
   5. Anticholinesterases ↓
B. Effect of Other Drugs on Activity of Quinidine
   1. Antacids ↑
   2. Anticholinergics ↑
   3. Carbonic anhydrase inhibitors ↑
   4. Phenothiazines ↑

References:
Alarcón-Segovia, D.: Drug-induced antinuclear antibodies and lupus syndromes. Drugs 12:69, 1976.
Argov, Z., and Mastaglia, F. L.: Disorders of neuromuscular transmission caused by drugs. N. Engl. J. Med. 301:409, 1979.
Is quinidine outdated?: Br. Med. J. 1:331, 1969.
Monninger, R., and Platt, D.: Toxic amblyopia due to quinidine. Am. J. Ophthalmol. 43:107, 1957.
Physicians' Desk Reference. 35th Ed., Oradell, N.J., Medical Economics Co., 1981, p. 1344.
Spitzberg, D. H.: Acute anterior uveitis secondary to quinidine sensitivity. Arch. Ophthalmol. 97:1993, 1979.
Taylor, D. R., and Potashnick, R.: Quinidine-induced exfoliative dermatitis. JAMA 145:641, 1951.

Class: Antihypertensive Agents

Generic Name: 1. Alkavervir; 2. Cryptenamine; 3. Protoveratrines A and B; 4. Veratrum Viride Alkaloids

Proprietary Name: 1. Veriloid; 2. Unitensen, Unitensyl (Canad.); 3. Pro-Amid, Puroverine (G.B.); 4. Gartrone, Vera-25/67

Primary Use: These veratrum alkaloids are used in the management of mild to moderate hypertension and various forms of renal dysfunction.

Ocular Side Effects:

A. Systemic Administration
   1. Decreased vision
   2. Mydriasis — may precipitate narrow-angle glaucoma
   3. Extraocular myotonia
   4. Constriction of visual fields (glaucoma patients)

Clinical Significance: Few ocular side effects have been reported for these drugs. All adverse ocular effects are reversible and rarely of clinical significance. However, in some glaucoma patients, a decrease in blood pressure can cause significant and even devastating loss of visual fields.

Interactions with Other Drugs:

A. Effect of Veratrum Alkaloids on Activity of Other Drugs
   1. Adrenergic blockers ↑
   2. General anesthetics ↑
   3. Monoamine oxidase inhibitors ↑
   4. Sympathomimetics ↑↓
   5. Tricyclic antidepressants ↓
B. Effect of Other Drugs on Activity of Veratrum Alkaloids
   1. Adrenergic blockers ↑
   2. Alcohol ↑
   3. Analgesics ↑
   4. General anesthetics ↑
   5. Monoamine oxidase inhibitors ↑
   6. Local anesthetics ↓
   7. Sympathomimetics ↓
   8. Tricyclic antidepressants ↓

References:

Beasley, J., and Robinson, K.: Intolerance to "verloid." Br. Med. J. *1*:316, 1954.
Bullock, J. D.: Antihypertensive drugs and danger to vision. JAMA 237:2186, 1977.
Dukes, M. N. G. (Ed.): Meyler's Side Effects of Drugs. Amsterdam, Excerpta Medica, Vol. VIII, 1975, p. 476.
Heilmann, K.: Glaukom und Hypertonie. MMW *116*:1821, 1974.

Kolb, E. J., and Korein, J.: Neuromuscular toxicity of veratrum alkaloids. Neurology 11:159, 1961.
Walsh, F. B., and Hoyt, W. F.: Clinical Neuro-Ophthalmology. 3rd Ed., Baltimore, Williams & Wilkins, Vol. III, 1969, p. 2655.

Generic Name: 1. Alseroxylon; 2. Deserpidine; 3. Rauwolfia Serpentina; 4. Rescinnamine; 5. Reserpine; 6. Syrosingopine

Proprietary Name: 1. Koglucoid, Raudolfin, Rau-Tab, Rautensin, Rauwiloid; 2. Harmonyl, Raunormine; 3. Austrawolf (Austral.), Hyper-Rauw, Hypertane (G.B.), Hypertensan (G.B.), Lesten (S. Afr.), Protium, Rau, Raudixin, Raufonol (Canad.), Rauja, Raumason, Rauneed, Raupena, Raupina (Germ.), Raupinetten (Germ.), Raupoid, Rauserfia, Rauserpa, Rausertina, Rautabs (Canad.), Rautensin (Austral., S. Afr.), Rautina, Rauval, Rauvolfia (G.B.), Rawfola, Rawlina (Austral.), Rivadescin (Germ.), Sarpagan (Fr.), Serfia, Serfolia, Serpetin (Jap.), T-Rau, Wolfina; 4. Cartric (Jap.), Cinnasil, Moderil; 5. Alkarau, Alserin (Canad.), Arcum R-S, Bonapene, Broserpine, De Serpa, Ebserpine (Canad.), Elserpine, Eskaserp, Hiserpia, Hyperine, Lemiserp, Maso-Serpine, Neo-Serp (Canad.), Rauloydin, Raurine, Rau-Sed, Rauserpin, Resedrex (Austral.), Resercen, Resercrine (Canad.), Reserjen, Reserpanca (Canad.), Reserpaneed, Reserpoid, Ryser (Austral.), Sandril, Sedaraupin (Germ.), Serfin, Serp, Serpalan, Serpaloid, Serpanray, Serpasil, Serpate, Serpax (Canad.), Serpena, Serpiloid (Austral.), Serpone (Canad.), Sertabs, Sertina, SK-Reserpine, Tenserp (Austral.), Tensin, T-Serp, Vio-Serpine, Zepine; 6. Syrosingopine

Primary Use: These rauwolfia alkaloids are used in the management of hypertension and agitated psychotic states.

Ocular Side Effects:

A. Systemic Administration
1. Conjunctival hyperemia
2. Horner's syndrome
    a. Miosis
    b. Ptosis
    c. Increased sensitivity to topical ocular epinephrine preparations
3. Nonspecific ocular irritation
    a. Lacrimation
    b. Hyperemia
4. Extraocular muscles
    a. Oculogyric crises

     b. Decreased spontaneous movements
     c. Abnormal conjugate deviations
     d. Jerky pursuit movements
  5. Decreased vision
  6. Retinal hemorrhages
  7. Decreased intraocular pressure
  8. Mydriasis — may precipitate narrow-angle glaucoma
  9. Problems with color vision
     a. Dyschromatopsia
     b. Objects have yellow tinge
  10. Eyelids or conjunctiva — lupoid syndrome
  11. Optic atrophy (?)
  12. Uveitis (?)

Clinical Significance: Most of the preceding ocular side effects have been primarily due to reserpine instead of the other rauwolfia alkaloids. However, the general toxicity of deserpidine and rescinnamine is said to be about the same as that of reserpine. The other drugs listed are probably less toxic. Ocular side effects are not uncommon, but nearly all are reversible.

Interactions with Other Drugs:

  A. Effect of Rauwolfia Alkaloids on Activity of Other Drugs
     1. Alcohol ↑
     2. Barbiturates ↑
     3. General anesthetics ↑
     4. Monoamine oxidase inhibitors ↑
     5. Sympathomimetics ↑↓
     6. Analgesics ↓
     7. Anticholinergics ↓
     8. Salicylates ↓
  B. Effect of Other Drugs on Activity of Rauwolfia Alkaloids
     1. Adrenergic blockers ↑
     2. Alcohol ↑
     3. Antihistamines ↑
     4. General anesthetics ↑
     5. Phenothiazines ↑
     6. Monoamine oxidase inhibitors ↑↓
     7. Sympathomimetics ↓
     8. Tricyclic antidepressants ↓

References:

Alarcón-Segovia, D.: Drug-induced antinuclear antibodies and lupus syndromes. Drugs *12*:69, 1976.

Freedman, D. X., and Benton, A. J.: Persisting effects of reserpine in man. N. Engl. J. Med. *264:*529, 1961.

Kaplan, M. R., and Pilger, I. S.: The effect of rauwolfia serpentina derivatives on intraocular pressure. Am. J. Ophthalmol. *43:*550, 1957.

Kline, N. S., Barsa, J., and Gosline, E.: Management of side effects of reserpine and combined reserpine-chlorpromazine treatment. Dis. Nerv. Syst. *17:*352, 1956.

Raymond, L. F.: Ocular pathology in reserpine sensitivity: Report of two cases. J. Med. Soc. N. J. *60:*417, 1963.

Walsh, F. B., and Hoyt, W. F.: Clinical Neuro-Ophthalmology. 3rd Ed., Baltimore, Williams & Wilkins, Vol. I and Vol. III, 1969, pp. 447, 2638, 2668.

Generic Name: Clonidine

Proprietary Name: *Systemic:* Catapres, Catapresan (Germ., Swed.), Catapressan (Fr.), Dixarit (G.B.) *Ophthalmic:* Isoglaucon (Germ.)

Primary Use: *Systemic:* This alpha-adrenergic agonist is used in the management of hypertension. *Ophthalmic:* Topical ocular clonidine has been used investigationally to reduce intraocular pressure.

Ocular Side Effects:

A. Systemic Administration
  1. Decreased vision
  2. Decreased intraocular pressure
  3. Eyelids or conjunctiva
    a. Angioneurotic edema
    b. Urticaria
    c. Pemphigoid lesion with or without symblepharon (?)
  4. Nonspecific ocular irritation
  5. Visual hallucinations
  6. Pupils
    a. Miosis — toxic states
    b. Absence of reaction to light — toxic states
  7. Diplopia (?)
  8. Keratoconjunctivitis sicca (?)
  9. Flashing lights (?)
  10. Retinal or macular
    a. Degeneration (?)
    b. Pigmentary changes (?)
B. Local Ophthalmic Use or Exposure
  1. Decreased intraocular pressure
  2. Eyelids or conjunctiva
    a. Angioneurotic edema
    b. Urticaria
  3. Mydriasis — may precipitate narrow-angle glaucoma

Clinical Significance: Clonidine has only recently been made commercially available in the United States. All reported side effects have been inconsequential and ceased after the removal of the drug or even while the drug was continued, except for possible retinal changes. Although retinal changes have been noted in laboratory animals, only 7 human cases have been reported to the Registry; it is difficult to say if these are just coincidental or in fact due to this agent. Retinal changes which have been reported in humans include depigmentation of the retinal and macular areas with decrease in vision. One additional case reported bilateral retinal tears which occurred within 2 days after starting this agent. There is a question whether glaucoma patients do indeed have progression of their visual fields, resulting from a decrease in the systolic and diastolic pressures, when started on systemic clonidine. Systemic clonidine has a minimal effect on pupillary changes, except in toxic dosages. Initially, there is marked constriction of the pupil at the toxic level; however, a toxic dose may cause pupillary dilatation in time. Since systemic clonidine has caused vulval pemphigoid, ocular signs of cicatricial pemphigoid must also be watched for. Topical ocular clonidine is well tolerated, causes minimal pupillary changes, and will decrease intraocular pressure 10 to 40 percent. An additional effect due to the drug may occur in the untreated contralateral eye, possibly from decrease in systemic blood pressure.

Interactions with Other Drugs:

A. Effect of Clonidine on Activity of other Drugs
 1. Adrenergic blockers ↑
 2. Alcohol ↑
 3. Barbiturates ↑
 4. Sedatives and hypnotics ↑
B. Effect of Other Drugs on Activity of Clonidine
 1. Adrenergic blockers ↑

References:

Harrison, R., and Kaufmann, C. S.: Clonidine. Effects of a topically administered solution on intraocular pressure and blood pressure in open-angle glaucoma. Arch. Ophthalmol. 95:1368, 1977.

Hodapp, E., et al.: The effect of topical clonidine on intraocular pressure. Arch. Ophthalmol. 99:1208, 1981.

Krieglstein, G. K., Langham, M. E., and Leydhecker, W.: The peripheral and central neural actions of clonidine in normal and glaucomatous eyes. Invest. Ophthalmol. Visual Sci. 17:149, 1978.

MacFaul, R., and Miller, G.: Clonidine poisoning in children. Lancet 1:1266, 1977.

Pai, G. S., and Lipsitz, D. J.: Clonidine poisoning. Pediatrics 58:749, 1976.

Van Joost, T. H., Faber, W. R., and Manuel, H. R.: Drug-induced anogenital pemphigoid. Br. J. Dermatol. 102:715, 1980.

Generic Name: Diazoxide

Proprietary Name: Eudemine (G.B.), Hyperstat, Proglicem (S. Afr.), Proglycem

Primary Use: This nondiuretic benzothiadiazine derivative is used in the emergency treatment of malignant hypertension.

Ocular Side Effects:

A. Systemic Administration
   1. Lacrimation
   2. Eyelids or conjunctiva
      a. Allergic reactions
      b. Erythema
   3. Decreased vision
   4. Cataracts
   5. Ring scotomas
   6. Diplopia
   7. Subconjunctival or retinal hemorrhages secondary to drug-induced anemia

Clinical Significance: Ocular side effects due to diazoxide are uncommon except for increased lacrimation, which occurs in up to 20 percent of patients taking this agent. In some instances, the lacrimation continued long after discontinued use of diazoxide. The cause of this unusual phenomenon is unknown. Acute reversible cataracts are extremely rare and are seen primarily in infants as a result of osmotic imbalance in hyperglycemia and hyperosmolar coma.

Interactions with Other Drugs:

A. Effect of Diazoxide on Activity of Other Drugs
   1. Tricyclic antidepressants ↑
B. Effect of Other Drugs on Activity of Diazoxide
   1. Adrenergic blockers ↑
   2. Alcohol ↑
   3. Analgesics ↑
   4. Monoamine oxidase inhibitors ↑
   5. Tricyclic antidepressants ↑

References:

AMA Drug Evaluations. 4th Ed., New York, John Wiley & Sons, 1980, pp. 580–581.
American Hospital Formulary Service. Washington, D.C., American Society of Hospital Pharmacists, Vol. I, 24:08, 1977.

Grant, W. M.: Toxicology of the Eye. 2nd Ed., Springfield, Charles C Thomas, 1974, p. 360.

Physicians' Desk Reference. 35th Ed., Oradell, N.J., Medical Economics Co., 1981, p. 1610.

Thomson, A., et al.: Clinical observations on an antihypertensive chlorothiazide analogue devoid of diuretic activity. Can. Med. Assoc. J. 87:1306, 1962.

Wade, A. (Ed.): Martindale: The Extra Pharmacopoeia. 27th Ed., London, Pharmaceutical Press, 1977, pp. 624–626.

Generic Name: Furosemide. See under *Diuretics*.

Generic Name: Guanethidine

Proprietary Name: *Systemic:* Ismelin *Ophthalmic:* Ismelin (G.B.)

Primary Use: *Systemic:* This adrenergic blocker is effective in the treatment of moderate to severe hypertension. *Ophthalmic:* This topical adrenergic blocker is used in the management of open-angle glaucoma and lid retraction due to thyroid disorders.

Ocular Side Effects:

A. Systemic Administration
1. Decreased vision
2. Nonspecific ocular irritation
   a. Hyperemia
   b. Photophobia
   c. Edema
3. Horner's syndrome
   a. Miosis
   b. Ptosis
   c. Enophthalmos (?)
4. Diplopia
5. Decreased intraocular pressure
6. Accommodative spasm
7. Flashing lights
8. Subconjunctival or retinal hemorrhages secondary to drug-induced anemia
9. Retinal vasospasms (?)
10. Loss of eyelashes or eyebrows (?)

B. Local Ophthalmic Use or Exposure
1. Irritation
   a. Hyperemia

        b. Photophobia
        c. Ocular pain
        d. Edema
        e. Burning sensation
   2. Horner's syndrome
        a. Miosis
        b. Ptosis
        c. Enophthalmos
   3. Decreased intraocular pressure
   4. Mydriasis
   5. Punctate keratitis
   6. Exacerbation of viral keratoconjunctivitis (?)

Clinical Significance: Topical ocular application or systemic administration of guanethidine frequently causes ocular side effects. These adverse ocular reactions are reversible and transitory with discontinued use of the drug. With time, the desired topical ocular response of decreased intraocular pressure may be lost.

Interactions with Other Drugs:

A. Effect of Guanethidine on Activity of Other Drugs
   1. General anesthetics ↑
   2. Monoamine oxidase inhibitors ↑
   3. Sympathomimetics ↑↓
   4. Anticholinergics ↓
B. Effect of Other Drugs on Activity of Guanethidine
   1. Alcohol ↑
   2. General anesthetics ↑
   3. Phenothiazines ↑↓
   4. Antihistamines ↓
   5. Local anesthetics ↓
   6. Monoamine oxidase inhibitors ↓
   7. Sympathomimetics ↓
   8. Tricyclic antidepressants ↓

References:

American Hospital Formulary Service. Washington, D.C., American Society of Hospital Pharmacists, Vol. I, 24:08, 1977.

Bonomi, L., and Di Comite, P.: Outflow facility after guanethidine sulfate administration. Arch. Ophthalmol. 78:337, 1967.

Cant, J. S., and Lewis, D. R. H.: Unwanted pharmacological effects of local guanethidine in the treatment of dysthyroid upper lid retraction. Br. J. Ophthalmol. 53:239, 1969.

Crombie, A. L., and Lawson, A. A. H.: Long-term trial of local guanethidine in treatment of eye signs of thyroid dysfunction and idiopathic lid retraction. Br. Med. J. 4:592, 1967.

Davidson, S. I.: Reports of ocular adverse reactions. Trans. Ophthalmol. Soc. U.K. 93:495, 1973.
Gay, A. J., and Wolkstein, M. A.: Topical guanethidine therapy for endocrine lid retraction. Arch. Ophthalmol. 76:364, 1966.
Gloster, J.: Guanethidine and glaucoma. Trans. Ophthalmol. Soc. U.K. 94:573, 1974.
Jones, D. E. P., Norton, D. A., and Davies, D. J. G.: Control of glaucoma by reduced dosage guanethidine-adrenaline formulation. Br. J. Ophthalmol. 63:813, 1979.

Generic Name: Hexamethonium

Proprietary Name: Hexamethonium

Primary Use: This ganglionic blocking agent is used primarily in emergency hypertensive crises.

Ocular Side Effects:

A. Systemic Administration
1. Decreased vision
2. Mydriasis — may precipitate narrow-angle glaucoma
3. Paralysis of accommodation
4. Macular edema
5. Decreased lacrimation
6. Decreased intraocular pressure
7. Visual fields
   a. Constriction
   b. Hemianopsia
8. Conjunctival edema
9. Retinal vasodilatation
10. Optic atrophy
11. Toxic amblyopia
12. Periorbital edema (?)

Clinical Significance: Hexamethonium frequently causes adverse ocular reactions, but the drug itself is rarely used except in severe end-stage hypertension or in a hypertensive crisis. While decreased vision, mydriasis, and paralysis of accommodation are common and reversible, most other ocular side effects are infrequent. Many of the drug-induced ocular side effects can be explained by a rapid change in the blood pressure.

Interactions with Other Drugs:

A. Effect of Hexamethonium on Activity of Other Drugs
1. Carbonic anhydrase inhibitors ↑
2. Sympathomimetics ↑
3. Anticholinesterases ↓

B. Effect of Other Drugs on Activity of Hexamethonium
1. Alcohol ↑
2. Monoamine oxidase inhibitors ↑

References:

Barnett, A. J.: Ocular effects of methonium compounds. Br. J. Ophthalmol. 36:593, 1952.
Bruce, G. M.: Permanent bilateral blindness following use of hexamethonium chloride. Arch. Ophthalmol. 54:422, 1955.
Cameron, A. J., and Burn, R. A.: Hexamethonium and glaucoma. Br. J. Ophthalmol. 36:482, 1952.
Goldsmith, A. J., and Hewer, A. J.: Unilateral amaurosis with partial recovery after using hexamethonium iodide. Br. Med. J. 2:759, 1952.
Walsh, F. B., and Hoyt, W. F.: Clinical Neuro-Ophthalmology. 3rd Ed., Baltimore, Williams & Wilkins, Vol. III, 1969, pp. 2667–2668.

Generic Name: Hydralazine

Proprietary Name: Aprelazine (Jap.), Apresoline, Dralzine, Hydrallazine (G.B.), Hydralyn, Hyperazin (Jap.)

Primary Use: This phthalazine derivative is effective in the management of essential or malignant hypertension, hypertensive complications of pregnancy, and hypertension associated with acute glomerulonephritis.

Ocular Side Effects:

A. Systemic Administration
1. Decreased vision
2. Nonspecific ocular irritation
   a. Lacrimation
   b. Photophobia
3. Eyelids or conjunctiva
   a. Allergic reactions
   b. Erythema
   c. Conjunctivitis — nonspecific
   d. Edema
   e. Urticaria
   f. Lupoid syndrome
4. Periorbital edema
5. Colored flashing lights
6. Subconjunctival or retinal hemorrhages secondary to drug-induced anemia

Clinical Significance: All ocular side effects due to hydralazine are reversible, transient, and seldom of clinical significance.

Interactions with Other Drugs:

A. Effect of Hydralazine on Activity of Other Drugs
   1. General anesthetics ↑
   2. Monoamine oxidase inhibitors ↑
   3. Sympathomimetics ↑↓
B. Effect of Other Drugs on Activity of Hydralazine
   1. Alcohol ↑
   2. Diuretics ↑
   3. General anesthetics ↑
   4. Monoamine oxidase inhibitors ↑↓
   5. Sympathomimetics ↓
   6. Tricyclic antidepressants ↓

References:

Grob, D., Langford, H. G., and Ziegler, B.: Further observations on the effects of autonomic blocking agents in patients with hypertension. 1. General systemic effects of Hexamethonine, Pentamethonium and Hydrazinophthalazine. Circulation 8:205, 1953.
Reidenberg, M. M.: Adverse drug reactions: Special cases of chemically-induced diseases. Trends Pharmacol. Sci. *1*:180, 1980.
von Oettingen, W. F.: Poisoning: A Guide to Clinical Diagnosis and Treatment. 2nd Ed., Philadelphia, W. B. Saunders, 1958.
Wade, A. (Ed.): Martindale: The Extra Pharmacopoeia. 27th Ed., London, Pharmaceutical Press, 1977, pp. 664–665.
Walsh, F. B., and Hoyt, W. F.: Clinical Neuro-Ophthalmology. 3rd Ed., Baltimore, Williams & Wilkins, Vol. III, 1969, p. 2668.

Generic Name: 1. Mecamylamine; 2. Pentolinium; 3. Tetraethylammonium; 4. Trimethaphan (Trimetaphan); 5. Trimethidinium

Proprietary Name: 1. Inversine, Mevasine (Austral., Germ., S. Afr., Swed.); 2. Ansolysen (G.B.); 3. Tetraethylammonium; 4. Arfonad; 5. Trimethidinium

Primary Use: These ganglionic blocking agents are used in the management of moderate to severe hypertension and are used to produce controlled hypotension for the reduction of surgical hemorrhage.

Ocular Side Effects:

A. Systemic Administration
   1. Decreased vision
   2. Mydriasis — may precipitate narrow-angle glaucoma
   3. Paralysis of accommodation
   4. Conjunctival edema
   5. Decreased intraocular pressure

  6. Myasthenic neuromuscular blocking effect (tetraethylammonium, trimethaphan)
    a. Ptosis
  7. Colored flashing lights (mecamylamine)
  8. Eyelids — urticaria (trimethaphan)

Clinical Significance: Although ocular side effects due to the ganglionic blocking agents are common, they are transitory, reversible, and seldom of major significance. Since these drugs can cause profound hypotensive episodes, visual complaints probably occur on a cerebral basis. Mydriasis and cycloplegic effects are probably due to the parasympatholytic effect of these drugs. Side effects tend to become less pronounced as administration of the drug is continued.

Interaction with Other Drugs:

  A. Effect of Ganglionic Blocking Agents on Activity of Other Drugs
    1. Carbonic anhydrase inhibitors ↑
    2. Diuretics ↑
    3. General anesthetics ↑
    4. Monoamine oxidase inhibitors ↑
    5. Sympathomimetics ↑↓
    6. Anticholinesterases ↓
  B. Effect of Other Drugs on Activity of Ganglionic Blocking Agents
    1. Adrenergic blockers ↑
    2. Alcohol ↑
    3. Carbonic anhydrase inhibitors ↑
    4. Diuretics ↑
    5. General anesthetics ↑
    6. Monoamine oxidase inhibitors ↑
    7. Phenothiazines ↑
    8. Sympathomimetics ↑↓
    9. Anticholinesterases ↓
    10. Tricyclic antidepressants ↓

References:

American Hospital Formulary Service. Washington, D.C., American Society of Hospital Pharmacists, Vol. I, 24:08, 1977.

Argov, Z., and Mastaglia, F. L.: Disorders of neuromuscular transmission caused by drugs. N. Engl. J. Med. 301:409, 1979.

Drucker, A. P., Sadove, M. S., and Unna, K.: Ocular manfiestations of intravenous tetraethylammonium chloride in man. Am. J. Ophthalmol. 33:1564, 1950.

von Oettingen, W. F.: Poisoning: A Guide to Clinical Diagnosis and Treatment. 2nd Ed., Philadelphia, W. B. Saunders, 1958.

Walsh, F. B., and Hoyt, W. F.: Clinical Neuro-Ophthalmology. 3rd Ed., Baltimore, Williams & Wilkins, Vol. III, 1969, p. 2668.

Windholz, M. (Ed.): The Merck Index: An Encyclopedia of Chemicals and Drugs. 9th Ed., Rahway, N.J., Merck and Co., Inc., 1976.

Generic Name: Methyldopa

Proprietary Name: Aldomet, Aldometil (Germ.), Co-Caps Methyldopa (G.B.), Dopamet (G.B.), Hyperpaxa (Swed.), Medomet (G.B.), Methoplain (Jap.), Presinol (Germ.), Sembrina (Germ.)

Primary Use: This adrenergic blocker is effective in the management of acute or severe hypertension.

Ocular Side Effects:

A. Systemic Administration
1. Decreased vision
2. Decreased intraocular pressure — minimal
3. Eyelids or conjunctiva
   a. Allergic reactions
   b. Hyperemia
   c. Conjunctivitis — nonspecific
   d. Edema
   e. Urticaria
   f. Lupoid syndrome
   g. Eczema
4. Subconjunctival or retinal hemorrhages secondary to drug-induced anemia
5. Paralysis of extraocular muscles
6. Keratoconjunctivitis sicca
7. Visual hallucinations
8. Hemianopsia
9. Decreased lacrimation

Clinical Significance: Adverse ocular side effects due to methyldopa are rare and usually insignificant. Lowering of intraocular pressure due to this drug has been documented; however, this decrease is only minimal. There have been a number of reports associating this drug with the onset of keratoconjunctivitis sicca. Although a cause-and-effect relationship is difficult to prove, some cases of keratoconjunctivitis sicca improved upon discontinuation of the drug. Only one case of Bell's palsy has been reported, and this may well have been coincidental.

Interactions with Other Drugs:

A. Effect of Methyldopa on Activity of Other Drugs
1. General anesthetics ↑
2. Monoamine oxidase inhibitors ↑
3. Sympathomimetics ↑↓
4. Tricyclic antidepressants ↓

B. Effect of Other Drugs on Activity of Methyldopa
    1. Adrenergic blockers ↑
    2. Alcohol ↑
    3. General anesthetics ↑
    4. Phenothiazines ↑
    5. Monoamine oxidase inhibitors ↑↓
    6. Barbiturates ↓
    7. Sympathomimetics ↓
    8. Tricyclic antidepressants ↓

References:

Alarcón-Segovia, D.: Drug-induced antinuclear antibodies and lupus syndromes. Drugs *12*:69, 1976.
AMA Drug Evaluations. 4th Ed., New York, John Wiley & Sons. 1980, pp. 570–571.
American Hospital Formulary Service. Washington, D.C., American Society of Hospital Pharmacists, Vol. I, *24*:08, 1977.
Chan, W.: Less common side effects of methyldopa. Med. J. Aust. 2:14, 1977.
Cove, D. H., et al.: Blindness after treatment for malignant hypertension. Br. Med. J. 2:245, 1979.
Davidson, S. I.: Reports of ocular adverse reactions. Trans. Ophthalmol. Soc. U.K. *93*:495, 1973.
Endo, M., Hirai, K., and Ohara, M.: Paranoid-hallucinatory state induced in a depressive patient by methyldopa: A case report. Psychoneuroendocrinology 3:211, 1978.
Okun, R., et al.: Long-term effectiveness of methyldopa in hypertension. Calif. Med. *104*:46, 1966.
Peczon, J. D.: Effect of methyldopa on intraocular pressure in human eyes. Am. J. Ophthalmol. *60*:82, 1965.
Suda, K., et al.: On the hypotensive effect of Aldomet. J. Clin. Ophthalmol. *18*:191, 1964.

Generic Name: Pargyline

Proprietary Name: Eutonyl

Primary Use: This nonhydrazine monoamine oxidase inhibitor is used in the treatment of moderate to severe hypertension.

Ocular Side Effects:

A. Systemic Administration
    1. Pupils
        a. Mydriasis
        b. Decreased reaction to light
    2. Decreased accommodation
    3. Visual hallucinations

4. Hyperactive eye movements
5. Problems with color vision — dyschromatopsia, red-green defect
B. Local Ophthalmic Use or Exposure
1. Decreased intraocular pressure

Clinical Significance: Significant ocular side effects due to pargyline are rare, and those reported are primarily in overdose situations. Optic nerve damage has not been found as a side effect of this drug, although it has been seen with other monoamine oxidase inhibitors. A well-documented study has reported a significant decrease in intraocular pressure in patients with chronic simple or absolute glaucoma following application of topical ocular pargyline.

Interactions with Other Drugs:

A. Effect of Pargyline on Activity of Other Drugs
1. Alcohol ↑
2. Analgesics ↑
3. Anticholinergics ↑
4. Antihistamines ↑
5. Barbiturates ↑
6. Carbonic anhydrase inhibitors ↑
7. General anesthetics ↑
8. Monoamine oxidase inhibitors ↑
9. Sedatives and hypnotics ↑
10. Sympathomimetics ↑
11. Tricyclic antidepressants ↑
12. Local anesthetics ↑↓
13. Phenothiazines ↑↓
14. Adrenergic blockers ↓
B. Effect of Other Drugs on Activity of Pargyline
1. Adrenergic blockers ↑
2. Diuretics ↑
3. General anesthetics ↑
4. Monoamine oxidase inhibitors ↑
5. Tricyclic antidepressants ↑
6. Analgesics ↑↓
7. Phenothiazines ↑↓
8. Alcohol ↓
9. Barbiturates ↓

References:

Grant, W. M.: Toxicology of the Eye. 2nd Ed., Springfield, Charles C Thomas, 1974, pp. 788–789.

Lipkin, D., and Kushnick, T.: Pargyline hydrochloride poisoning in a child. JAMA *201*:135, 1967.

Mehra, K. S., Roy, P. N., and Singh, R.: Pargyline drops in glaucoma. Arch. Ophthalmol. *92*:453, 1974.

Sutnick, A. I., et al.: Psychotic reactions during therapy with pargyline. JAMA *188*: 610, 1964.

Walsh, F. B., and Hoyt, W. F.: Clinical Neuro-Ophthalmology. 3rd Ed., Baltimore, Williams & Wilkins, Vol. III, 1969, p. 2628.

Class: Digitalis Glycosides

Generic Name: 1. Acetyldigitoxin; 2. Deslanoside; 3. Digitoxin; 4. Digoxin; 5. Gitalin; 6. Lanatoside C; 7. Ouabain

Proprietary Name: 1. Acylanid, Acylanide (Fr.); 2. Cedilanid-D, Desace (Fr.); 3. Crystodigin, De-Tone, Digilong (Germ.), Digimed (Germ.), Digimerck (Germ.), Digisidin, Digitaline, Digitox (Austral.), Digitrin (Swed.), Ditaven (Germ.), Maso-Toxin, Purodigin, Unidigin; 4. Cardiox (Austral.), Coragoxine (Fr.), Davoxin, Dialoxin (Austral.), Digacin (Germ.), Diganox (G.B.), Digolan (Austral.), Digoxine (Fr.), Fibroxin (Austral.), Lanacrist (Swed.), Lanatoxin (Germ.), Lanicor (Germ.), Lanoxin, Masoxin, Natigoxin (Austral.), Natigoxine (Canad.), Novodigal (Germ.), Prodigox (Austral.), Rougoxin (Canad.), SK-Digoxin, Winoxin (Canad.); 5. Cristaloxine (Fr.), Gitaligin; 6. Cedilanid, Celadigal (Germ.), Ceto Sanol (Germ.), Lanimerck (Austral., Germ.), Lanocide (Austral.); 7. Ouabaine (G.B.), Purostrophan (Germ.), Strodival (Germ.), Strophoperm (Germ.)

Primary Use: Digitalis glycosides are effective in the control of congestive heart failure and certain arrhythmias.

Ocular Side Effects:

A. Systemic Administration
 1. Problems with color vision
   a. Dyschromatopsia, blue-yellow defect
   b. Objects have yellow, green, blue, or red tinge
   c. Colored haloes around lights — mainly blue
 2. Visual sensations
   a. Flickering vision — often yellow or green
   b. Colored borders to objects
   c. Glare phenomenon — objects appear covered with brown, orange, or white snow

      d. Light flashes
      e. Scintillating scotomas
      f. Frosted appearance of objects
    3. Scotomas — central or paracentral
    4. Decreased vision
    5. Abnormal ERG
    6. Diplopia
    7. Decreased intraocular pressure
    8. Retrobulbar neuritis
    9. Eyelids or conjunctiva
      a. Allergic reactions
      b. Angioneurotic edema
  10. Mydriasis (digoxin)
  11. Visual hallucinations (digoxin)
  12. Paresis of extraocular muscles (digitoxin)
  13. Photophobia (digitoxin)

Clinical Significance: Nearly all of the ocular side effects due to the digitalis glycosides are reversible. They are most frequently seen with the long-acting agents such as digoxin or digitoxin, and least often with short-acting agents such as ouabain. The most unique adverse ocular reaction to this group of drugs is the glare phenomenon or the snowy appearance of objects. While common to all the drugs in this group, it is severest and most frequent with acetyldigitoxin. Adjustment of the clinical dose may be done in part with color vision testing. Since one of the first signs of digitalis glycoside toxicity is disturbance of the yellow-blue axis of color vision, testing in this area can aid in the adjustments of therapy. However, since possibly only about 25 percent of patients in the toxic range have ocular manifestations, one should not rely too heavily on this test. Alterations in both light- and dark-adapted cone-mediated ERG amplitudes have been described as a retinal toxic reaction from cardiac glycosides. Individuals in whom cone dysfunction is diagnosed should be carefully questioned regarding cardiac medications, especially since digitalis glycoside toxicity can be made worse by concomitant quinidine. Intraocular pressure may be decreased by deslanoside, digitoxin, digoxin, gitalin, and lanatoside C. Clinical use of these drugs for the treatment of glaucoma is not practical since the required therapeutic systemic dose is very near toxic levels. Topical ocular application of these agents causes keratopathy.

Interactions with Other Drugs:
A. Effect of Digitalis Glycosides on Activity of Other Drugs
    1. Adrenergic blockers ↑
    2. Sympathomimetics ↑

B. Effect of Other Drugs on Activity of Digitalis Glycosides
1. Adrenergic blockers ↑
2. Quinidine ↑
3. Sympathomimetics ↑
4. Antacids ↓
5. Barbiturates ↓
6. Phenylbutazone ↓

References:

AMA Drug Evaluations. 4th Ed., New York, John Wiley & Sons, 1980, pp. 497–506.
Grant, W. M.: Toxicology of the Eye. 2nd Ed., Springfield, Charles C Thomas, 1974, p. 244.
Lely, A. H., and Van Enter, C. H. J.: Large scale digitoxin intoxication. Br. Med. J. 3:737, 1970.
Manninen, V.: Impaired colour vision in diagnosis of digitalis intoxication. Br. Med. J. 4:653, 1974.
Physicians' Desk Reference. 35th Ed., Oradell, N.J., Medical Economics Co., 1981, pp. 755, 1571, 1609.
Robertson, D. M., Hollenhorst, R. W., and Callahan, J. A.: Ocular manifestations of digitalis toxicity. Arch. Ophthalmol. 76:640, 1966.
Taylor, W. O. G.: Impaired colour vision in diagnosis of digitalis intoxication. Br. Med. J. 1:271, 1975.
Weleber, R. G., and Shults, W. T.: Digoxin retinal toxicity. Clinical and electrophysiologic evaluation of a cone dysfunction syndrome. Arch. Ophthalmol. 99:1568, 1981.

Generic Name: Digitalis

Proprietary Name: Digifortis, Digiglusin, Digiplex (Fr.), Digitalysat (Germ.), Pil-Digis

Primary Use: The active constituents of digitalis are the glycosides which are effective in the control of congestive heart failure and certain arrhythmias.

Ocular Side Effects:

A. Systemic Administration
1. Problems with color vision
    a. Dyschromatopsia, blue-yellow or red-green defect
    b. Objects have yellow, green, blue, or red tinge
    c. Colored haloes around lights — mainly blue
2. Visual sensations
    a. Flickering vision — often yellow or green
    b. Colored borders to objects
    c. Glare phenomenon — objects appear covered with brown, orange, or white snow

      d. Light flashes
      e. Scintillating scotomas
      f. Frosted appearance of objects
  3. Decreased vision
  4. Visual fields
      a. Scotomas — central or paracentral
      b. Constriction
  5. Photophobia
  6. Abnormal ERG
  7. Mydriasis
  8. Visual hallucinations — especially bright floating spots
  9. Diplopia
10. Ptosis
11. Paresis of extraocular muscles
12. Accommodative spasm
13. Eyelids or conjunctiva
      a. Allergic reactions
      b. Angioneurotic edema
      c. Urticaria
      d. Lupoid syndrome
14. Toxic amblyopia
15. Retrobulbar or optic neuritis
16. Myopia (?)

Clinical Significance: Ocular side effects are common with digitalis and are probably seen more frequently with it than with all the other digitalis glycosides combined. Most of the ocular side effects are transitory and reversible. The glare phenomenon and disturbances with color vision are the most striking and the most common adverse ocular reactions seen. Most patients on digitalis therapy are also taking numerous other drugs, and it may be difficult to decide which side effect is due to which medication. A recent report suggests that after long-term digitalis therapy, a reversible red-green color defect occurs in the majority of patients. Adjusting one's clinical dose may be done in part by color vision testing. Since one of the first signs of digitalis toxicity is disturbance of the yellow-blue axis of color vision, testing in this area can aid the adjustment of therapy. However, although at least 25 percent of patients in the toxic range have ocular manifestations, this test is not infallible and has limited clinical importance.

Interactions with Other Drugs:

  A. Effect of Digitalis on Activity of Other Drugs
     1. Adrenergic blockers ↑
     2. Sympathomimetics ↑

B. Effect of Other Drugs on Activity of Digitalis
1. Adrenergic blockers ↑
2. Sympathomimetics ↑
3. Antacids ↓
4. Barbiturates ↓
5. Phenylbutazone ↓

References:

American Hospital Formulary Service. Washington, D.C., American Society of Hospital Pharmacists, Vol. I, 24:04, 1978.
Cluff, L. E., Caranasos, G. J., and Stewart, R. B.: Clinical Problems with Drugs. Philadelphia, W. B. Saunders, 1975, pp. 207–212.
Crews, S. J.: Ocular adverse reactions to drugs. Practitioner 219:72, 1977.
Gilman, A. G., Goodman, L. S., and Gilman, A. (Eds.): The Pharmacological Basis of Therapeutics. 6th Ed., New York, Macmillan, 1980, pp. 729–760.
Manninen, V.: Impaired colour vision in diagnosis of digitalis intoxication. Br. Med. J. 4:653, 1974.
Peczon, J. D.: Clinical evaluation of digitalization in glaucoma. Arch. Ophthalmol. 71:500, 1964.
Sprague, H. B., White, P. D., and Kellogg, J. F.: Disturbances of vision due to digitalis. JAMA 85:716, 1925.
White, P. D.: An important toxic effect of digitalis overdosage on the vision. N. Engl. J. Med. 272:904, 1965.

Class: Diuretics

Generic Name: 1. Bendroflumethiazide; 2. Benzthiazide; 3. Chlorothiazide; 4. Chlorthalidone; 5. Cyclothiazide; 6. Hydrochlorothiazide; 7. Hydroflumethiazide; 8. Methyclothiazide; 9. Metolazone; 10. Polythiazide; 11. Quinethazone; 12. Trichlormethiazide

Proprietary Name: 1. Aprinox (G.B.), Aprinox-M (Austral.), Bendrofluazide (G.B.), Berkozide (G.B.), Bristuric (Austral.), Centyl (G.B.), Naturetin, Naturine (Fr.), Neo-NaClex (G.B.), Pluryl (Austral.), Salures (Swed.); 2. Aquapres, Aqua-Scrip, Aquasec, Aquatag, Aquex, Diucen, Exna, Fovane (Fr.), Hydrex, Hy-Drine, Lemazide, Marazide, Proaqua, Rid-ema, S-Aqua, Urazide; 3. Diuril, Diurilix (Fr.), Flumen (Ital.), Minzil (Ital.), Salisan (Denm.), Saluren (Ital.), Saluric (G.B.), SK-Chlorothiazide, Yadalan (Span.); 4. Hygroton, Igroton (Ital.), Uridon (Canad.); 5. Anhydron, Doburil (Austral.), Fluidil; 6. Aquarius (Canad.), Chemhydrazide (Canad.), Chlorzide, Delco-Retic, Direma (G.B.), Diucen-H, Diuchlor H (Canad.), Diu-Scrip, Esidrex

(G.B.), Esidrix, Hydrazide (Canad.), Hydrid (Canad.), Hydro-Aquil (Canad.), Hydrodiuretex (Canad.), HydroDiuril, Hydromal, Hydrosaluret (Canad.), HydroSaluric (G.B.), Hydrozide, Hyeloril, Hyperetic, Kenazide, Lexxor, Loqua, Mictrin, Neo-Codema (Canad.), Neo-Flumen (Austral.), Novohydrazide (Canad.), Oretic, Ro-Hydrazide, SK-Hydrochlorothiazide, Thiuretic, Urozide (Canad.), Zide; 7. Di-Ademil (Austral.), Diucardin, Hydol (S. Afr.), Hydrenox (G.B.), Leodrine (Fr.), NaClex (Austral.), Robezon (Jap.), Rontyl (Denm.), Saluron; 8. Aquatensen, Duretic (Canad.), Enduron; 9. Diulo, Zaroxolyn; 10. Drenusil (Germ., S. Afr.), Nephril (G.B.), Renese; 11. Aquamox (G.B.), Hydromox; 12. Aquex, Esmarin (Germ.), Fluitran (N.Z.), Flutra (Swed.), Metahydrin, Naqua, Rochlomethiazide

Primary Use: These thiazides and related diuretics are effective in the maintenance therapy of edema associated with chronic congestive heart failure, essential hypertension, renal dysfunction, cirrhosis, pregnancy, premenstrual tension, and hormonal imbalance.

Ocular Side Effects:

A. Systemic Administration
　1. Decreased vision
　2. Myopia
　3. Problems with color vision
　　a. Objects have yellow tinge
　　b. Large yellow spots on white background
　4. Retinal edema
　5. Eyelids or conjunctiva
　　a. Allergic reactions
　　b. Photosensitivity
　　c. Urticaria
　　d. Purpura
　　e. Lupoid syndrome
　　f. Erythema multiforme
　　g. Stevens-Johnson syndrome
　6. Decreased intraocular pressure — minimal
　7. Paralysis of accommodation
　8. Subconjunctival or retinal hemorrhages secondary to drug-induced anemia
　9. Cortical blindness (?)

Clinical Significance: Ocular side effects due to these diuretics occur only occasionally and are usually transitory. Myopia is probably caused by an increase in the anteroposterior diameter of the lens which may be reversible even if use of the drug is continued.

9

Interactions with Other Drugs:

A. Effects of Thiazides on Activity of Other Drugs
1. Adrenergic blockers ↑
2. Monoamine oxidase inhibitors ↑
3. Phenothiazines ↑
4. Tricyclic antidepressants ↑
5. Sympathomimetics ↑↓
B. Effect of Other Drugs on Activity of Thiazides
1. Alcohol ↑
2. Analgesics ↑
3. Barbiturates ↑
4. General anesthetics ↑
5. Monoamine oxidase inhibitors ↑
6. Tricyclic antidepressants ↑↓
7. Sympathomimetics ↓

References:

Beasley, F. J.: Transient myopia and retinal edema during hydrochlorothiazide (Hydrodiuril) therapy. Arch. Ophthalmol. 65:212, 1961.
Ericson, L. A.: Hygroton-induced myopia and retinal edema. Acta Ophthalmol. 41:538, 1963.
Pallin, O., and Ericson, R.: Ultrasound studies in a case of Hygroton-induced myopia. Acta Ophthalmol. 43:692, 1965.
Peczon, J. D., and Grant, W. M.: Diuretic drugs in glaucoma. Am. J. Ophthalmol. 66:680, 1968.
Weinstock, F. J.: Transient severe myopia. JAMA 217:1245, 1971.

Generic Name: Ethacrynic Acid (Etacrynic Acid)

Proprietary Name: Crinuryl (Isr.), Edecril (Austral., Jap.), Edecrin, Hydromedin (Germ.)

Primary Use: This phenoxyacetic acid derivative is effective as a short-acting diuretic in all types of edema.

Ocular Side Effects:

A. Systemic Administration
1. Decreased vision
2. Nystagmus
3. Subconjunctival or retinal hemorrhages secondary to drug-induced anemia.

Clinical Significance: Few ocular side effects have been reported due to ethacrynic acid therapy. Although blurring of vision is not uncommon, it is seldom of major significance. Ethacrynic acid in dust form is highly irritating to the eyes.

Interactions with Other Drugs:

A. Effect of Ethacrynic Acid on Activity of Other Drugs
   1. Alcohol ↑
   2. Carbonic anhydrase inhibitors ↑

References:

AMA Drug Evaluations. 4th Ed., New York, John Wiley & Sons, 1980, pp. 598–599.
Peczon, J. D., and Grant, W. M.: Diuretic drugs in glaucoma. Am. J. Ophthalmol. 66:680, 1968.
Pillay, V. K. G., et al.: Transient and permanent deafness following treatment with ethacrynic acid in renal failure. Lancet 1:77, 1969.
Schneider, W. J., and Becker, E. L.: Acute transient hearing loss after ethacrynic acid therapy. Arch. Intern. Med. 117:715, 1966.
Schwartz, F. D., Pillay, V. K. G., and Kark, R. M.: Ethacrynic acid: Its usefulness and untoward effects. Am. Heart J. 79:427, 1970.

Generic Name: Furosemide

Proprietary Name: Arasemide (Jap.), Dryptal (G.B.), Franyl (Jap.), Frusemide (G.B.), Frusid (G.B.), Furantral (Pol.), Impugan (Swed.), Lasilix (Fr.), Lasix, Seguril (Span.)

Primary Use: This potent sulfonamide diuretic is effective primarily in the treatment of hypertension complicated by congestive heart failure or renal impairment.

Ocular Side Effects:

A. Systemic Administration
   1. Decreased vision
   2. Problems with color vision — dyschromatopsia
   3. Eyelids or conjunctiva
      a. Allergic reactions
      b. Photosensitivity
      c. Urticaria
      d. Erythema multiforme
      e. Exfoliative dermatitis
   4. Visual hallucinations
   5. Decreased intraocular pressure — minimal
   6. Decreased tolerance to contact lenses

7. Subconjunctival or retinal hemorrhages secondary to drug-induced anemia
8. Decreased accommodation (?)
9. Photophobia (?)
10. Ocular teratogenic effects (?)

Clinical Significance: Furosemide has potent systemic side effects and is not commonly used. Ocular side effects are rare and seldom of significance. One instance of a baby born blind after the mother took 40 mg of furosemide 3 times daily during her second trimester has been reported.

Interactions with Other Drugs:

A. Effect of Furosemide on Activity of Other Drugs
   1. Adrenergic blockers ↑
   2. Monoamine oxidase inhibitors ↑
   3. Phenothiazines ↑
   4. Tricyclic antidepressants ↑
B. Effect of Other Drugs on Activity of Furosemide
   1. Adrenergic blockers ↑
   2. Monoamine oxidase inhibitors ↑
   3. Phenothiazines ↑
   4. Tricyclic antidepressants ↑
C. Cross Sensitivity
   1. Sulfonamides

References:

AMA Drug Evaluations. 4th Ed., New York, John Wiley & Sons, 1980, pp. 597–598.
Davidson, S. I.: Reports of ocular adverse reactions. Trans. Ophthalmol. Soc. U.K. 93:495, 1973.
Peczon, J. D., and Grant, W. M.: Diuretic drugs in glaucoma. Am. J. Ophthalmol. 66:680, 1968.
Physicians' Desk Reference. 35th Ed., Oradell, N.J., Medical Economics Co., 1981, p. 938.

Generic Name: Spironolactone

Proprietary Name: Aldactone

Primary Use: This aldosterone antagonist is effective in the treatment of edema associated with cirrhosis, nephrotic syndrome, congestive heart failure, and essential hypertension. It is also used in the diagnosis of hyperaldosteronism.

Ocular Side Effects:

A. Systemic Administration
    1. Decreased vision
    2. Myopia
    3. Decreased intraocular pressure — minimal

Clinical Significance: Few significant ocular side effects due to spirono-lactone have been reported, and all are transitory and reversible.

Interactions with Other Drugs:

A. Effect of Other Drugs on Activity of Spironolactone
    1. General anesthetics ↑
    2. Monoamine oxidase inhibitors ↑
    3. Other diuretics ↑
    4. Salicylates ↓

References:

AMA Drug Evaluations. 4th Ed., New York, John Wiley & Sons, 1980, p. 600.

Belci, C.: Miopia transitoria in corso di terapia con diuretici. Boll. Oculist 47:24, 1968.

Duke-Elder, S.: System of Ophthalmology. St. Louis, C. V. Mosby, Vol. XIV, Part 2, 1972, p. 1343.

Dukes, M. N. G. (Ed.): Meyler's Side Effects of Drugs. Amsterdam, Excerpta Medica, Vol. IX, 1980, pp. 356–358.

Grant, W. M.: Toxicology of the Eye. 2nd Ed., Springfield, Charles C Thomas, 1974, p. 939.

Class: Osmotics

Generic Name: Glycerin (Glycerol)

Proprietary Name: *Systemic:* Glyrol, Luxoral (Ital.), Osmoglyn *Ophthalmic:* Ophthalgan

Primary Use: *Systemic:* This trihydric alcohol is a hyperosmotic agent used to decrease intraocular pressure in various acute glaucomas and in preoperative intraocular procedures. *Ophthalmic:* This topical trihydric alcohol is a hyperosmotic used to reduce corneal edema for diagnostic procedures, increased comfort, or improved vision.

Ocular Side Effects:

A. Systemic Administration
    1. Decreased intraocular pressure
    2. Subconjunctival or retinal hemorrhages
    3. Visual hallucinations
    4. Retinal tear
    5. Decreased vision
    6. Expulsive hemorrhage (?)
B. Local Ophthalmic Use or Exposure
    1. Irritation
        a. Lacrimation
        b. Hyperemia
        c. Ocular pain
        d. Burning sensation
    2. Subconjunctival hemorrhages

Clinical Significance: Systemic glycerin causes decreased intraocular pressure, which is an intended ocular response, and has surprisingly few other ocular effects. However, severe vitreal dehydration with resultant shrinkage of the vitreous possibly may cause traction on the adjacent retina, resulting in a tear. This principle has been described as well with cerebral dehydration causing intracranial hemorrhages. In addition, visual hallucinations are thought to occur probably due to cerebral dehydration. There have been reports of expulsive hemorrhages occurring during intraocular surgery due to strong osmotic agents. The postulated mechanism is that a sudden drop in intraocular pressure may rupture sclerotic posterior ciliary arteries.

Interactions with Other Drugs:

A. Effect of Glycerin on Activity of Other Drugs
    1. Ascorbic acid ↑
B. Effect of Other Drugs on Activity of Glycerin
    1. Anticholinesterases ↑
    2. Ascorbic acid ↑
    3. Carbonic anhydrase inhibitors ↑

References:

AMA Drug Evaluations. 4th Ed., New York, John Wiley & Sons, 1980, pp. 365–366, 403.

Chang, S., Abramson, D. H., and Coleman, D. J.: Diabetic ketoacidosis with retinal tear. Ann. Ophthalmol. 9:1507, 1977.

Cogan, D. G.: Clearing of edematous corneas by glycerine. Am. J. Ophthalmol. 26: 551, 1943.

Havener, W. H.: Ocular Pharmacology. 4th Ed., St. Louis, C. V. Mosby, 1978, pp. 453–459.

Hovland, K. R.: Effects of drugs on aqueous humor dynamics. Int. Ophthalmol. Clin. 11(2):99, 1971.

Virno, M., et al.: Oral glycerol in ophthalmology. Am. J. Ophthalmol. 55:1133, 1963.

Generic Name: 1. Isosorbide; 2. Mannitol

Proprietary Name: 1. Isosorbide; 2. Manicol (Fr.), Osmitrol, Osmosol (Austral.), Resectisol

Primary Use: These hyperosmotic agents are used to decrease intraocular pressure in various acute glaucomas and in preoperative intraocular procedures. Mannitol is also used in the management of oliguria and anuria.

Ocular Side Effects:

A. Systemic Administration
  1. Decreased intraocular pressure
  2. Decreased vision
  3. Subconjunctival or retinal hemorrhages
  4. Visual hallucinations
  5. Eyelids or conjunctiva
     a. Blepharitis (?)
     b. Urticaria
  6. Retinal tear
  7. Expulsive hemorrhage (?)

Clinical Significance: Isosorbide is excreted unchanged in the urine so that both systemic and ocular side effects are rare. Adverse ocular reactions are more frequent with mannitol since it is administered parenterally and is a more potent agent. Probably all ocular side effects listed are secondary to dehydration effects. Severe vitreal dehydration with resultant shrinkage of the vitreous possibly may cause traction on the adjacent retina, resulting in a tear. This principle has been described as well with cerebral dehydration causing intracranial hemorrhage. Expulsive hemorrhages have been reported to occur during surgery in which strong osmotic agents were used. The postulated mechanism for this is a sudden decrease in intraocular pressure, which may rupture sclerotic posterior ciliary arteries.

References:

Barry, K., Khoury, A. H., and Brooks, M. H.: Mannitol and isosorbide. Arch. Ophthalmol. 81:695, 1969.

Becker, B., Kolker, A. E., and Krupin, T.: Isosorbide. An oral hyperosmotic agent. Arch. Ophthalmol. 78:147, 1967.

Chang, S., Abramson, D. H., and Coleman, D. J.: Diabetic ketoacidosis with retinal tear. Ann. Ophthalmol. 9:1507, 1977.

Havener, W. H.: Ocular Pharmacology. 4th Ed., St. Louis, C. V. Mosby, 1978, pp. 451–453, 459–460.

Smith, E. W., and Drance, S. M.: Reduction of human intraocular pressure with intravenous mannitol. Arch. Ophthalmol. 68:734, 1962.

Weiss, D., Shaffer, R. N., and Wise, B. L.: Mannitol infusion to reduce intraocular pressure. Arch. Ophthalmol. 68:341, 1962.

Generic Name: Urea

Proprietary Name: Ureaphil, Urevert (G.B.)

Primary Use: This hyperosmotic agent is used to decrease temporarily intracranial, cerebrospinal, or intraocular pressure.

Ocular Side Effects:

A. Systemic Administration
   1. Decreased intraocular pressure
   2. Rebound glaucoma
   3. Subconjunctival or retinal hemorrhages
   4. Visual hallucinations
   5. Decreased vision
   6. Retinal tear
   7. Nystagmus (?)
   8. Expulsive hemorrhage (?)

Clinical Significance: Urea rarely causes ocular side effects other than the intended response of decreased intraocular pressure. However, on occasion a "rebound glaucoma" may occur, possibly caused by the following proposed mechanism. Urea lowers intraocular pressure by drawing intraocular fluid into the vascular system. In rare instances, when the urea concentration is higher within the eye than intravascularly, an increased amount of extravascular fluid flows into the eye. The vitreous may then expand, causing the anterior chamber to precipitate a narrow-angle attack. In addition, retinal tears may possibly develop secondary to severe vitreal dehydration with resultant shrinkage of the vitreous. This principle has been described as well with cerebral dehydration causing intracranial hemorrhage. There have been reports of expulsive hemorrhage occurring during surgery due to strong osmotic agents. A sudden decrease in intraocular pressure, which may rupture sclerotic posterior ciliary arteries, is postulated as the mechanism.

Interactions with Other Drugs:

A. Effect of Other Drugs on Activity of Urea
1. Anticholinesterases ↑
2. Carbonic anhydrase inhibitors ↑

References:

American Hospital Formulary Service. Washington, D.C., American Society of Hospital Pharmacists, Vol. II, *40*:28, 1976.
Chang, S., Abramson, D. H., and Coleman, D. J.: Diabetic ketoacidosis with retinal tear. Ann. Ophthalmol. *9*:1507, 1977.
Havener, W. H.: Ocular Pharmacology. 4th Ed., St. Louis, C. V. Mosby, 1978, pp. 449–450.
Hill, K., Whitney, J. B., and Trotter, R. R.: Intravenous hypertonic urea in the management of acute angle-closure glaucoma. Arch. Ophthalmol. *65*:497, 1961.
Kwito, M. L., Kronenberg, B., and Galin, M. A.: The effect of intravenous urea on ocular fluid dynamics. Ann. Ottal. *94*:1039, 1968.

Class: Peripheral Vasodilators

Generic Name: 1. Aluminum Nicotinate; 2. Niacin (Nicotinic Acid); 3. Niacinamide (Nicotinamide); 4. Nicotinyl Alcohol

Proprietary Name: 1. Nicalex; 2. Acidemel (S. Afr.), Diacin, Efacin, Niac, Nicangin (Swed.), Nico-400, Nicobid, Nicocap, Nicolar, Niconacid (Germ.), Ni Cord, Nico-Span, Nicotinex, Nicyl (Fr.), Ni-Span, SK-Niacin, Span Niacin, Vasotherm, Wampocap; 3. Nicamid (Switz.), Nicobion (Fr., Germ.), Nicotamide (Fr.); 4. Roniacol

Primary Use: Nicotinic acid and its derivatives are used as peripheral vasodilators, as vitamins, and in the treatment of hyperlipidemia.

Ocular Side Effects:

A. Systemic Administration
1. Decreased vision
2. Cystoid macular edema
3. Eyelids or conjunctiva
   a. Allergic reactions
   b. Hyperpigmentation
   c. Angioneurotic edema
   d. Urticaria
   e. Loss of eyelashes or eyebrows (?)

4. Proptosis
5. Toxic amblyopia
6. Scotomas — paracentral (?)
7. Increased intraocular pressure (?)

Clinical Significance: Massive dosages of these drugs have been shown to cause ocular side effects, all of which have been reversible after use is discontinued. An atypical cystoid macular edema is believed to be attributable to nicotinic acid. The macular disorder improves or disappears completely following discontinuance of nicotinic acid therapy. If the macular edema persists for a long period of time, one would expect permanent changes; however, this has yet to be reported.

Interactions with Other Drugs:

A. Effect of Nicotinic Acid Derivatives on Activity of Other Drugs
   1. Phenothiazines ↑

References:

AMA Drug Evaluations. 4th Ed., New York, John Wliey & Sons, 1980, pp. 931–932.
Chazin, B. J.: Effect of nicotinic acid on blood cholesterol. Geriatrics *15*:423, 1960.
Gass, J. D.: Nicotinic acid maculopathy. Am. J. Ophthalmol. *76*:500, 1973.
Harris, J. L.: Toxic amblyopia associated with administration of nicotinic acid. Am. J. Ophthalmol. *55*:133, 1963.
Parsons, W. B., Jr., and Flinn, J. H.: Reduction in elevated blood cholesterol levels by large doses of nicotinic acid. JAMA *165*:234, 1957.

———————————

Generic Name: Phenoxybenzamine

Proprietary Name: Dibenyline (G.B.), Dibenzyline

Primary Use: This alpha-adrenergic blocking agent is used in the management of pheochromocytoma and sometimes in the treatment of vasospastic peripheral vascular disease other than the obstructive types.

Ocular Side Effects:

A. Systemic Administration
   1. Miosis
   2. Ptosis
   3. Conjunctival hyperemia
   4. Decreased intraocular pressure (?)

Clinical Significance: Ocular side effects such as miosis due to phenoxybenzamine are common, but they are seldom a problem except when associated with posterior subcapsular or central lens changes. Ptosis and conjunctival hyperemia are seldom clinically significant although they are frequently seen. All adverse ocular reactions are reversible and transitory after discontinued drug use.

Interactions with Other Drugs:

A. Effect of Phenoxybenzamine on Activity of Other Drugs
  1. Sympathomimetics ↓

References:

AMA Drug Evaluations. 4th Ed., New York, John Wiley & Sons, 1980, p. 540.
Gilman, A. G., Goodman, L. S., and Gilman, A. (Eds.): The Pharmacological Basis of Therapeutics. 6th Ed., New York, Macmillan, 1980, pp. 178–183.
Grant, W. M.: Toxicology of the Eye. 2nd Ed., Springfield, Charles C Thomas, 1974, p. 814.
Walsh, F. B., and Hoyt, W. F.: Clinical Neuro-Ophthalmology. 3rd Ed., Baltimore, Williams & Wilkins, Vol. 1, 1969, p. 447.

Generic Name: Tolazoline

Proprietary Name: Priscol (G.B.), Priscoline, Tazol, Toline (Austral.), Toloxan, Tolzol, Zoline (Austral.)

Primary Use: This alpha-adrenergic blocking agent is used in the management of spastic peripheral vascular disorders and as a diagnostic test for open-angle glaucoma.

Ocular Side Effects:

A. Systemic Administration
  1. Intraocular pressure
    a. Increased
    b. Decreased — especially in hypertensive individuals
  2. Subconjunctival or retinal hemorrhages secondary to drug-induced anemia
B. Local Ophthalmic Use or Exposure — Subconjunctival Injection
  1. Increased intraocular pressure — especially in open-angle glaucoma
  2. Ptosis
  3. Miosis
  4. Conjunctival hyperemia

Clinical Significance: In general, the ocular pressure response from systemic tolazoline is of little clinical significance because of its variability and small amplitude. However, in hypertensive individuals the transient decreased intraocular pressure induced by tolazoline may be significant. Ocular side effects from subconjunctival injections are common but rarely significant. Increased intraocular pressure may be attributable in part to vasodilatation.

Interactions with Other Drugs:

A. Effect of Tolazoline on Activity of Other Drugs
   1. General anesthetics ↑
   2. Monoamine oxidase inhibitors ↑
B. Effect of Other Drugs on Activity of Tolazoline
   1. General anesthetics ↑
   2. Monoamine oxidase inhibitors ↑

References:

Duke-Elder, S.: System of Ophthalmology. St. Louis, C. V. Mosby, Vol. XIV, Part 2, 1972, p. 1046.
Newell, F. W., Ridgway, W. L., and Zeller, R. W.: The treatment of glaucoma with dibenamine. Am. J. Ophthalmol. 34:527, 1951.
Sugar, S., and Santos, R.: The Priscoline provocative test. Am. J. Ophthalmol. 40:510, 1955.
Walsh, F. B., and Hoyt, W. F.: Clinical Neuro-Ophthalmology. 3rd Ed., Baltimore, Williams & Wilkins, Vol. I, 1969, p. 447.
Zarrabi, M.: Quelques observations sur le Priscol en ophtalmologie. Ophthalmologica 122:76, 1951.

Class: Vasopressors

Generic Name: Ephedrine

Proprietary Name: *Systemic:* Bofedrol, Ectasule Minus, Efedrinetter (Swed.), Ephedroides (Fr.), Isofedrol, Nefrytol-Junior (S. Afr.), Slo-Fedrin, Spaneph (G.B.) *Ophthalmic:* Ephedrine

Primary Use: *Systemic:* This sympathomimetic amine is effective as a vasopressor, a bronchodilator, and a nasal decongestant. *Ophthalmic:* This topical sympathomimetic amine is used as a conjunctival vasoconstrictor.

Ocular Side Effects:

A. Systemic Administration
   1. Mydriasis — may precipitate narrow-angle glaucoma
   2. Visual hallucinations

3. Decreased intraocular pressure
4. Rebound miosis (?)
B. Local Ophthalmic Use or Exposure
  1. Conjunctival vasoconstriction
  2. Decreased vision
  3. Eyelids or conjunctiva
    a. Allergic reactions
    b. Conjunctivitis — nonspecific
  4. Irritation
    a. Lacrimation
    b. Rebound hyperemia
    c. Photophobia
  5. Mydriasis — may precipitate narrow-angle glaucoma
  6. Aqueous floaters — pigment debris
  7. Decreased intraocular pressure (?)

Clinical Significance: Ocular side effects from systemic administration of ephedrine are rare and topical ocular ephedrine solutions are seldom used in concentrations sufficient to cause significant side effects other than the intended response of vasoconstriction. Repeated use, however, may cause rebound conjunctival hyperemia or, in some instances, loss of the drug's vasoconstrictive effect.

Interactions with Other Drugs:

A. Effect of Ephedrine on Activity of Other Drugs
  1. Sympathomimetics ↑
  2. Adrenergic blockers ↓
  3. Local anesthetics ↓
B. Effect of Other Drugs on Activity of Ephedrine
  1. Monoamine oxidase inhibitors ↑
  2. Sympathomimetics ↑
  3. Adrenergic blockers ↓
C. Contraindications
  1. Ophthalmic lotions containing polyvinyl alcohol

References:

AMA Drug Evaluations. 4th Ed., New York, John Wiley & Sons, 1980, pp. 454–455, 484.
Hardesty, J. F.: Control of intraocular hypertension by systemic medication. Trans. Am. Ophthalmol. Soc. 32:497, 1934.
Havener, W. H.: Ocular Pharmacology. 4th Ed., St. Louis, C. V. Mosby, 1978, p. 243.
Mitchell, D. W. A.: The effect of ephedrine instillations on intraocular pressure. Br. J. Physiol. Opt. NS 14:38, 1957.
Walsh, F. B., and Hoyt, W. F.: Clinical Neuro-Ophthalmology. 3rd Ed., Baltimore, Williams & Wilkins, Vol. I, 1969, p. 446.

Generic Name: Epinephrine

Proprietary Name: *Systemic:* Adremad (Fr.), Adrenalin, Adrenaline (G.B.), Adrenatrate, Asmatane, Asmolin, Asthma Meter, Bronkaid, Dysne-Inhal (Canad.), Dyspne (Austral.), Glin-Epin (Austral.), Glycirenan (Germ.), Intranefrin (Canad.), Liadren (Ital.), Medihaler-Epi, Micronefrin, Primatene, Suprarenin, Sus-Phrine, Vaponefrin *Ophthalmic:* Adrenaline (G.B.), E1/2, E2, Epifrin, Epinal, Epitrate, Eppy, Glaucon, Glauconin (Swed.), Glaufrin (Swed.), Lyophrin (G.B.), Mistura E, Mytrate, Simplene (G.B.)

Primary Use: *Systemic:* This sympathomimetic amine is effective as a vasopressor, a bronchodilator, and a vasoconstrictor in prolonging the action of anesthetics. *Ophthalmic:* This topical sympathomimetic amine is used in the management of open-angle glaucoma.

Ocular Side Effects:

A. Systemic Administration
   1. Mydriasis — may precipitate narrow-angle glaucoma
   2. Problems with color vision
       a. Dyschromatopsia, red-green defect
       b. Objects have green tinge
   3. Hemianopsia
   4. Lacrimation
B. Local Ophthalmic Use or Exposure
   1. Decreased intraocular pressure
   2. Decreased vision
   3. Mydriasis — may precipitate narrow-angle glaucoma
   4. Eyelids or conjunctiva
       a. Allergic reactions
       b. Blepharoconjunctivitis — follicular
       c. Vasoconstriction
       d. Poliosis
       e. Pemphigoid lesion
       f. Hyperplasia of sebaceous glands
   5. Irritation
       a. Lacrimation
       b. Rebound hyperemia
       c. Photophobia
       d. Ocular pain
       e. Burning sensation
   6. Adrenochrome deposits
       a. Conjunctiva (cysts)

    b. Cornea
    c. Nasolacrimal system (cast formation)
 7. Cystoid macular edema
 8. Punctate keratitis
 9. Corneal edema
10. Narrowing or occlusion of lacrimal canaliculi
11. Subconjunctival or retinal hemorrhages
12. Loss of eyelashes or eyebrows
13. Paradoxical pressure elevation in open-angle glaucoma
14. Scotomas
15. Aqueous floaters — pigment debris
16. Periorbital edema
17. Iris
    a. Iritis
    b. Cysts
18. Black discoloration of soft contact lenses
19. Reactivation of corneal herpes simplex

Clinical Significance: Ocular side effects from systemic epinephrine are uncommon; however, topical ocular application may commonly cause significant side effects other than the intended responses of decreased intraocular pressure and conjunctival vasoconstriction. In over 20 percent of patients, the drug must be stopped after prolonged use because of ocular discomfort and rebound conjunctival hyperemia. Over 50 percent of patients develop reactive hyperemia with long term use. While most epinephrine-induced macular edemas are reversible, there are rare cases of advanced cystoid macular edema due to continued topical epinephrine use, which may have irreversible macular changes. Once the medication is discontinued, it may, in some cases, still take over 6 months to clear cystoid maculopathy. Cystoid macular changes secondary to epinephrine occur more frequently in aphakic patients but have been seen in phakic eyes as well. This drug is now recognized to cause a clinical picture not unlike ocular pemphigoid; it can also cause conjunctival epidermalization and loss of eyelashes. Most ocular adverse reactions due to epinephrine resolve or significantly improve with discontinuation of the drug. There are data to suggest that topical ocular epinephrine may cause significant corneal edema due to a toxic response on the endothelium, resulting in increased corneal hydration. This primarily occurs in corneas with damaged epithelium, which allows for increased penetration of this drug through the cornea. Timolol and epinephrine occasionally have an additive effect on reactive hyperemia. Systemic side effects from topical ocular epinephrine preparations may be of major clinical importance with direct effects on the cardiovascular and indirect effects on the central nervous system. There are numerous case reports in the Registry concerning adverse systemic effects from topical ocular epinephrine preparations.

Interactions with Other Drugs:

A. Effect of Epinephrine on Activity of Other Drugs
  1. Local anesthetics ↑
  2. Urea ↑
  3. Anticholinesterases ↓
B. Effect of Other Drugs on Activity of Epinephrine
  1. Antihistamines ↑
  2. Monoamine oxidase inhibitors ↑
  3. Sympathomimetics ↑
  4. Tricyclic antidepressants ↑
  5. Adrenergic blockers ↓
  6. Alcohol ↓
  7. Phenothiazines ↓
C. Synergistic Activity
  1. Adrenergic blockers

References:

Becker, B., and Morton, W. R.: Topical epinephrine in glaucoma suspects. Am. J. Ophthalmol. *62*:272, 1966.
Drance, S. M., and Ross, R. A.: The ocular effects of epinephrine. Surv. Ophthalmol. *14*:330, 1970.
Hull, D. S., et al.: Effect of epinephrine on the corneal endothelium. Am. J. Ophthalmol. *79*:245, 1975.
Kass, M. A., Stamper, R. L., and Becker, B.: Madarosis in chronic epinephrine therapy. Arch. Ophthalmol. *88*:429, 1972.
Norn, M. S.: Pemphigoid related to epinephrine treatment. Am. J. Ophthalmol. *83*: 138, 1977.
Obstbaum, S. A., Kolker, A. E., and Phelps, C. D.: Low-dose epinephrine. Arch. Ophthalmol. *92*:118, 1974.
Reinecke, R. D., and Kuwabara, T.: Corneal deposits secondary to topical epinephrine. Arch. Ophthalmol. *70*:170, 1963.
Spaeth, G. L.: Nasolacrimal duct obstruction caused by topical epinephrine. Arch. Ophthalmol. *77*:355, 1967.
Waltman, S. R., et al.: Corneal endothelial changes with long-term topical epinephrine therapy. Arch. Ophthalmol. *95*:1357, 1977.
Wright, P.: Squamous metaplasia or epidermalization of the conjunctiva as an adverse reaction to topical medication. Trans. Ophthalmol. Soc. U.K. *99*:244, 1979.

Generic Name: Hydroxyamphetamine

Proprietary Name: Paredrine (*Systemic* and *Ophthalmic*)

Primary Use: *Systemic:* This sympathomimetic amine is effective as a vasopressor and is used in the treatment of heart block and postural hypotension. *Ophthalmic:* This topical sympathomimetic amine is used as a mydriatic.

Ocular Side Effects:

A. Local Ophthalmic Use or Exposure
1. Mydriasis — may precipitate narrow-angle glaucoma
2. Decreased vision
3. Irritation
   a. Lacrimation
   b. Photophobia
   c. Ocular pain
4. Paradoxical pressure elevation in open-angle glaucoma
5. Eyelids or conjunctiva — allergic reactions
6. Paralysis of accommodation — minimal
7. Problems with color vision — objects have a blue tinge

Clinical Significance: Other than precipitating narrow-angle glaucoma, ocular side effects from topical ocular administration of hydroxyamphetamine are insignificant and reversible. Some feel this may be the safest mydriatic to use with a shallow anterior chamber since it is slow-acting and possibly more easily counteracted by miotics. Administration of 1 percent hydroxyamphetamine eyedrops causes a more pronounced mydriasis in patients with mongolism or Down's syndrome than in normal patients.

Interactions with Other Drugs:

A. Effect of Hydroxyamphetamine on Activity of Other Drugs
1. Analgesics ↑
2. Tricyclic antidepressants ↑
3. Adrenergic blockers ↓
4. Alcohol ↓
5. Antihistamines ↓
B. Effect of Other Drugs on Activity of Hydroxyamphetamine
1. Local anesthetics ↑
2. Monoamine oxidase inhibitors ↑
3. Tricyclic antidepressants ↑
4. Adrenergic blockers ↓
5. Phenothiazines ↓

References:

Gartner, S., and Billet, E.: Mydriatic glaucoma. Am. J. Ophthalmol. 43:975, 1957.
Grant, W. M.: Toxicology of the Eye. 2nd Ed., Springfield, Charles C Thomas, 1974, pp. 567–568.

Kronfeld, P. C., McGarry, H. I., and Smith, H. E.: The effect of mydriatics upon the intraocular pressure in so-called primary wide-angle glaucoma. Am. J. Ophthalmol. 26:245, 1943.
Priest, J. H.: Atropine response of the eyes in mongolism. Am. J. Dis. Child. 100:869, 1960.
Walsh, F. B., and Hoyt, W. F.: Clinical Neuro-Ophthalmology. 3rd Ed., Baltimore, Williams & Wilkins, Vol. I, 1969, p. 446.

Generic Name: 1. Mephentermine; 2. Metaraminol; 3. Methoxamine; 4. Norepinephrine (Levarterenol)

Proprietary Name: 1. Wyamine; 2. Aramine, Pressonex; 3. Vasoxine (G.B.), Vasoxyl, Vasylox (G.B.); 4. Arterenol (Germ.), Levophed, Noradrenaline (G.B.), Nordren (Austral.)

Primary Use: These sympathomimetic amines are used in the management of hypotension and shock.

Ocular Side Effects:

A. Systemic Administration
    1. Mydriasis — may precipitate narrow-angle glaucoma
    2. Horizontal nystagmus
    3. Decreased intraocular pressure (norepinephrine)
    4. Photophobia (norepinephrine)
    5. Diplopia (norepinephrine)
    6. Rebound conjunctival hyperemia (norepinephrine)
    7. Visual hallucinations (mephentermine)

Clinical Significance: Ocular side effects due to these sympathomimetic amines are reversible and transitory. Seldom are adverse ocular reactions seen due to these drugs except in overdose situations.

Interactions with Other Drugs:

A. Effect of Sympathomimetics on Activity of Other Drugs
    1. Monoamine oxidase inhibitors ↑ (norepinephrine)
    2. Tricyclic antidepressants ↑
    3. Adrenergic blockers ↑↓
    4. Analgesics ↓
    5. Anticholinesterases ↓
    6. Phenothiazines ↓ (norepinephrine)
B. Effect of Other Drugs on Activity of Sympathomimetics
    1. Alcohol ↑
    2. Anticholinergics ↑

3. Antihistamines ↑
4. General anesthetics ↑ (norepinephrine)
5. Monoamine oxidase inhibitors ↑
6. Tricyclic antidepressants ↑
7. Adrenergic blockers ↑↓
8. Phenothiazines ↑↓
9. Anticholinesterases ↓

References:

American Hospital Formulary Service. Washington, D.C., American Society of Hospital Pharmacists, Vol. I, *12*:12, 1977.

Gilman, A. G., Goodman, L. S., and Gilman, A. (Eds.): The Pharmacological Basis of Therapeutics. 6th Ed., New York, Macmillan, 1980, pp. 151–153, 164–166.

Horler, A. R., and Wynne, N. A.: Hypertensive crises due to pargyline and metaraminol. Br. Med. J. 2:460, 1965.

Pollack, I. P., and Rossi, H.: Norepinephrine in the treatment of ocular hypertension and glaucoma. Arch. Ophthalmol. 93:173, 1975.

Watillon, M., and Robe-Vanwijck, A.: Les medicaments cardiovasculaires. Bull. Soc. Belge Ophtalmol. *160*:174, 1972.

Generic Name: Phenylephrine

Proprietary Name: *Systemic:* Neo-Synephrine *Ophthalmic:* Ak-Dilate, Alcon-Efrin, Degest (Austral., Canad.), Efricel, I-Care (Austral.), Isopto Frin, Isopto Phenylephrine (Austral.), Mistura D, Mydfrin, Neo-Synephrine, Prefrin, Tear-Efrin

Primary Use: *Systemic:* This sympathomimetic amine is effective as a vasopressor and is used in the management of hypotension, shock, and tachycardia. *Ophthalmic:* This topical sympathomimetic amine is used as a vasoconstrictor and a mydriatic.

Ocular Side Effects:

A. Local Ophthalmic Use or Exposure
1. Mydriasis — may precipitate narrow-angle glaucoma
2. Decreased vision
3. Conjunctival vasoconstriction
4. Rebound miosis
5. Irritation
   a. Lacrimation
   b. Rebound hyperemia
   c. Photophobia
   d. Ocular pain
6. Punctate keratitis

7. Eyelids or conjunctiva — allergic reactions
8. Aqueous floaters — pigment debris
9. Corneal edema
10. Paradoxical pressure elevation in open-angle glaucoma
11. Cystoid macular edema (?)

Clinical Significance: Other than the possibility of precipitating narrow-angle glaucoma, the ocular side effects due to phenylephrine are usually of little significance. Although this is one of the more toxic drugs to the epithelium, the primary reason for its low level of toxicity is that it is seldom used for prolonged periods of time. A 10-percent concentration of phenylephrine can cause significant keratitis. Pupillary dilatation lasting for prolonged periods has been reported, especially in patients on guanethidine. Mydriasis varies with iris pigmentation and depth of the anterior chamber. Blue irides and shallow anterior chambers produce the greatest mydriasis, and dark irides or deep chambers the least. A diminished mydriatic response has been seen after subsequent use of phenylephrine. Data suggest that 10-percent concentrations of phenylephrine should be used with caution or not at all in patients with cardiac disease, significant hypertension, aneurysms, and advanced arteriosclerosis. It also should be used with caution in the elderly and in patients on monoamine oxidase inhibitors, tricyclic antidepressants, or atropine. Data in the Registry suggest that 2.5 percent, just as 10 percent, phenylephrine can also cause significant adverse systemic reactions in rare patients.

Interactions with Other Drugs:

A. Effect of Phenylephrine on Activity of Other Drugs
   1. Local anesthetics ↑↓
   2. Adrenergic blockers ↓
   3. Phenothiazines ↓
B. Effect of Other Drugs on Activity of Phenylephrine
   1. Adrenergic blockers ↑
   2. Monoamine oxidase inhibitors ↑
   3. Tricyclic antidepressants ↑

References:

Fraunfelder, F. T., and Scafidi, A. F.: Possible adverse effects from topical ocular 10% phenylephrine. Am. J. Ophthalmol. 85:447, 1978.
Haddad, N. J., Moyer, N. J., and Riley, F. C., Jr.: Mydriatic effect of phenylephrine hydrochloride. Am. J. Ophthalmol. 70:729, 1970.
Harris, L. S.: Cycloplegic-induced intraocular pressure elevations. Arch. Ophthalmol. 79:242, 1968.
Holtman, H. W., and Meyer, W.: Problems of the side effects of neosynephrine. Albrecht von Graefes Arch. Klin. Ophthalmol. 185:221, 1972.

Lansche, R. K.: Systemic reactions to topical epinephrine and phenylephrine. Am. J. Ophthalmol. *61*:95, 1966.

Mathias, C. G. T., et al.: Allergic contact dermatitis to echothiophate iodide and phenylephrine. Arch. Ophthalmol. *97*:286, 1979.

McReynolds, W. U., Havener, W. H., and Henderson, J. W.: Hazards of the use of sympathomimetic drugs in ophthalmology. Arch. Ophthalmol. *56*:176, 1956.

Meyer, S. M., and Fraunfelder, F. T.: 3. Phenylephrine hydrochloride. Ophthalmology *87*:1177, 1980.

Mitsui, Y., and Takagi, Y.: Nature of aqueous floaters due to sympathomimetic mydriatics. Arch. Ophthalmol. *65*:626, 1961.

VII

Hormones and Agents Affecting Hormonal Mechanisms

Class: Adrenal Corticosteroids

Generic Name: 1. Adrenal Cortex Injection; 2. Aldosterone; 3. Betamethasone; 4. Cortisone; 5. Desoxycorticosterone (Desoxycortone); 6. Dexamethasone; 7. Fludrocortisone; 8. Fluorometholone; 9. Fluprednisolone; 10. Hydrocortisone; 11. Medrysone; 12. Meprednisone; 13. Methylprednisolone; 14. Paramethasone; 15. Prednisolone; 16. Prednisone; 17. Triamcinolone

Proprietary Name: *Systemic:* 1. Cortadren (Canad.), Cortine Naturelle (Fr.), Eschatin (Canad.), Lipo-Adrenal Cortex, Novocortex (Fr.), Supracort (G.B.); 2. Aldocorten (G.B.), Aldocortin; 3. Bentelan (Ital.), Betapred (Swed.), Betnelan (Austral.), Betnesol (G.B.), Bextasol Inhaler (G.B.), Celestan (Germ.), Celestene (Fr.), Celestona (Swed.), Celestone; 4. Adricort, Cortal (Swed.), Cortate (Austral.), Cortelan (G.B.), Cortemel (S. Afr.), Cortilen (Ital.), Cortistab (G.B.), Cortistan, Cortisyl (G.B.), Cortogen (S. Afr.), Cortone, Pantisone; 5. Cortiron (Germ.), Deoxycortone (G.B.), Doca, Percorten, Syncorta (Jap.), Syncortyl (Fr.); 6. Acidocort (Fr.), Auxiloson (Germ.), Auxison (Aust., Fr.), Carulon (Jap.), Cebedex (Fr.), Corson (Jap.), Cortisumman (Germ.), Dalaron, Decacort (Swed.), Decadron, Decaesadril (Ital.), Decaject, Decameth, Decasone (Austral.), Decasterolone (Ital.), Decofluor (Ital.), Dectan (Jap.), Dectancyl (Fr.), Deksone, Delladec, Deronil, Desacort (Ital.), Desacortone (Ital.), Desalark (Ital.), Desameton (Ital.), Deseronil (Ital.), Dethamedin (Jap.), Dexacen, Dexacortal (Swed.), DexaCortisyl (Austral., G.B.), Dexamed (Germ.), Dexamethadrone (Canad.), Dexaport, Dexa-Scheroson (Germ.), Dexa-Sine (Germ.), Dexasone, Dexinolon (Germ.), Dexmethsone (Austral.), Dexon, Dexone, Dezone, Egocort (Austral.), Fluormone (Ital.), Fluorocort (Ital.), Fortecortin (Germ.), Hexadrol, Luxazone (Ital.), Metasolon (Jap.), Millicorten (Germ.), Miral, Moco (Jap.), Oradexon (Austral., G.B.), Orgadrone (Jap.), Penthasone (Canad.), Predni-F (Germ.), Savacort-D, Sawasone (Jap.), SK-Dexamethasone, Soludecadron (Fr.), Solurex, Spersadex (Germ., S. Afr.), Tendron; 7. Astonin-H (Germ.), Cortineff (Pol.), Florinef, Scherofluron (Germ.); 9. Alphadrol, Etadrol (Ital.); 10. Actocortin (Germ., Swed.), A-Hydrocort, Anusol-HC, Barriere-HC (Canad.), Bio-Cort (Canad.), Bio-Cortex, Biosone, Cetacort, Corlan (G.B.), Corphos, Cortamed (Canad.), Cortef, Cortenema, Cortiment (Canad., Swed.), Cortomister (Fr.), Efcortelan (G.B.), Efcortesol (G.B.), Eldecort, Emo-Cort (Canad.), Ficortril (Germ., Swed.), Flebocortid (Austral., Ital.), Heb-Cort, Hycor (Austral.), Hycorace, Hydrocort, Hydrocortal (Swed.), Hydrocortemel (S. Afr.), Hydrocortistab (G.B.), Hydrocortone, Hydrosone, Hynax (Austral.), Hysone-A (Austral.), Idrocortisone (Ital.), Intracort (Austral.), Komed HC, Manticor (Canad.), Microcort (Canad.), Nordicort (Austral.), Novohydrocort (Canad.), Nutracort, Pabracort (G.B.), Panhydrosone, Phiacort (Austral.), Polycort (S. Afr.), Scheroson (Austral.), Scheroson F (Germ.), Sigmacort (Austral.), Siguent Hycor (Austral.), Solu-Cortef, Solu-Glyc (Swed.), Span-Ster, Squibb-HC (Austral.), Sterocort (Canad.), Tega-cort, Unicort (Canad.), Venocort (Austral.), Venocortin (S. Afr.), Wincort (Canad.); 12. Betapar; 13. A-Methapred, Depo-Medrate (Germ.), Depo-Medrol, Depo-Medrone (G.B.), Depo-Pred, Dura-Meth, Medralone, Medrate (Germ.), Medrol, Medules, Mepred, Rep-Pred, Solu-Medrol, Solu-Medrone (G.B.), Urbason (Germ., Swed.); 14. Alondra (Arg.), Dilar (Fr.), Haldrate (G.B.), Haldrone, Metilar (G.B.), Monocortin, Paramesone (Jap.), Stemex; 15. Adnisolone (Austral.), Alto-Pred (G.B.), Bio-Pred, Codelcortone (G.B.), Codelsol (G.B.), Cordrol, Dacortin H (Span.), Decortin-H (Germ.), Delcort-E, Delcortol (Denm.), Delta-Cortef, Deltacortenolo (Ital.), Delta-cortilen (Ital.), Deltacortril (G.B.), Deltalone (G.B.), Delta Phoricol (G.B.), Deltasolone (Austral.), Deltastab (G.B.), Deltidrosol (Ital.), Di-Adreson-F (G.B.), Di-Pred, Donisolone (Jap.), Dua-Pred, Duo-Cort, Durapred, Encortolone (Pol.), Endoprenovis (Ital.), Erbacort (Fr.), Fernisolone-P, Hostacortin-H (Germ.), Hydeltra, Hydeltrasol, Hydrocortancyl (Fr.), Hydrosol, Jectasone, Keteocort H (Germ.), Key-Pred, Lenisolone (S. Afr.), Marsolone (G.B.), Mecortolon (Pol.), Meticortelone, Metreton, Nisolone, Nor-Pred, Nova-Pred (Canad.), Panacort, Panafcortelone (Austral.), Panisolone, Paracortol (Austral.), Phortisolone (Fr.), Poly-Pred (S. Afr.), Precortalon (Swed.), Pre-Cortisyl (G.B.), Predalone, Pred-Clysma (Swed.), Predeltilone (S. Afr.), Predenema (G.B.), Predicort, Prednelan (N.Z.), Prednesol (G.B.), Predni-Coelin (Germ.), Predni-H (Germ.), Predniretard (Fr.), Prednisol (Ital.), Predonine (Jap.), Predoxine, Predsol (G.B.), Prelone (Austral.), PSP-IV, Rolesone (Fr.), Ropredlone, Savacort-50/100, Scherisolon (Austral., Germ.), Sigpred, Sintisone (G.B.), Sodasone,

Solone (Austral.), Sol-Pred, Solucort (Fr.), Solu-Dacortin (Aust., Austral., Swed.), Solu-Decortin-H (Germ.), Solu-Pred, Solu-Predalone, Ster-5, Steraject-50, Sterane, Sterofrin (Austral.), Ulacort, Ultracorten-H (Germ.), Ultracortenol (Austral., Germ.); 16. Adasone (Austral.), Ancortone (Ital.), Colisone (Canad.), Cortancyl (Fr.), Dabroson (Germ.), Dacortin (Span.), Decortin (Germ.), DeCortisyl (G.B.), Delcortin (Denm.), Deltacortene (Ital.), Deltacortone (G.B.), Delta Prenovis (Ital.), Deltasone, Deltison (Swed.), Di-Adreson (G.B.), Encorton (Pol.), Erftopred (Germ.), Hostacortin (Germ.), Inocortyl (Fr.), Keteocort (Germ.), Keysone, Lisacort, Marsone (G.B.), Maso-Pred, Meticorten, Nisone (Span.), Orasone, Panafcort (Austral., S. Afr.), Pan-Sone, Paracort (Canad.), Parmenison (Aust.), Pred-5, Predeltin (S. Afr.), Prednicen-M, Prednilong (S. Afr.), Prednilonga (Germ.), Predniment (Germ.), Predni-Tablinen (Germ.), Prednital (Ital.), Presone (Austral.), Propred (Austral.), Rectodelt (Germ.), Ropred, Sarogesic, Servisone, SK-Prednisone, Sone (Austral.), Sterapred, Ultracorten (Germ.), Urtilone (Fr.), Wescopred (Canad.), Winpred (Canad.); 17. Acetospan, Adcortyl (G.B.), Amcort, Aristocort, Aristo-Pak, Aristosol, Aristospan, Cenocort, Cino-40, Delphicort (Germ.), Kenacomb (Austral.), Kenacort, Kenalog, Kenalone (Austral.), Ledercort (G.B.), Lederspan (G.B.), Rocinolone, SK-Triamcinolone, Solodelf (Germ.), Solutedarol (Fr.), Spencort, Tedarol (Fr.), Tracilon, Triamalone (Canad.), Triamcin, Triamcort (Ital.), Triam Forte, Triamolone, Tri-Kort, Vetalog, Volon (Germ.), Volonimat (Germ.) *Ophthalmic:* 3. Betnesol (G.B.); 4. Cortistab (G.B.); 6. Decadron, Isopto-Maxidex (Swed.), Maxidex; 8. FML Liquifilm, Oxylone; 10. Cortef, Hydrocortistab (G.B.), Hydrocortone; 11. HMS Liquifilm; 15. Ak-Pred, Ak-Tate, Econopred, Hydeltrasol, Inflamase, Metreton, Optocort (Austral.), Pred Forte, Pred Mild, Predsol (G.B.), Predulose

Primary Use: *Systemic:* These corticosteroids are effective in the replacement therapy of adrenocortical insufficiency and in the treatment of inflammatory and allergic disorders. *Ophthalmic:* These corticosteroids are effective in the treatment of ocular inflammatory and allergic disorders.

Ocular Side Effects:

A. Systemic Administration
   1. Decreased vision
   2. Posterior subcapsular cataracts (some may be reversible)
   3. Increased intraocular pressure
   4. Decreased resistance to infection
   5. Mydriasis — may precipitate narrow-angle glaucoma

6. Myopia
7. Exophthalmos
8. Papilledema secondary to pseudotumor cerebri
9. Diplopia
10. Myasthenic neuromuscular blocking effect
    a. Paresis or paralysis of extraocular muscles
    b. Ptosis
11. Problems with color vision — dyschromatopsia
12. Delayed healing of corneal wound
13. Visual fields
    a. Scotomas
    b. Constriction
    c. Enlarged blind spot
    d. Glaucoma field defect
14. Retinal edema
15. Translucent blue sclera
16. Eyelids or conjunctiva
    a. Hyperemia
    b. Edema
    c. Angioneurotic edema
    d. Lyell's syndrome
17. Microcysts — nonpigment epithelium of ciliary body and pigment epithelium of iris
18. Subconjunctival or retinal hemorrhages
19. Decreased tear lysozymes
20. Toxic amblyopia
21. Ocular teratogenic effect—cataracts (?)
B. Local Ophthalmic Use or Exposure — Topical Application or Subconjunctival or Retrobulbar Injection
    1. Increased intraocular pressure
    2. Decreased resistance to infection
    3. Delayed healing of corneal or scleral wounds
    4. Mydriasis — may precipitate narrow-angle glaucoma
    5. Ptosis
    6. Posterior subcapsular cataracts
    7. Decreased vision
    8. Enhances lytic action of collagenase
    9. Paralysis of accommodation
    10. Visual fields
        a. Scotomas
        b. Constriction
        c. Enlarged blind spot
        d. Glaucoma field defect

11. Problems with color vision
    a. Dyschromatopsia
    b. Colored haloes around lights
12. Eyelids or conjunctiva
    a. Allergic reactions
    b. Persistent erythema
    c. Telangiectasis
    d. Depigmentation
    e. Poliosis
    f. Scarring (subconjunctival injection)
    g. Fat atrophy (retrobulbar or subcutaneous injection)
    h. Skin atrophy (subcutaneous injection)
13. Punctate keratitis
14. Irritation
    a. Lacrimation
    b. Photophobia
    c. Ocular pain
    d. Burning sensation
    e. Anterior uveitis
15. Corneal or scleral thickness
    a. Increased — initial
    b. Decreased
16. Toxic amblyopia
17. Optic atrophy
18. Granulomas
19. May aggravate the following diseases
    a. Scleromalacia perforans
    b. Corneal "melting" diseases
    c. Behcet's disease
    d. Eales' disease
    e. Presumptive ocular toxoplasmosis
20. Retinal embolic phenomenon (injection)
21. Enhances facultative intraocular pathogens
C. Inadvertent Ocular Exposure — Intraocular Injection
    1. Ocular pain
    2. Decreased vision
    3. Intraocular pressure
       a. Increased — initial
       b. Decreased
    4. Retinal hemorrhages
    5. Retinal degeneration
    6. Ascending optic atrophy
    7. Toxic amblyopia
    8. Retinal detachment

9. Global atrophy
10. Endophthalmitis

Clinical Significance: Ocular side effects due to systemic or ocular administration of steroids are common and have significant clinical importance. Possibly of all the medications used by ophthalmologists, this
group of drugs causes the most side effects, perhaps because of frequency of drug use. The idea of "safe" oral, subconjunctival, or topical
ocular dosage is now in jeopardy, and patients must be evaluated on
individual susceptibility. This is characterized by a study in which
there was no significant correlation between patients on oral steroids
and posterior subcapsular cataracts, based on total dosage, weekly dosage (intensity), duration of dosage, or age of patients. Recently, it was
shown that 50 percent of the patients using 800 drops of 0.1 percent
dexamethasone will develop some lens changes. Generally, steroid-
induced posterior subcapsular cataracts are irreversible, but data support the reversibility of cataracts in some lenses of nephrotic children.
While age alone may not be a prominent factor in causing lens changes,
the young patient is more susceptible to systemic steroid effects, especially topical ocular and subconjunctival administration of fluorinated
corticosteroids. In fact, the fluorinated compounds given by the periocular and topical ophthalmic routes have been implicated in the death
of an infant. Race is also a factor, since steroid-induced glaucoma from
topical ocular medication is less frequent in blacks than in Caucasians
and depigmentation from subcutaneous steroid injection is more frequent in blacks. Even the withdrawal of steroids can cause significant
adverse effects, as seen in a 7-month-old child who developed benign
intracranial hypertension with severe visual loss following withdrawal
of topical cutaneous steroids. Although individual variation to steroid
exposure may be marked, steroid responders with elevated intraocular
pressure secondary to topical ocular corticosteroids have more field loss
than steroid nonresponders. Steroids affect changes in almost all ocular
structures. This has been reconfirmed recently by showing that steroids
can cause microcysts of the iris pigment epithelium and of the ciliary
body nonpigment epithelium. The time required for onset of a major
adverse effect from topical ocular steroids varies greatly. Effects to enhance epithelial herpes simplex may be days, while it may take years
for posterior subcapsular cataracts to develop. Topical ocular cortico-
steroid-induced glaucoma may take a number of weeks to develop, yet
most patients administered the stronger steroid dosages will develop
elevated intraocular pressure in time. The recent popularity of subconjunctival injections of steroids has brought additional drug reactions.
Subconjunctival injections of steroids placed over a diseased cornea or
sclera can cause a thinning, and possibly rupture, at the site of the in-

jection. Posterior subcapsular cataracts and subconjunctival granulomas have also been induced due to this mode of drug administration. Inadvertent intraocular steroid injections have caused blindness; this is probably due to the drug vehicle since the drug itself is nontoxic to the retina and optic nerve in most cases. However, depot steroids are toxic; complications from inadvertent intraocular depot injections are numerous and include significant toxicity of the associated agents due to prolonged release of the steroid.

Interactions with Other Drugs:

A. Effect of Corticosteroids on Activity of Other Drugs
1. Barbiturates ↑
2. Sedatives and hypnotics ↑
3. Tricyclic antidepressants ↑
4. Anticholinesterases ↓
5. Antiviral eye preparations ↓
6. Salicylates ↓
B. Effect of Other Drugs on Activity of Corticosteroids
1. Salicylates ↑
2. Antihistamines ↓
3. Barbiturates ↓
4. Phenylbutazone ↓
5. Sedatives and hypnotics ↓

References:

Armaly, M. F.: Effect of corticosteroids on intraocular pressure and fluid dynamics. I. Effect of dexamethasone in the normal eye. Arch. Ophthalmol. 70:482, 1963.

Becker, B.: The side effects of corticosteroids. Invest. Ophthalmol. 3:492, 1964.

Burch, P. G., and Migeon, C. J.: Systemic absorption of topical steroids. Arch. Ophthalmol. 79:174, 1968.

Crews, S. J.: Adverse reactions to corticosteroid therapy in the eye. Proc. R. Soc. Med. 58:533, 1965.

David, D. S., and Berkowitz, J. S.: Ocular effects of topical and systemic corticosteroids. Lancet 2:149, 1969.

Ey, R. C., et al.: Prevention of corneal vascularization. Am. J. Ophthalmol. 66:1118, 1968.

Forman, A. R., Loreto, J. A., and Tina, L. U.: Reversibility of corticosteroid-associated cataracts in children with the nephrotic syndrome. Am. J. Ophthalmol. 84:75, 1977.

Fraunfelder, F. T., and Watson, P. G.: Evaluation of eyes enucleated for scleritis. Br. J. Ophthalmol. 60:227, 1976.

Kraus, A. M.: Congenital cataract and maternal steroid ingestion. J. Pediatr. Ophthalmol. 12:107, 1975.

McKay, D. A. R., Watson, P. G., and Lyne, A. J.: Relapsing polychondritis and eye disease. Br. J. Ophthalmol. 58:600, 1974.

Miller, B., and Ellis, P. P.: Conjunctival flora in patients receiving immunosuppressive drugs. Arch. Ophthalmol. 95:2012, 1977.

Nozik, R. A.: Orbital rim fat atrophy after repository periocular corticosteroid injection. Am. J. Ophthalmol. 82:928, 1976.

O'Connor, G. R.: Periocular corticosteroid injections: Uses and abuses. Eye Ear Nose Throat Month. 55:83, 1976.
Pavlin, C. R., et al.: Ocular complications in renal transplant recipients. Can. Med. Assoc. J. 117:360, 1977.
Romano, P. E., Traisman, H. S., and Green, O. C.: Fluorinated corticosteroid toxicity in infants. Am. J. Ophthalmol. 84:247, 1977.
Schlagel, T. F., Jr., and Wilson, F. M.: Accidental intraocular injection of depot corticosteroids. Trans. Am. Acad. Ophthalmol. Otolaryngol. 78:847, 1974.
Selmanowitz, V., and Orentreich, N.: Cutaneous corticosteroid injection and amaurosis. Analysis for cause and prevention. Arch. Dermatol. 110:729, 1974.
Yablonski, M., et al.: Cataracts induced by topical dexamethasone in diabetics. Arch. Ophthalmol. 96:474, 1978.

Class: Antithyroid Agents

Generic Name: 1. Carbimazole; 2. Methimazole (Thiamazole); 3. Methylthiouracil; 4. Propylthiouracil

Proprietary Name: 1. Carbazole (Austral.), Neo-Mercazole (G.B.), Neo-Morphazole (Germ.), Neo-Thyreostat (Germ.); 2. Favistan (Germ.), Tapazole, Thacapzol (Swed.); 3. Muracin, Thyreostat (Germ.); 4. Propacil, Propycil (Germ.), Propyl-Thyracil (Canad.), Thyreostat II (Germ.), Tiotil (Swed.)

Primary Use: These thioamides are effective in the treatment of hyperthyroidism and angina pectoris.

Ocular Side Effects:

A. Systemic Administration
   1. Nystagmus (methylthiouracil)
   2. Keratitis
   3. Eyelids or conjunctiva
      a. Allergic reactions
      b. Conjunctivitis — nonspecific
      c. Depigmentation
      d. Urticaria
      e. Lupoid syndrome
      f. Exfoliative dermatitis
   4. Decreased lacrimation (methylthiouracil)
   5. Exophthalmos
   6. Subconjunctival or retinal hemorrhages secondary to drug-induced anemia
   7. Loss of eyelashes or eyebrows (?)

Clinical Significance: Ocular side effects secondary to these thioamides are rare. Nystagmus and decreased lacrimation have only been reported with methylthiouracil. Adverse ocular reactions are reversible and transitory after discontinued use of these drugs.

References:

Frawley, T. F., and Koepf, G. F.: Neurotoxicity due to thiouracil and thiourea derivatives. J. Clin. Endocrinol. *10*:623, 1950.
Papadopoulos, S., and Harden, R. McG.: Hair loss in patients treated with carbimazole. Br. Med. J. 2:1502, 1966.
Prowse, C. B.: A toxic effect of thiouracil hitherto undescribed. Br. Med. J. 2:1312, 1960.
Schneeberg, N. G.: Loss of sense of taste due to methylthiouracil therapy. JAMA *149*:1091, 1952.
Willcox, P. H.: Antithyroid treatment. A personal series. Postgrad. Med. J. *43*:146, 1967.
Windholz, M. (Ed.): The Merck Index: An Encyclopedia of Chemicals and Drugs. 9th Ed., Rahway, N.J., Merck and Co., Inc., 1976.

Generic Name: 1. Iodide and iodine solutions and compounds; 2. Radioactive iodides

Proprietary Name: *Systemic:* 1. Aqueous Iodine Solution (G.B.), Compound Iodine Solution, Iodex (G.B.), Jodex (Germ.), Lugol's Solution, Pima, Solute Iodo-Iodure Fort (Fr.), Strong Iodine Solution, Teinture d'Iode (Fr.), Trivajodan (Germ.), Weak Iodine Solution (G.B.); 2. Iodotope I-125, Iodotope I-131, Iodotope Therapeutic, Sodium Iodide (I^{125}), Sodium Iodide (I^{131}) *Ophthalmic:* 1. Iodine Solution

Primary Use: *Systemic:* Iodide and iodine are effective in the diagnosis and management of thyroid disease, in the short-term management of respiratory tract disease, and in some instances, of fungal infections. *Ophthalmic:* Topical iodide and iodine solutions are used primarily as a chemical cautery in the treatment of herpes simplex.

Ocular Side Effects:

A. Systemic Administration — Oral
  1. Decreased vision
  2. Decreased accommodation
  3. Exophthalmos
  4. Nonspecific ocular irritation
     a. Lacrimation
     b. Ocular pain
     c. Burning sensation

    5. Eyelids or conjunctiva
      a. Allergic reactions
      b. Hyperemia
      c. Conjunctivitis — nonspecific
      d. Edema
      e. Angioneurotic edema
      f. Urticaria
      g. Exfoliative dermatitis
      h. Nodules
    6. Punctate keratitis
    7. Hemorrhagic iritis
    8. Hypopyon
    9. Vitreous floaters
   10. Ocular teratogenic effects (radioactive iodides)
B. Systemic Administration — Intravenous
    1. Those mentioned for oral administration
    2. Visual fields
      a. Scotomas
      b. Constriction
      c. Hemianopsia
    3. Paralysis of accommodation
    4. Problems with color vision
      a. Dyschromatopsia
      b. Objects have green tinge
    5. Visual hallucinations
    6. Mydriasis
    7. Retinal degeneration
    8. Retinal or macular edema
    9. Retinal vasoconstriction
   10. Retrobulbar neuritis
   11. Toxic amblyopia
   12. Optic atrophy
C. Local Ophthalmic Use or Exposure
    1. Decreased vision
    2. Keratitis bullosa
    3. Eyelids or conjunctiva
      a. Allergic reactions
      b. Blepharoconjunctivitis
      c. Edema
      d. Urticaria
    4. Irritation
      a. Lacrimation
      b. Hyperemia

        c. Ocular pain
        d. Edema
    5. Brown corneal discoloration
    6. Corneal vascularization
    7. Stromal scarring
    8. Delayed corneal wound healing

Clinical Significance: Few serious irreversible ocular side effects secondary to iodide or iodine administration have been reported except when these agents have been given intravenously. When they are given orally, retinal findings are exceedingly rare or maybe even nonexistent. Allergic reactions to these agents are of rapid onset and not uncommon. Most ocular side effects are dose-related.

References:

Balázs, G., Kincses, É., and Kósa, C.: Iatrogenic diseases caused by iodine. Orv. Hetil. *108*:407, 1967.
Gerber, M.: Ocular reactions following iodide therapy. Am. J. Ophthalmol. *43*:879, 1957.
Goldberg, H. K.: Iodism with severe ocular involvement. Report of a case. Am. J. Ophthalmol. *22*:65, 1939.
Havener, W. H.: Ocular Pharmacology. 4th Ed., St. Louis, C. V. Mosby, 1978, pp. 438–439.
Inman, W. H. W.: Iododerma. Br. J. Dermatol. *91*:709, 1974.
Walsh, F. B., and Hoyt, W. F.: Clinical Neuro-Ophthalmology. 3rd Ed., Baltimore, Williams & Wilkins, Vol. III, 1969, pp. 2558–2560.

Class: Oral Contraceptives

Generic Name: Combination products of estrogens and progestogens.

Proprietary Name: Anovlar (G.B.), Brevicon, Conovid (G.B.), Controvlar (G.B.), Demulen, Enavid (G.B.), Enovid, Eugynon (G.B.), Gynovlar (G.B.), Loestrin, Lo/Ovral, Microgynon (G.B.), Micronor, Minovlar (G.B.), Modicon, Norinyl, Norlestrin, Norluten (Fr.), Norlutin, Orlest (G.B.), Ortho-Novin (G.B.), Ortho-Novum, Ovanon (G.B.), Ovcon, Ovral, Ovran (G.B.), Ovranette (G.B.), Ovulen, Ovysmen (G.B.)

Primary Use: These hormonal agents are used in the treatment of amenorrhea, dysfunctional uterine bleeding, premenstrual tension, dysmenorrhea, hypogonadism, and most commonly, as oral contraceptives.

Ocular Side Effects:

A. Systemic Administration
   1. Decreased vision
   2. Retinal vascular disorders
      a. Occlusion
      b. Hemorrhage
      c. Retinal or macular edema
      d. Spasms
   3. Visual fields
      a. Scotomas — central or paracentral
      b. Constriction
      c. Quadrantanopsia or hemianopsia
   4. Retrobulbar or optic neuritis
   5. Diplopia
   6. Papilledema secondary to pseudotumor cerebri
   7. Pupils
      a. Mydriasis — may precipitate narrow-angle glaucoma
      b. Anisocoria
   8. Decreased tolerance to contact lenses
   9. Problems with color vision
      a. Dyschromatopsia, yellow-blue defect
      b. Objects have blue tinge
      c. Colored haloes around lights — mainly blue
   10. Eyelids or conjunctiva
      a. Allergic reactions
      b. Edema
      c. Photosensitivity
      d. Angioneurotic edema
      e. Urticaria
      f. Lupoid syndrome
      g. Erythema multiforme
      h. Ptosis
   11. Myopia
   12. Exophthalmos
   13. Paralysis of extraocular muscles
   14. Aggravates retinitis pigmentosa (?)

Clinical Significance: Because of moral, religious, legal, and social implications of oral contraceptives, the incidence and types of adverse effects due to this group of drugs have taken years to be filtered out. Only now are toxicologists getting a true feeling for what harmful effects may develop. A higher incidence of migraine, thrombophlebitis, and pseudotumor cerebri occurs in women taking oral contraceptives

10

than in a comparable population. A higher incidence of ocular side effects associated with these three entities is therefore probable. There is some evidence that combination oral contraceptives which contain more progestins have fewer side effects than those which contain mainly estrogens, but this is still conjecture. There is little proved relationship between these drugs and other diseases of the eye even though a minimum of 100 reports in the literature concern themselves with this possibility. There may be a relationship between women taking oral contraceptives and a decreased tolerance to wearing contact lenses. Most of the other ocular side effects listed are based on clinical reports of possible adverse reactions. Probably many of these are true ocular side effects, but at present most must be assumed to be only possibilities and await further documentation. With long-term use, there are data that suggest decreased color perception, mainly blue and yellow, and prolonged photostress recovery times. If a patient has a transient ischemic attack, the oral contraceptive should be discontinued since the incidence of strokes is significantly increased. In the Registry and the literature, there are cases which implicate these drugs in causing macular edema. A number of these patients have been rechallenged with recurrence of the edema. There is a suggestion without definite proof that pregnancy causes progression of retinitis pigmentosa. Since these oral contraceptives cause a "pseudo-pregnancy", there is a question whether they may also cause progression of this retinal disease. In a few cases, the courts have ruled that a cause-and-effect relationship between the use of oral contraceptives and retinal vascular abnormalities exists. Therefore, in most instances patients with retinal vascular abnormalities probably should not be given these medications. If retinal vascular abnormalities develop, the use of these drugs in that patient may need to be re-evaluated.

Interactions with Other Drugs:

  A. Effect of Oral Contraceptives on Activity of Other Drugs
    1. Analgesics ↑
    2. Corticosteroids ↑
    3. Adrenergic blockers ↓
    4. Tricyclic antidepressants ↓
  B. Effect of Other Drugs on Activity of Oral Contraceptives
    1. Antihistamines ↓
    2. Barbiturates ↓
    3. Mineral oil ↓
    4. Phenylbutazone ↓
    5. Sedatives and hypnotics ↓

References:

Andelman, M. B., et al.: Family planning and public health. Int. J. Fertil. *13*:405, 1968.

Chizek, D. J., and Franceschetti, A. T.: Oral contraceptives: Their side effects and ophthalmological manifestations. Surv. Ophthalmol. *14*:90, 1969.

Connell, E. B., and Kelman, C. D.: Eye examinations in patients taking oral contraceptives. Fertil. Steril. *20*:67, 1969.

Connell, E. B., and Kelman, C. D.: Ophthalmologic findings with oral contraceptives. Obstet. Gynecol. *31*:456, 1968.

Davidson, S. I.: Reported adverse effects of oral contraceptives on the eye. Trans. Ophthalmol. Soc. U.K. *91*:561, 1971.

Department of Health, Education, and Welfare. Food and Drug Administration: Oral contraceptives. Fed. Register *43*:4214, 1978.

Faust, J. M., and Tyler, E. T.: Ophthalmologic findings in patients using oral contraception. Fertil. Steril. *17*:1, 1966.

Follmann, P.: Ophthalmodynamometric values during treatment with oral contraceptives. Szemeszet *112*:212, 1975.

Fulmek, R.: Occlusion of a branch of the central retinal artery after prolonged use of ovulation inhibitors. Klin. Monatsbl. Augenheilkd. *164*:371, 1974.

Goren, S. B.: Retinal edema secondary to oral contraceptives. Am. J. Ophthalmol. *64*:447, 1967.

Lakowski, R., and Morton, A.: The effect of oral contraceptives on colour vision in diabetic women. Can. J. Ophthalmol. *12*:89, 1977.

Marre, M., Neubauer, O., and Nemetz, U.: Colour vision and the "pill." Mod. Probl. Ophthalmol. *13*:345, 1974.

McGrand, J. C., and Cory, C. C.: Ophthalmic disease and the pill. Br. Med. J. *2*:187, 1969.

Pearlman, J. T., and Saxton, J.: Retinitis pigmentosa and birth control pills. JAMA *231*:810, 1975.

Petursson, G. J., Fraunfelder, F. T., and Meyer, S. M.: 6. Oral contraceptives. Ophthalmology *88*:368, 1981.

Reilingh, A. D. V., Reinera, M. D., and Van Bijsterveld, O. P.: Contact lens tolerance and oral contraceptives. Ann. Ophthalmol. *10*:947, 1978.

Salmon, M. L., Winkelman, J. Z., and Gay, A. J.: Neuro-ophthalmic sequelae in users of oral contraceptives. JAMA *206*:85, 1968.

Walsh, F. B., et al.: Oral contraceptives and neuro-ophthalmologic interest. Arch. Ophthalmol. *74*:628, 1965.

Class: Ovulatory Agents

Generic Name: Clomiphene (Clomifene)

Proprietary Name: Clomid, Clomivid (Swed.), Dyneric (Germ.)

Primary Use: This synthetic nonsteroidal agent is effective in the treatment of anovulation.

Ocular Side Effects:

A. Systemic Administration
   1. Decreased vision

   2. Mydriasis
   3. Visual sensations
      a. Flashing lights
      b. Scintillating scotomas
      c. Distortion of images secondary to sensations of waves or glare
      d. Various colored lights — mainly silver
      e. Phosphene stimulation
      f. Prolongation of after image
   4. Visual fields
      a. Scotomas — central
      b. Constriction
   5. Photophobia
   6. Diplopia
   7. Eyelids or conjunctiva
      a. Allergic reactions
      b. Urticaria
      c. Loss of eyelashes or eyebrows (?)
   8. Decreased tolerance to contact lenses
   9. Retinal vasospasms (?)
  10. Detachment posterior vitreous (?)
  11. Posterior subcapsular cataracts (?)

Clinical Significance: Ocular side effects are seen in 1.5 to 10 percent of patients taking clomiphene. Ocular symptoms are severe enough to require some patients to discontinue the use of the drug. A patient who had worn contact lenses for years was reported to have developed decreased tolerance to contact lenses once this agent was started. Except for detachment of the posterior vitreous and posterior subcapsular cataracts, which are both questionable and not proved side effects, all others are reversible within a few days after discontinuation of the drug.

References:

Asch, R. H., and Greenblatt, R. B.: Update on the safety and efficacy of clomiphene citrate as a therapeutic agent. J. Reprod. Med. 17:175, 1976.
Beck, P., et al.: Induction of ovulation with clomiphene. Report of a study including comparison with intravenous estrogen and human chorionic gonadotropin. Obstet. Gynecol. 27:54, 1966.
Kistner, R. W.: The use of clomiphene citrate in the treatment of anovulation. Semin. Drug Treatment 3(2):159, 1973.
Piskazeck, V. K., and Leitsmann, H.: Über die Behandlung der funktionellen Sterilität mit Clostylbegyt. Zentralbl. Gynaekol. 98:904, 1976.
Roch, L. M., II, et al.: Visual changes associated with clomiphene citrate therapy. Arch. Ophthalmol. 77:14, 1967.
Today's Drugs. Clomiphene citrate. Br. Med. J. 1:363, 1968.

Class: Thyroid Hormones

Generic Name: 1. Dextrothyroxine; 2. Levothyroxine; 3. Liothyronine; 4. Liotrix; 5. Thyroglobulin; 6. Thyroid

Proprietary Name: 1. Biotirmone (Fr.), Choloxin, Debetrol (Fr.), Dethyron (Denm.), Dynothel (Germ.), Nadrothyron (Germ.); 2. Cytolen, Eltroxin (G.B.), Euthyrox (Germ.), Letter, Levaxin (Swed.), Levoid, Levothroid, Noroxine, Oroxine (Austral.), Percutacrine Thyroxinique (Fr.), Synthroid, Thyratabs (Swed.), Thyrine (Austral.), Thyroxevan (Austral.), Thyroxinal (Austral.), Thyroxine (G.B.); 3. Cynomel (Fr.), Cytomel, Tertroxin (G.B.), Triiodothyronine (G.B.), Trithyrone (Fr.); 4. Euthroid, Thyrolar; 5. Proloid, Thyractin; 6. Arco Thyroid, Armour Thyroid, Dathroid, Delcoid, S-P-T, Thermoloid, Thy, Thyranon (Swed.), Thyrar, Thyroboline (Fr.), Thyrocrine, Thy-Span-3, Tuloidin, Tulopac

Primary Use: These thyroid hormones are effective in the replacement therapy of thyroid deficiencies such as hypothyroidism and simple goiter. Dextrothyroxine is also effective in the management of hypercholesterolemia.

Ocular Side Effects:

A. Systemic Administration
  1. Decreased vision
  2. Eyelids or conjunctiva
     a. Hyperemia
     b. Edema
     c. Loss of eyelashes or eyebrows (?) (dextrothyroxine)
  3. Diplopia
  4. Myasthenic neuromuscular blocking effect
     a. Paralysis of extraocular muscles
     b. Ptosis
  5. Exophthalmos
  6. Scotomas — central (?)
  7. Optic neuritis (?)
  8. Optic atrophy (?)
  9. Cataracts (?) (dextrothyroxine)

Clinical Significance: There have been no reports in the past three decades of ocular side effects of any consequence related to these drugs. Generally, all these eye symptoms clear within a few months after discontinuing the medication.

Interactions with Other Drugs:

   A. Effect of Thyroid Hormones on Activity of Other Drugs
      1. Analgesics ↑
      2. Sympathomimetics ↑
      3. Tricyclic antidepressants ↑
      4. Adrenergic blockers ↓
      5. Barbiturates ↓
   B. Effect of Other Drugs on Activity of Thyroid Hormones
      1. Barbiturates ↑
      2. Tricyclic antidepressants ↑

References:

Argov, Z., and Mastaglia, F. L.: Disorders of neuromuscular transmission caused by drugs. N. Engl. J. Med. *301*:409, 1979.

Brain, W. R.: Exophthalmos following administration of thyroid extract. Lancet *1*:182, 1936.

Grant, W. M.: Toxicology of the Eye. 2nd Ed., Springfield, Charles C Thomas, 1974, pp. 1014–1015.

Smith, J. L.: Neuro-Ophthalmology. St. Louis, C. V. Mosby, Vol. VI, 1972, pp. 5–6.

Uenoyama, E.: Atrophia nervi optici after taking an anti-fat remedy. (Thyreoidine ?) Jahresbericht Ophthalmol. *63*:147, 1936.

Walsh, F. B., and Hoyt, W. F.: Clinical Neuro-Ophthalmology. 3rd Ed., Baltimore, Williams & Wilkins, Vol. III, 1969, p. 2592.

VIII

Agents Affecting Blood Formation and Coagulability

Class: Agents Used to Treat Deficiency Anemias

Generic Name: Cobalt

Proprietary Name: Cobalt

Primary Use: This agent is used in the treatment of iron-deficiency anemia.

Ocular Side Effects:

A. Systemic Administration
1. Decreased vision
2. Cataracts
3. Visual fields (?)
   a. Scotomas — central or paramacular
   b. Constriction
4. Retinal hemorrhages (?)
5. Optic atrophy (?)
6. Retinal edema (?)
7. Choroidal pigmentary changes (?)
8. Decreased choroidal profusion (?)

Clinical Significance: Cobalt is now only occasionally used since significant systemic side effects occur and safer drugs are currently available. Only rarely are ocular side effects due to cobalt therapy seen, and decreased vision is the most common complaint. One case suggestive of cobalt-induced optic atrophy with retinal and choroidal changes has been reported.

References:

Gilman, A. G., Goodman, L. S., and Gilman, A. (Eds.): The Pharmacological Basis of Therapeutics. 6th Ed., New York, Macmillan, 1980, pp. 1326–1327.
Light, A., Oliver, M., and Rachmilewitz, E. A.: Optic atrophy following treatment with cobalt chloride in a patient with pancytopenia and hypercellular marrow. Isr. J. Med. Sci. 8:61, 1972.
Smith, J. D., Odom, R. B., and Maibach, H. I.: Contact urticaria from cobalt chloride. Arch. Dermatol. *111*:1610, 1975.
Walsh, F. B., and Hoyt, W. F.: Clinical Neuro-Ophthalmology. 3rd Ed., Baltimore, Williams & Wilkins, Vol. III, 1969, pp. 2686–2687.

Generic Name: 1. Ferrocholinate; 2. Ferrous Fumarate; 3. Ferrous Gluconate; 4. Ferrous Succinate; 5. Ferrous Sulfate; 6. Iron Dextran; 7. Iron Sorbitex; 8. Polysaccharide-Iron Complex

Proprietary Name: 1. Chel-Iron, Ferrolip, Kelex; 2. Arne-C, Cefera, Children, Eldofe, El-Ped-Ron, Erco-Fer (Swed.), Farbegen, Feco-T, FemIron, Feostat, Feramal (Austral.), Ferrofume (Canad.), Ferrokapsul (Germ.), Ferro-Sequels, Ferrum Hausmann (Belg.), Fersaday (G.B.), Fersamal (G.B.), Firon, Fumafer (Fr., Swed.), Fumasorb, Fumerin, Fumiron (Austral., Canad.), Galfer (G.B.), Hematon (Canad.), Hemocyte, Ircon, Laud-Iron, Maniron, Novofumar (Canad.), Palafer (Canad.), Span-FF, Toleron, Tolifer (Canad.); 3. Entron, Fergon, Ferralet, Ferro-G (Austral.), Ferronicum (S. Afr.), Ferrous-G, Fersin (Austral.), Fertinic (Canad.), Glucohaem (Austral.), Iron, Ironate (Austral.), Nionate (S. Afr.), Novoferrogluc (Canad.), Simron; 4. Cerevon (Canad.), Ferromyn (G.B.); 5. Duroferon (Swed.), Feosol, Feospan (G.B.), Fer-in-Sol, Feritard (Austral.), FeroGradumet, Ferolix, Ferralyn, Ferr-O$_2$ (Germ.), Ferro 66 DL (Germ.), Ferro-Gradumet (G.B.), Ferrophor-Dragees (Germ.), Ferrosan-Tydales (S. Afr.), Fesofor (Canad., S. Afr.), Fesotyme, Fespan (Austral.), Haemofort (Austral.), Irospan, Mol-Iron, Novoferrosulfa (Canad.), Resoferix (Germ.), Slow-Fe (G.B.), Sorbifer Durules (Austral.), Telefon, Toniron (G.B.); 6. Direx (G.B.), Ferrodex, Ferrospan, Hydextran, Imferon, Iron Hy-Dex (S. Afr.), Ironorm (G.B.); 7. Jectofer (G.B.); 8. Hytinic, Niferex, Nu-Iron

Primary Use: These iron preparations are effective in the prophylaxis and treatment of iron-deficiency anemias.

Ocular Side Effects:

A. Systemic Administration
1. Decreased vision (iron dextran)
2. Yellow-brown discoloration

        a. Sclera
        b. Choroid
    3. Eyelids or conjunctiva (iron dextran)
        a. Erythema
        b. Edema
        c. Angioneurotic edema
        d. Urticaria
    4. Retinal degeneration
    5. Optic neuritis (?)
    6. Optic atrophy (?)
    7. Problems with color vision — dyschromatopsia (?)
B. Inadvertent Ocular Exposure
    1. Irritation
        a. Hyperemia
        b. Photophobia
    2. Yellow-brown discoloration or deposits
        a. Eyelids
        b. Conjunctiva
        c. Cornea
        d. Sclera
    3. Hypopyon
    4. Ulceration
        a. Eyelids
        b. Conjunctiva
        c. Cornea

Clinical Significance: Systemically administered iron preparations seldom cause ocular side effects. Adverse ocular reactions have been reported after multiple blood transfusions (over 100), unusually large amounts of iron in the diet, or markedly prolonged iron therapy. A few cases of retinitis pigmentosa-like fundal degeneration have been reported. Direct ocular exposure to acidic ferrous salts can cause ocular irritation, but significant ocular side effects rarely occur.

Interactions with Other Drugs:

A. Effect of Iron on Activity of Other Drugs
    1. Tetracyclines ↓
B. Effect of Other Drugs on Activity of Iron
    1. Antacids ↓
    2. Chloramphenicol ↓

References:

Chisholm, J. F.: Iron pigmentation of the palpebral conjunctiva. Am. J. Ophthalmol. 33:1108, 1950.

Duke-Elder, S.: System of Ophthalmology. St. Louis, C. V. Mosby, Vol. XIV, Part 2, 1972, p. 1099.

Dukes, M. N. G. (Ed.): Meyler's Side Effects of Drugs. Amsterdam, Excerpta Medica, Vol. IX, 1980, pp. 374–377.

Grant, W. M.: Toxicology of the Eye. 2nd Ed., Springfield, Charles C Thomas, 1974, pp. 594–605.

Lane, R. S.: Intravenous infusion of iron-dextran complex for iron-deficiency anaemia. Lancet 1:852, 1964.

Zuckerman, B. D., and Lieberman, T. W.: Corneal rust ring. Arch. Ophthalmol. 63:254, 1960.

Generic Name: Methylene Blue (Methylthionine)

Proprietary Name: Desmoidpillen (Germ.), M-B Tabs, Urolene Blue, Wright's Stain

Primary Use: *Systemic:* Methylene blue is a weak germicidal agent used in the treatment of methemoglobinemia and "cyanosis anemia" and as a urinary or gastrointestinal antiseptic. It is also used as a dye to demonstrate cerebrospinal fluid fistulae or blocks. *Ophthalmic:* Methylene blue is used as a tissue marker during ocular or lacrimal surgery and has been applied to the conjunctiva to decrease glare during microsurgery.

Ocular Side Effects:

A. Systemic Administration
   1. Decreased vision
   2. Decreased accommodation
   3. Mydriasis
   4. Papilledema
   5. Diplopia
   6. Paresis of extraocular muscles
   7. Accommodative spasm
   8. Optic atrophy
   9. Blue-gray discoloration of ocular tissue — especially vitreous and retina
   10. Problems with color vision — objects have blue tinge
   11. Subconjunctival or retinal hemorrhages secondary to drug-induced anemia
B. Local Ophthalmic Use or Exposure
   1. Burning sensation
   2. Stains corneal nerves

Clinical Significance: Severe ocular side effects due to methylene blue have only been reported with intrathecal or intraventricular injections.

The most common ocular side effects after intravenous administration other than cyanopsia or blue-gray discoloration of ocular tissue are decreased vision, mydriasis, and decreased accommodation. Topical ocular application in low concentrations (1%) is almost free of ocular side effects; however, irritation is so severe that a local anesthetic is required for the patient's comfort.

References:

Evans, J. P., and Keegan, H. R.: Danger in the use of intrathecal methylene blue. JAMA *174*:856, 1960.
Gerber, A., and Lambert, R. K.: Blue appearance of fundus caused by prolonged ingestion of methylthionine chloride. Arch. Ophthalmol. *16*:443, 1936.
Lubeck, M. J.: Effects of drugs on ocular muscles. Int. Ophthalmol. Clin. *11*(2):35, 1971.
Norn, M. S.: Methylene blue (Methylthionine) vital staining of the cornea and conjunctiva. Acta Ophthalmol. *45*:347, 1967.
Walsh, F. B., and Hoyt, W. F.: Clinical Neuro-Ophthalmology. 3rd Ed., Baltimore, Williams & Wilkins, Vol. III, 1969, pp. 2706–2707.

Class: Anticoagulants

Generic Name: 1. Acenocoumarol; 2. Dicumarol (Dicoumarol); 3. Ethyl Biscoumacetate; 4. Phenprocoumon; 5. Warfarin

Proprietary Name: 1. Nicoumalone (G.B.), Sinthrom (Austral., Canad., Germ.), Sinthrome (G.B.); 2. AP (Swed.), Dufalone (Canad.); 3. Stabilene (Fr.), Tromexan (G.B.); 4. Liquamar, Marcumar (Canad., Germ.); 5. Athrombin-K, Coumadin, Coumadine (Fr.), Marevan (G.B.), Panwarfin, Waran (Swed.), Warfilone (Canad.), Warnerin (Canad.)

Primary Use: These coumarin derivatives are used as anticoagulants in the prophylaxis and treatment of venous thrombosis.

Ocular Side Effects:

A. Systemic Administration
1. Subconjunctival or retinal hemorrhages
   a. Secondary to drug-induced anticoagulation
   b. Secondary to drug-induced anemia
2. Eyelids or conjunctiva
   a. Allergic reactions

      b. Conjunctivitis — nonspecific
      c. Urticaria
      d. Necrosis
      e. Loss of eyelashes or eyebrows (?)
  3. Problems with color vision — dyschromatopsia (acenocoumarol)
  4. Lacrimation (dicumarol, warfarin)
  5. Decreased vision (dicumarol, warfarin)
  6. Ocular teratogenic effect (warfarin)
      a. Optic atrophy
      b. Cataracts
      c. Microphthalmia
      d. Blindness

Clinical Significance: Ocular side effects due to coumarin anticoagulants are rare. Massive retinal hemorrhages, especially in diseased tissue with possible capillary fragility (diabetic disciform degeneration of the macula), have been reported. Even so, as extensively as this group of agents has been used, only a few major adverse ocular side effects have been reported. These drugs should be discontinued prior to ocular surgery to prevent increased hemorrhaging in patients with diabetes or hypertension; however, it is now questioned if this is necessary for most other patients. There are data to suggest that this group of drugs can cause teratogenic effects. Although the teratogenic effects appear to be most severe when warfarin is taken during the first trimester, the effects can occur anytime during gestation. Chondrodysplasia punctata with its associated ocular defects has been reported in offspring of patients receiving warfarin therapy throughout their pregnancies.

Interactions with Other Drugs:

A. Effect of Other Drugs on Activity of Coumarins
  1. Adrenergic blockers ↑
  2. Analgesics ↑
  3. Antibiotics ↑
     (Chloramphenicol, Kanamycin, Neomycin, Penicillins, Streptomycin, Sulfonamides, Tetracyclines)
  4. Chymotrypsin-trypsin ↑
  5. General anesthetics ↑
  6. Monoamine oxidase inhibitors ↑
  7. Oxyphenbutazone ↑
  8. Phenylbutazone ↑
  9. Salicylates ↑
  10. Urea ↑

11. Alcohol ↑↓
12. Corticosteroids ↑↓
13. Antacids ↓
14. Antihistamines ↓
15. Barbiturates ↓
16. Diuretics ↓
17. Phenothiazines ↓
18. Sedatives and hypnotics ↓

References:

Feman, S. S., et al.: Intraocular hemorrhage and blindness associated with systemic anticoagulation. JAMA 220:1354, 1972.

Hall, D. L., Steen, W. H., Jr., and Drummond, J. W.: Anticoagulants and cataract surgery. Ann. Ophthalmol. 12:759, 1980.

Hall, J. G.: Embryopathy associated with oral anticoagulant therapy. Birth Defects 12(5):33, 1976.

Laroche, J., and Laroche, C.: Nouvelles recherches sur la modification de la vision des couleurs sous l'action des médicaments à dose thérapeutique. Ann. Pharm. Fr. 35:173, 1977.

Maddox, K.: Blindness due to an anticoagulant. Med. J. Aust. 1:420, 1977.

Renick, A. M., Jr.: Anticoagulant-induced necrosis of skin and subcutaneous tissues: Report of two cases and review of the English literature. South. Med. J. 69:775, 1978.

Walsh, F. B., and Hoyt, W. F.: Clinical Neuro-Ophthalmology. 3rd Ed., Baltimore, Williams & Wilkins, Vol. III, 1969, pp. 2683-2684.

Warkany, J.: Warfarin embryopathy. Teratology 14:205, 1976.

Generic Name: 1. Anisindione; 2. Diphenadione; 3. Phenindione

Proprietary Name: 1. Miradon, Unidone (Fr.); 2. Diphenadione; 3. Danilone, Dindevan (G.B.), Eridione, Haemopan (Austral.), Hedulin, Pindione (Fr.)

Primary Use: These indandione derivatives are used as anticoagulants in the prophylaxis and treatment of venous thrombosis.

Ocular Side Effects:

A. Systemic Administration
    1. Subconjunctival or retinal hemorrhages
       a. Secondary to drug-induced anticoagulation
       b. Secondary to drug-induced anemia ·
    2. Decreased vision
    3. Problems with color vision — dyschromatopsia (phenindione)
    4. Paralysis of accommodation
    5. Eyelids or conjunctiva
       a. Allergic reactions

b. Conjunctivitis — nonspecific
c. Urticaria
d. Exfoliative dermatitis
e. Necrosis
f. Loss of eyelashes or eyebrows (?)

Clinical Significance: The most common adverse ocular reaction due to these indandione anticoagulants is ocular hemorrhage, which is just an extension of the intended pharmacologic activity of these drugs. This is probably more common in ocular conditions with associated capillary fragility such as disciform macular degeneration. Most other ocular side effects are uncommon, insignificant, and reversible. To date, no ocular teratogenic effects have been reported with this group of anticoagulants.

Interactions with Other Drugs:

A. Effect of Other Drugs on Activity of Indandiones
    1. Adrenergic blockers ↑
    2. Analgesics ↑
    3. Antibiotics ↑
        (Chloramphenicol, Kanamycin, Neomycin, Penicillins, Streptomycin, Sulfonamides, Tetracyclines)
    4. Chymotrypsin-trypsin ↑
    5. General anesthetics ↑
    6. Monoamine oxidase inhibitors ↑
    7. Oxyphenbutazone ↑
    8. Phenylbutazone ↑
    9. Salicylates ↑
    10. Urea ↑
    11. Alcohol ↑↓
    12. Corticosteroids ↑↓
    13. Antacids ↓
    14. Antihistamines ↓
    15. Barbiturates ↓
    16. Diuretics ↓
    17. Phenothiazines ↓
    18. Sedatives and hypnotics ↓

References:

American Hospital Formulary Service. Washington, D.C., American Society of Hospital Pharmacists, Vol. 1, 20:12.04, 1981.
Gilman, A. G., Goodman, L. S., and Gilman, A. (Eds.): The Pharmacological Basis of Therapeutics. 6th Ed., New York, Macmillan, 1980, p. 1359.

Laroche, J., and Laroche, C.: Nouvelles recherches sur la modification de la vision des couleurs sous l'action des médicaments à dose thérapeutique. Ann. Pharm. Fr. 35:173, 1977.

Renick, A. M., Jr.: Anticoagulant-induced necrosis of skin and subcutaneous tissues: Report of two cases and review of the English literature. South. Med. J. 69:775, 1978.

Wade, A. (Ed.): Martindale: The Extra Pharmacopoeia. 27th Ed., London, Pharmaceutical Press, 1977, pp. 726–731.

Generic Name: Heparin

Proprietary Name: Calciparin (Germ.), Calciparine (Austral., Fr.), Cutheparine (Fr.), Depo-Heparin, Disebrin (Ital.), Hamocura (Germ.), Hepacarin (Jap.), Hepalean (Canad.), Hepathrom, Hep-Lock, Heprinar, Lipo-Hepin, Liquaemin, Liquemin (Germ.), Liquemine (Fr.), Norheparin (Germ.), Panheprin, Thrombophob (Germ.), Thrombo-Vetren (Germ.), Vetren (Germ.)

Primary Use: This complex organic acid inhibits the blood clotting mechanism and is used in the prophylaxis and treatment of venous thrombosis.

Ocular Side Effects:

A. Systemic Administration
   1. Subconjunctival or retinal hemorrhages
      a. Secondary to drug-induced anticoagulation
      b. Secondary to drug-induced anemia
   2. Eyelids or conjunctiva
      a. Allergic reactions
      b. Conjunctivitis — nonspecific
      c. Angioneurotic edema
      d. Urticaria
      e. Loss of eyelashes or eyebrows (?)
   3. Decreased vision
   4. Lacrimation
   5. Hyphema
B. Local Ophthalmic Use or Exposure — Subconjunctival Injection
   1. Subconjunctival or periocular hemorrhages
   2. Subconjunctival scarring
   3. Exacerbation of primary disease
   4. Decreased intraocular pressure — minimal

Clinical Significance: Ocular side effects due to systemic heparin are few and usually of little consequence. Ocular hemorrhage is the most serious adverse reaction and is probably more common in ocular conditions with increased capillary fragility. Subconjunctival or periocular hemorrhage is the most common adverse reaction due to subconjunctival heparin injections. It is more common after the third or fourth injection and seldom prevents continuation of this mode of heparin therapy. Although reports of decreased vision are rare, the etiology of such is unknown. A single case of sudden onset severe keratoconjunctivitis sicca associated with the use of intravenous and subcutaneous heparin injections has been received by the Registry. In addition, a single case of a hyphema in an otherwise normal eye was seen 1 hour after 10,000 units of heparin were administered intravenously.

Interactions with Other Drugs:
   A. Effect of Other Drugs on Activity of Heparin
      1. EDTA ↑
      2. Salicylates ↑
      3. Antihistamines ↓
      4. Penicillins ↓
      5. Phenothiazines ↓
      6. Tetracyclines ↓
   B. Effect of Heparin on Activity of Other Drugs
      1. Hyaluronidase ↓

References:

Aronson, S. B., and Elliott, J. H.: Ocular Inflammation. St. Louis, C. V. Mosby, 1972, pp. 91–92.
Gilman, A. G., Goodman, L. S., and Gilman, A. (Eds.): The Pharmacological Basis of Therapeutics. 6th Ed., New York, Macmillan, 1980, pp. 1348–1353.
Lipson, M. L.: Toxicity of systemic agents. Int. Ophthalmol. Clin. 11(2):159, 1971.
Physicians' Desk Reference. 35th Ed., Oradell, N.J., Medical Economics Co., 1981, p. 1067.
Slusher, M. M., and Hamilton, R. W.: Spontaneous hyphema during hemodialysis. N. Engl. J. Med. 293:561, 1975.
Turcotte, J. G., Kraft, R. O., and Fry, W. J.: Heparin reactions in patients with vascular disease. Arch. Surg. 90:375, 1965.

Class: Blood Substitutes

Generic Name: Dextran

Proprietary Name: Dextraven (G.B.), Gentran, Hyskon, LMD, LMWD, Lomodex (G.B.), Macrodex, Perfadex (Swed.), Rheomacrodex, Rheotran

Primary Use: This water soluble glucose polymer is used for early fluid replacement and for plasma volume expansion in the adjunctive treatment of certain types of shock.

Ocular Side Effects:

A. Systemic Administration
1. Eyelids or conjunctiva
   a. Erythema
   b. Conjunctivitis — nonspecific
   c. Angioneurotic edema
   d. Urticaria
2. Nonspecific ocular irritation
   a. Lacrimation
   b. Edema
   c. Burning sensation
3. Keratitis

Clinical Significance: The most common adverse ocular reaction due to dextran is irritation. An allergic keratitis, which disappeared when the drug was discontinued, has also been reported in several patients.

References:

Blake, J., and Cassidy, H.: Ocular hypersensitivity to dextran. Ir. J. Med. Sci. *148*: 249, 1979.
Fothergill, R., and Heaney, G. A.: Reactions to dextran. Br. Med. J. 2:1502, 1976.
Krenzelok, E. P., and Parker, W. A.: Dextran 40 anaphylaxis. Minn. Med. 58:454, 1975.
Ledoux-Corbusier, M.: L'urticaire medicamenteuse. Brux. Med. 55:629, 1975.
Richter, W., et al.: Adverse reactions to plasma substitutes: Incidence and pathomechanisms. In Watkins, J., and Wand, A. (Eds.): Adverse Response to Intravenous Drugs. New York, Grune & Stratton, 1978, pp. 49–70.

Class: Oxytocic Agents

Generic Name: Ergot

Proprietary Name: Ergot

Primary Use: This drug is used to control postpartum and illegal abortion hemorrhages.

Ocular Side Effects:

A. Systemic Administration
    1. Decreased vision
    2. Paralysis of accommodation
    3. Hypermetropia
    4. Pupils
      a. Mydriasis — acute
      b. Miosis
      c. Decreased reaction to light
    5. Toxic amblyopia
    6. Visual fields
      a. Scotomas
      b. Constriction
      c. Enlarged blind spot
    7. Retinal edema
    8. Retinal vasoconstriction
    9. Scintillating scotomas (?)
    10. Diplopia (?)
    11. Nystagmus (?)
    12. Optic atrophy (?)
    13. Cataracts (?)

Clinical Significance: Ergot preparations have caused numerous ocular side effects, primarily in overdose situations for attempted abortions. In general, these adverse ocular reactions are usually transitory and rarely permanent. While amblyopia may occur, it is reversible in most instances. To date, no solid data have incriminated medically administered ergot in causing lens changes; however, cataracts, diplopia, nystagmus, and scintillating scotomas were reported in an epidemic ergot intoxication due to contaminated grain.

Interactions with Other Drugs:

A. Synergistic Activity
    1. Sympathomimetics

References:

Grant, W. M.: Toxicology of the Eye. 2nd Ed., Springfield, Charles C Thomas, 1974, pp. 454–456.
Kohn, B. A.: The differential diagnosis of cataracts in infancy and childhood. Am. J. Dis. Child. 130:184, 1976.
Kravitz, D.: Neuroretinitis associated with symptoms of ergot poisoning: Report of a case. Arch. Ophthalmol. 13:201, 1935.

Schneider, P.: Beiderseitige Ophthalmoplegia interna, hervorgerufen durch Extractum Secalis cornuti. Munch. Med. Wochenschr. *49*:1620, 1902.

Scott, J. G.: Does ergot cause cataract? Med. Proc. *8*:4, 1962.

Wade, A. (Ed.): Martindale: The Extra Pharmacopoeia. 27th Ed., London, Pharmaceutical Press, 1977, pp. 589–590.

IX

Homeostatic and Nutrient Agents

Class: Agents Used to Treat Hyperglycemia

Generic Name: 1. Acetohexamide; 2. Chlorpropamide; 3. Tolazamide; 4. Tolbutamide

Proprietary Name: 1. Dimelor (G.B.), Dymelor, Ordimel (Swed.); 2. Chloromide (Canad.), Chloronase (Canad., Germ.), Diabetal (Swed.), Diabetoral (Germ.), Diabett, Diabines (Swed.), Diabinese, Melitase (G.B.), Novopropamide (Canad.), Stabinol (Canad.); 3. Diabewas (Ital.), Norglycin (Germ.), Tolanase (G.B.), Tolinase; 4. Arcosal (Denm.), Artosin (Austral., Germ., S. Afr., Sweden.), Chembutamide (Canad.), Dolipol (Fr.), Insilange-D (Jap.), Ipoglicone (Ital.), Mellitol (Canad.), Mobenol (Canad.), Neo-Dibetic (Canad.), Nigloid (Jap.), Novobutamide (Canad.), Oramide (Canad.), Oribetic, Orinase, Pramidex (G.B.), Rastinon (G.B.), SK-Tolbutamide, Tolbutol (Canad.), Tolbutone (Canad.), Wescotol (Canad.)

Primary Use: These oral hypoglycemic sulfonylureas are effective in the management of selected cases of diabetes mellitus.

Ocular Side Effects:

A. Systemic Administration
1. Decreased vision
2. Paresis of extraocular muscles
3. Diplopia
4. Eyelids or conjunctiva
   a. Allergic reactions
   b. Hyperemia
   c. Conjunctivitis — nonspecific
   d. Edema
   e. Photosensitivity

     f. Purpura
     g. Lupoid syndrome (tolazamide)
     h. Erythema multiforme
     i. Stevens-Johnson syndrome
     j. Exfoliative dermatitis
     k. Loss of eyelashes or eyebrows (?)
  5. Photophobia
  6. Problems with color vision — dyschromatopsia, red-green defect
  7. Subconjunctival or retinal hemorrhages secondary to drug-induced anemia
  8. Scotomas — central or centrocecal (chlorpropamide, tolbutamide)
  9. Retrobulbar or optic neuritis
 10. Hypermetropia (?) (tolbutamide)

Clinical Significance: As with other hypoglycemics, the sulfonylureas have few documented toxic effects on the eyes. Adverse ocular reactions are mainly due to drug-induced hypoglycemic attacks. Overall, chlorpropamide has a 6 percent incidence of untoward reactions, while the incidence of acetohexamide, tolazamide, and tolbutamide is around 3 percent. Cutaneous reactions due to these drugs are not unusual. While optic nerve disease has been reported in the literature and to the Registry, differentiation of which changes are due to diabetes and which are due to a toxic drug effect is difficult and may be impossible. Regardless, these changes are usually reversible.

Interactions with Other Drugs:

 A. Effect of Sulfonylureas on Activity of Other Drugs
    1. Barbiturates ↑
    2. Phenylbutazone ↑
    3. Salicylates ↑
    4. Sedatives and hypnotics ↑
    5. Sulfonamides ↑
 B. Effect of Other Drugs on Activity of Sulfonylureas
    1. Adrenergic blockers ↑
    2. Analgesics ↑
    3. Chloramphenicol ↑
    4. Monoamine oxidase inhibitors ↑
    5. Oxyphenbutazone ↑
    6. Phenylbutazone ↑
    7. Salicylates ↑
    8. Sulfonamides ↑
    9. Alcohol ↑↓

10. Phenothiazines ↑↓
11. Corticosteroids ↓
12. Diuretics ↓
13. Sympathomimetics ↓

References:

Alarcón-Segovia, D.: Drug-induced antinuclear antibodies and lupus syndrome. Drugs *12*:69, 1976.

Birch, J., et al.: Acquired color vision defects. In Pokorny, J., et al. (Eds.): Congenital and Acquired Color Vision Defects. New York, Grune & Stratton, 1979, p. 243.

Catros, A., et al.: Nevrite optique axiale bilaterale au cours d'un traitement par le D860. Rev. Otoneuroophtalmol. *30*:253, 1958.

Davidson, S. I.: Report of ocular adverse reactions. Trans. Ophthalmol. Soc. U.K. *93*:495, 1973.

Dukes, M. N. G. (Ed.): Meyler's Side Effects of Drugs. Amsterdam, Excerpta Medica, Vol. IX, 1980, pp. 710–714.

George, C. W.: Central scotomata due to chlorpropamide (Diabenese). Arch. Ophthalmol. *69*:773, 1963.

Givner, I.: Centrocecal scotomas due to chlorpropamide. Arch. Ophthalmol. *66*:64, 1961.

Kapetansky, F. M.: Refractive changes with tolbutamide. Ohio State Med. J. *59*:275, 1963.

Generic Name: Insulin

Proprietary Name: Actrapid, Deposulin (Germ.), Endopancrine (Fr.), Insulatard NPH, Lentard, Lente (Iletin or Insulin), Mixtard, Monotard, NPH Iletin, Protamine (Zinc and Iletin), Regular (Iletin or Insulin), Semilente (Iletin or Insulin), Semitard, Ultralente (Iletin or Insulin), Ultratard, Velosulin

Primary Use: This hypoglycemic agent is effective in the management of diabetes mellitus.

Ocular Side Effects:

A. Systemic Administration
1. Decreased vision
2. Nystagmus
3. Paresis of extraocular muscles
4. Diplopia
5. Pupils
    a. Mydriasis
    b. Absence of reaction to light
6. Eyelids or conjunctiva
    a. Allergic reactions

  b. Erythema
  c. Blepharoconjunctivitis
  d. Angioneurotic edema
  e. Urticaria
 7. Decreased tear lysozymes
 8. Strabismus
 9. Intraocular pressure
  a. Increased
  b. Decreased
 10. Immunogenic retinopathy (?)

Clinical Significance: Since most of the adverse ocular effects attributed to insulin normally occur with diabetes mellitus, the condition for which insulin is used, it is most difficult to state a cause-and-effect relationship. Generally, if an adverse insulin-related event occurs, it is reversible and primarily due to a drug-related hypoglycemic attack. In some cases, the reversibility is slow and may take many weeks to occur. It has been recently suggested that some diabetic retinopathy is insulin-induced and immunogenic in nature. While data in primates support this, it will be difficult to prove in humans. A separate report has also suggested that insulin caused or aggravated lipemic retinitis in a patient with possible hyperlipoproteinemia type V.

Interactions with Other Drugs:

A. Effect of Insulin on Activity of Other Drugs
  1. Sympathomimetics ↓
B. Effect of Other Drugs on Activity of Insulin
  1. Alcohol ↑
  2. Analgesics ↑
  3. Chloramphenicol ↑
  4. Monoamine oxidase inhibitors ↑
  5. Oxyphenbutazone ↑
  6. Phenylbutazone ↑
  7. Salicylates ↑
  8. Sulfonamides ↑
  9. Corticosteroids ↓
  10. Diuretics ↓
  11. Sympathomimetics ↓

References:

AMA Drug Evaluations. 4th Ed., New York, John Wiley & Sons, 1980, pp. 742–750.
Dukes, M. N. G. (Ed.): Meyler's Side Effects of Drugs. Amsterdam, Excerpta Medica, Vol. IX, 1980, pp. 705–708.

Gralnick, A.: The retina and intraocular tension during prolonged insulin coma with autopsy eye findings. Am. J. Ophthalmol. *24*:1174, 1941.

Grant, W. M.: Toxicology of the Eye. 2nd Ed., Springfield, Charles C Thomas, 1974, pp. 579–580.

Moses, R. A. (Ed.): Adler's Physiology of the Eye. 6th Ed., St. Louis, C. V. Mosby, 1975, p. 21.

Shabo, A. L., and Maxwell, D. S.: Insulin-induced immunogenic retinopathy resembling the retinitis proliferans of diabetes. Trans. Am. Acad. Ophthalmol. Otolaryngol. *81*:497, 1976.

Vermeer, B. J., and Polano, M. K.: A case of xanthomatosis and hyperlipoproteinemia type V probably induced by overdosage of insulin. Dermatologica *151*:43, 1975.

Walsh, F. B., and Hoyt, W. F.: Clinical Neuro-Ophthalmology. 3rd Ed., Baltimore, Williams & Wilkins, Vol. III, 1969, pp. 2684–2685.

Class: Vitamins

Generic Name: 1. Calcitriol; 2. Cholecalciferol, Vitamin D$_3$; 3. Ergocalciferol, Vitamin D$_2$

Proprietary Name: 1. Rocaltrol; 2. D-Mulsin (Germ.), Provitina D$_3$ (Germ.), Ultra "D", Vigorsan D$_3$ (Germ.); 3. Calciferol, Deltalin, Deltavit (Ital.), Drisdol, Ostelin (Austral.), Ostoforte (Canad.), Radiostol (Canad.), Savitol (Germ.), Sterogyl (G.B.)

Primary Use: Vitamin D is used as a dietary supplement and in the management of vitamin D-deficient states and hypoparathyroidism.

Ocular Side Effects:

  A. Systemic Administration
1. Strabismus
2. Epicanthus
3. Calcium deposits or band keratopathy
    a. Conjunctiva
    b. Cornea
    c. Sclera
4. Nystagmus
5. Decreased pupillary reaction to light
6. Narrowed optic foramina
7. Papilledema
8. Optic atrophy
9. Small optic discs
10. Visual hallucinations

11. Subconjunctival or retinal hemorrhages secondary to drug-induced anemia
12. Paresis of extraocular muscles (?)
13. Optic neuritis (?)
14. Cataracts (?)
15. Hemianopsia (?)

Clinical Significance: Severe adverse ocular reactions due to vitamin D are either caused by a direct toxicity or an unusual sensitivity and are primarily seen in infants. Calcium deposits in or around the optic canal cause narrowing of the optic foramina, which may in turn cause papilledema. If the vitamin intake is not discontinued, optic atrophy may result. Children with these toxic effects often have elfin-like faces and prominent epicanthal folds. In adults, the toxic effects are few and the calcium deposits in ocular tissue appear to be the main adverse reaction. One case of a presumed basilar artery insufficiency with hemianopsia due to vitamin D intake has been reported.

References:

Cogan, D. G., Albright, F., and Bartter, F. C.: Hypercalcemia and band keratopathy. Arch. Ophthalmol. *40*:624, 1948.

Dukes, M. N. G. (Ed.): Meyler's Side Effects of Drugs. Amsterdam, Excerpta Medica, Vol. IX, 1980, pp. 637–639.

Gartner, S., and Rubner, K.: Calcified scleral nodules in hypervitaminosis D. Am. J. Ophthalmol. *39*:658, 1955.

Harley, R. D., et al.: Idiopathic hypercalcemia of infancy: Optic atrophy and other ocular changes. Trans. Am. Acad. Ophthalmol. Otolaryngol. *69*:977, 1965.

Wagener, H. P.: The ocular manifestations of hypercalcemia. Am. J. Med. Sci. *231*: 218, 1956.

Generic Name: Vitamin A (Retinol)

Proprietary Name: A 313 (Fr.), Acon, Alphalin, A-Mulsin (Germ.), Anatola (Canad.), Arovit (Fr., Germ., Swed.), Aquasol A, Atamin Forte (Austral.), Avibon (Fr.), A-Vicotrat (Germ.), Avita (S. Afr.), A-Vitan, Carotin (Austral.), Dispatabs, Fab-A-Vit (S. Afr.), Halivite (Fr.), Ido-A (Swed.), Ro-A-Vit (G.B.), Solatene, Solu-A, Vi-Alpha, Vogan (Germ.)

Primary Use: Vitamin A is used as a dietary supplement and in the management of vitamin A-deficient states and in the treatment of acne.

Ocular Side Effects:

A. Systemic Administration
   1. Nystagmus

2. Loss of eyelashes or eyebrows
3. Paresis or paralysis of extraocular muscles
4. Diplopia
5. Yellow discoloration of eyelids
6. Papilledema secondary to pseudotumor cerebri
7. Miosis
8. Exophthalmos
9. Strabismus
10. Decreased intraocular pressure
11. Enlarged blind spot
12. Problems with color vision
    a. Objects have yellow tinge
    b. Improves red dyschromatopsia
13. Subconjunctival or retinal hemorrhages secondary to drug-induced anemia
14. Cataracts (?)
15. Ocular teratogenic effect (?)

Clinical Significance: With increased interest in diet and popularization of vitamin therapy, an increased incidence of vitamin intoxication is occurring. Ocular manifestations from hypervitaminosis A are varied and dose-related. While some direct effects are evident, such as loss of eyelashes, many of the central effects, such as diplopia and strabismus, are due to increased intracranial pressure. To date, the mechanism of how excess vitamin A causes intracranial hypertension is not known. Ocular side effects due to hypervitaminosis A are much more frequent and extensive in infants and children than in adults. Nearly all ocular side effects are rapidly reversible if recognized early and the vitamin therapy discontinued; however, in some instances, it may be several months before these effects are completely resolved. This probably occurs because of the extensive storage of vitamin A in the liver. If exophthalmos is present, it may be secondary to thyroid changes since vitamin A has antithyroid activity.

Interactions with Other Drugs:

A. Effect of Vitamin A on Activity of Other Drugs
   1. Corticosteroids ↓

References:

DiBenedetto, R. J.: Chronic hypervitaminosis A in an adult. JAMA *201*:700, 1967.
Lascari, A. D., and Bell, W. E.: Pseudotumor cerebri due to hypervitaminosis A. Clin. Pediatr. *9*:627, 1970.
Lombaert, A., and Carton, H.: Benign intracranial hypertension due to A-hypervitaminosis in adults and adolescents. Eur. Neurol. *14*:340, 1976.

Muenter, M. D., Perry, H. O., and Ludwig, J.: Chronic vitamin A intoxication in adults. Hepatic, neurologic and dermatologic complications. Am. J. Med. *50*:129, 1971.

Oliver, T. K., and Havener, W. H.: Eye manifestations of chronic vitamin A intoxication. Arch. Ophthalmol. *60*:19, 1958.

Overbach, A. M., and Rodman, M. J.: Drugs Used with Neonates and during Pregnancy. Oradell, N. J., Medical Economics Co., 1975, pp. 7–24.

Turtz, C. A., and Turtz, A. I.: Vitamin-A intoxication. Am. J. Ophthalmol. *50*:165, 1960.

X

Agents Used to Treat Allergic and Neuromuscular Disorders

Class: Agents Used to Treat Myasthenia Gravis

Generic Name: 1. Ambenonium; 2. Edrophonium; 3. Pyridostigmine

Proprietary Name: 1. Mysuran, Mytelase; 2. Tensilon; 3. Mestinon, Regonol

Primary Use: These anticholinesterase agents are effective in the treatment of myasthenia gravis. Edrophonium is primarily used as an antidote for curariform agents and as a diagnostic test for myasthenia gravis.

Ocular Side Effects:

A. Systemic Administration
1. Miosis
2. Decreased vision
3. Diplopia
4. Lacrimation
5. Blepharoclonus — toxic states
6. Paradoxical response (ptotic eye up and nonptotic eye down)
B. Local Ophthalmic Use or Exposure — Edrophonium
1. Photophobia
2. Eyelids or conjunctiva
   a. Allergic reactions
   b. Conjunctivitis — nonspecific
3. Iritis
4. Iris cysts
5. Decreased anterior chamber depth
6. Vitreous hemorrhages
7. Cataracts

Clinical Significance: Ocular side effects due to these anticholinesterase agents are rare and seldom of clinical significance. All adverse ocular reactions are reversible with discontinued drug use. Blepharoclonus is only seen in overdose situations. In rare instances, edrophonium may cause a paradoxical response when used in myasthenia gravis testing. In these cases, the ptotic eyelid goes up, while the normal eyelid goes down.

Interactions with Other Drugs:

A. Effect of Anticholinesterases on Activtiy of Other Drugs
  1. Succinylcholine ↑ (edrophonium)
  2. Antibiotics ↓ (edrophonium)
     (Kanamycin, Neomycin, Streptomycin)
B. Effect of Other Drugs on Activity of Anticholinesterases
  1. Antihistamines ↑
  2. Monoamine oxidase inhibitors ↑
  3. Phenothiazines ↑
  4. Tricyclic antidepressants ↑

References:

AMA Drug Evaluations. 4th Ed., New York, John Wiley & Sons, 1980, pp. 280–282.
American Hospital Formulary Service. Washington, D.C., American Society of Hospital Pharmacists, Vol. I 12:04, 1977, Vol. II 36:56, 1977.
Dukes, M. N. G. (Ed.): Meyler's Side Effects of Drugs. Amsterdam, Excerpta Medica, Vol. IX, 1980, p. 227.
Gilman, A. G., Goodman, L. S., and Gilman, A. (Eds.): The Pharmacological Basis of Therapeutics. 6th Ed., New York, Macmillan, 1980, pp. 112–116.
Leopold, I. H. (Ed.): Glaucoma Drug Therapy: Monograph 1, Parasympathetic Agents. Irvine, Calif., Allergan Pharmaceuticals, 1975, pp. 19–21.
Physicians' Desk Reference. 35th Ed., Oradell, N.J., Medical Economics Co., 1981, pp. 1518, 2013.
Van Dyk, H. J. L., and Florence, L.: The Tensilon test. A safe office procedure. Ophthalmology 87:210, 1980.

Class: Antihistamines

Generic Name: 1. Antazoline; 2. Pyrilamine (Mepyramine); 3. Tripelennamine

Proprietary Name: 1. Antasten (Swed.), Arithmin; 2. Allergon (S. Afr.), Anthisan (G.B.), Dorantamin, Enrumay, Histan, Kriptin, Neo-Antergan (Canad.), Paraminyl, Pymal (S. Afr.), Stamine, Statomin; 3. PBZ, Pyribenzamine, Ro-Hist

Primary Use: These ethylenediamines are indicated for the treatment of allergic or vasomotor rhinitis, allergic conjunctivitis, and allergic skin manifestations of urticaria and angioneurotic edema.

Ocular Side Effects:

A. Systemic Administration
    1. Decreased vision
    2. Pupils
       a. Mydriasis — may precipitate narrow-angle glaucoma
       b. Decreased or absent reaction to light
       c. Anisocoria
    3. Decreased accommodation
    4. Decreased tolerance to contact lenses
    5. Diplopia
    6. Decreased lacrimation
    7. Eyelids or conjunctiva
       a. Erythema
       b. Photosensitivity
       c. Urticaria
       d. Blepharospasm
    8. Visual hallucinations
    9. Nystagmus (tripelennamine) — toxic states
   10. Strabismus (tripelennamine) — toxic states
   11. Subconjunctival or retinal hemorrhages secondary to drug-induced anemia
   12. Constriction of visual fields — variable

Clinical Significance: Ocular side effects due to these antihistamines are uncommon and frequently disappear even if the use of the drug is continued. These antihistamines have a weak atropine action which accounts for pupillary changes. However, with long-term use, these effects can accumulate so that unilateral or bilateral signs such as anisocoria, decreased accommodation, and blurred vision can occur. These drugs maybe cause a decrease in mucoid or lacrimal secretions, which possibly accounts for decreased contact lens tolerance and aggravation or induction of keratoconjunctivitis sicca in some patients. Recently, it has been shown that these drugs in large dosages or with chronic therapy can produce facial dyskinesia which may start as a unilateral or bilateral blepharospasm. Total lack of pupillary responses and visual hallucinations usually only occur in toxic states. There is, however, a report of visual hallucinations occurring in a 5-year-old child after only the third oral dose of tripelennamine.

Interactions with Other Drugs:

A. Effect of Antihistamines on Activity of Other Drugs
1. Alcohol ↑
2. Anticholinergics ↑
3. Sedatives and hypnotics ↑
4. Sympathomimetics ↑
5. Adrenergic blockers ↓
6. Barbiturates ↓
7. Corticosteroids ↓
8. Phenylbutazone ↓

B. Effect of Other Drugs on Activity of Antihistamines
1. Monoamine oxidase inhibitors ↑
2. Phenothiazines ↑
3. Adrenergic blockers ↓
4. Barbiturates ↓
5. Phenylbutazone ↓

References:

Dukes, M. N. G. (Ed.): Meyler's Side Effects of Drugs. Amsterdam, Excerpta Medica, Vol. IX, 1980, pp. 265–268.

Hays, D. P., Johnson, B. F., and Perry, R.: Prolonged hallucinations following a modest overdose of tripelennamine. Clin. Toxicol. *16*:331, 1980.

Physicians' Desk Reference. 35th Ed., Oradell, N.J., Medical Economics Co., 1981, p. 912.

Rinker, J. R., and Sullivan, J. H.: Drug reactions following urethral instillation of tripelennamine (Pyribenzamine). J. Urol. *91*:433, 1964.

Schipior, P. G.: An unusual case of antihistamine intoxication. J. Pediatr. *71*:589, 1967.

Generic Name: 1. Azatadine; 2. Cyproheptadine

Proprietary Name: 1. Idulian (Fr.), Optimine; 2. Antegan (Austral.), Nuran (Germ.), Periactin, Periactinol (Germ.), Vimicon (Canad.)

Primary Use: These chemically related antihistamines are used in the symptomatic relief of allergic or vasomotor rhinitis, allergic conjunctivitis, and allergic skin manifestations.

Ocular Side Effects:

A. Systemic Administration
1. Decreased vision
2. Mydriasis — may precipitate narrow-angle glaucoma
3. Decreased tolerance to contact lenses
4. Diplopia

5. Decreased lacrimation
6. Photosensitivity
7. Visual hallucinations
8. Subconjunctival or retinal hemorrhages secondary to drug-induced anemia

Clinical Significance: Ocular side effects due to these agents are rare and frequently disappear even if use of the drug is continued. Both agents have atropine-like effects such as mydriasis and decreased secretions. Possible decreased lacrimal or mucoid secretion has been suggested as the cause of decreased tolerance to contact lenses and aggravation of keratoconjunctivitis sicca.

Interactions with Other Drugs:

A. Effect of Antihistamines on Activity of Other Drugs
   1. Alcohol ↑
   2. Anticholinergics ↑
   3. Sedatives and hypnotics ↑
   4. Sympathomimetics ↑
   5. Adrenergic blockers ↓
   6. Analgesics ↓
   7. Barbiturates ↓
   8. Corticosteroids ↓
   9. Phenylbutazone ↓
B. Effect of Other Drugs on Activity of Antihistamines
   1. Monoamine oxidase inhibitors ↑
   2. Phenothiazines ↑
   3. Adrenergic blockers ↓
   4. Barbiturates ↓
   5. Phenylbutazone ↓

References:

American Hospital Formulary Service. Washington, D.C., American Society of Hospital Pharmacists, Vol. I, 4:00, 1979.

Gilman, A. G., Goodman, L. S., and Gilman, A. (Eds.): The Pharmacological Basis of Therapeutics. 6th Ed., New York, Macmillan, 1980, p. 639.

Grant, W. M.: Toxicology of the Eye. 2nd Ed., Springfield, Charles C Thomas, 1974, p. 346.

Miller, D.: Role of the tear film in contact lens wear. Int. Ophthalmol. Clin. 13(1): 247, 1973.

Physicians' Desk Reference. 35th Ed., Oradell, N.J., Medical Economics Co., 1980, p. 1228.

Generic Name: 1. Brompheniramine; 2. Chlorpheniramine; 3. Dexbrompheniramine; 4. Dexchlorpheniramine; 5. Dimethindene; 6. Pheniramine; 7. Triprolidine

Proprietary Name: 1. Dimegan (Fr.), Dimetane, Dimotane (G.B.), Ebalin (Germ.), Ilvin (Germ., Swed.), Rolabromophen, Symptom 3, Veltane; 2. Alermine, Allerbid, Allergex (Austral., S. Afr.), Allergisan (Swed.), Allerhist (S. Afr.), Allertab, Al-R, Antagonate, Ardehist, Barachlor, Chestamine, Chlo-Amine, Chlor-4/100, Chloraman, Chloramate, Chloramin (Austral.), Chloren, Chlormene, Chlorohist, Chlorophen, Chloroton, Chlor-pen, Chlor-Span, Chlortab, Chlor-Trimeton, Chlor-Tripolon (Canad.), Chlortrone (Canad.), Cosea, Drize, Haynon (G.B.), Histacon, Histadur, Histaids (Austral.), Histalon (Canad.), Histaspan, Histex, Histol, H-Stadur, Lorphen, Malachlor, Nasahist, Niratron, Panahist, Phenetron, Piranex (Austral.), Piriton (G.B.), Pyranistan, Rhinihist, Teldrin, Trymegen; 3. Dexbrompheniramine; 4. Polaramine, Polaronil (Germ.); 5. Fenistil (Germ., Swed.), Fenostil (G.B.), Forhistal, Triten; 6. Avil (Austral., Germ., S. Afr.), Aviletten (Germ.), Avilettes (Austral.), Daneral-SA (G.B.), Inhiston; 7. Actidil, Actidilon (Fr.), Pro-Actidil (G.B.), Pro-Actidilon (Fr.)

Primary Use: These alkylamine antihistamines are used in the symptomatic relief of allergic or vasomotor rhinitis, allergic conjunctivitis, and allergic skin manifestations.

Ocular Side Effects:

A. Systemic Administration
   1. Decreased vision
   2. Pupils
      a. Mydriasis — may precipitate narrow angle glaucoma
      b. Decreased or absent reaction to light
      c. Anisocoria
   3. Decreased tolerance to contact lenses
   4. Diplopia
   5. Decreased lacrimation
   6. Eyelids or conjunctiva
      a. Erythema
      b. Photosensitivity
      c. Urticaria
      d. Blepharospasm
   7. Visual hallucinations
   8. Subconjunctival or retinal hemorrhages secondary to drug-induced anemia
   9. Constriction of visual fields — variable

11

Clinical Significance: Ocular side effects due to these antihistamines are rare and frequently disappear even if use of the drug is continued. These antihistamines have a weak atropine action which accounts for the pupillary changes. With chronic use, anisocoria, decreased accommodation, and blurred vision can also occur. These agents possibly decrease both mucoid and lacrimal secretions, which may account for decreased contact lens tolerance and aggravation or even induction of keratoconjunctivitis sicca in some patients. Recently, it has been shown that these drugs in large dosages or with chronic therapy can produce facial dyskinesia, which may start with unilateral or bilateral blepharospasms. Lack of pupillary responses or visual hallucinations occur only in toxic states. The alkylamines seem to have a lower incidence of ocular side effects than do other antihistamines, with dexchlorpheniramine having the fewest reported side effects.

Interactions with Other Drugs:

A. Effect of Antihistamines on Activity of Other Drugs
   1. Alcohol ↑
   2. Anticholinergics ↑
   3. Sedatives and hypnotics ↑
   4. Sympathomimetics ↑
   5. Adrenergic blockers ↓
   6. Barbiturates ↓
   7. Corticosteroids ↓
   8. Phenylbutazone ↓
B. Effect of Other Drugs on Activity of Antihistamines
   1. Monoamine oxidase inhibitors ↑
   2. Phenothiazines ↑
   3. Adrenergic blockers ↓
   4. Barbiturates ↓
   5. Phenylbutazone ↓

References:

Davis, W. A.: Dyskinesia associated with chronic antihistamine use. N. Engl. J. Med. *294*:113, 1976.
General Practitioner Research Group: A new antihistaminic and mucoinhibitory drug. Practitioner *192*:682, 1964.
Gilman, A. G., Goodman, L. S., and Gilman, A. (Eds.): The Pharmacological Basis of Therapeutics. 6th Ed., New York, Macmillan, 1980, pp. 622–629.
Granacher, R. P., Jr.: Facial dyskinesia after antihistamines. N. Engl. J. Med. *296*: 516, 1977.
Grant, W. M.: Toxicology of the Eye. 2nd Ed., Springfield, Charles C Thomas, 1974, pp. 281, 355.
Koffler, B. H., and Lemp, M. A.: The effect of an antihistamine (chlorpheniramine maleate) on tear production in humans. Ann. Ophthalmol. *12*:217, 1980.
Miller, D.: Role of the tear film in contact lens wear. Int. Ophthalmol. Clin. *13*(1): 247, 1973.

Soleymanikashi, Y., and Weiss, N. S.: Antihistaminic reaction: A review and presentation of two unusual examples. Ann. Allergy 28:486, 1970.
Sovner, R. D.: Dyskinesia associated with chronic antihistamine use. N. Engl. J. Med. 294:113, 1976.

Generic Name: 1. Carbinoxamine; 2. Clemastine; 3. Diphenhydramine; 4. Diphenylpyraline; 5. Doxylamine

Proprietary Name: 1. Allergefon (Fr.), Clistin, Histex (Austral.); 2. Tavegil (G.B.), Tavegyl, Tavist; 3. Alergicap (Austral.), Allerdryl, Baramine, Bax, Benachior, Benadryl, Benahist, Ben-Allergin, Bendylate, Benhydramil (Canad.), Bentrac, Benylin, Bonyl, Bidramine (Austral.), Dabylen (Germ.), Desentol (Swed.), Dihydral (S. Afr.), Diphen-Ex, Dyhydramine (S. Afr.), Eldadryl, Fenylhist, Histergan (G.B.), Histine, Hyrexin, Lensen, Nordryl, Notose, Phen-Amin 50, Phenamine, Rodryl, Rohydra, SK-Diphenhydramine, Span-Lanin, Tusstat; 4. Allerzine (Austral.), Anti-Hist (Austral.), Belfene (Fr.), Diafen, Eskayol (Swed.), Hispril, Histalert (Austral., S. Afr.), Histryl (G.B.), Kolton-Gelee (Germ.), Lergoban (G.B.), Neo-Lergic (Canad.); 5. Decapryn, Mereprine (Fr., Germ.), Unisom

Primary Use: These ethanolamine antihistamines are used in the symptomatic relief of allergic or vasomotor rhinitis, allergic conjunctivitis, and allergic skin manifestations.

Ocular Side Effects:

A. Systemic Administration
  1. Decreased vision
  2. Pupils
     a. Mydriasis — may precipitate narrow-angle glaucoma
     b. Decreased or absent reaction to light
     c. Anisocoria
  3. Decreased tolerance to contact lenses
  4. Eyelids or conjunctiva
     a. Erythema
     b. Photosensitivity
     c. Urticaria
     d. Blepharospasm
  5. Decreased lacrimation
  6. Diplopia
  7. Visual hallucinations
  8. Decrease or paralysis of accommodation
  9. Nystagmus

10. Subconjunctival or retinal hemorrhages secondary to drug-induced anemia
11. Constriction of visual fields — variable

Clinical Significance: Ocular side effects due to these antihistamines are rare and frequently disappear even if use of the drug is continued. These ethanolamines have a weak atropine action which accounts for the pupillary and ciliary body changes. However, with chronic long-term use, these effects can build so that unilateral or bilateral signs such as anisocoria, loss of accommodation, and decreased vision can occur. A suspected decrease in mucoid and lacrimal secretions may account for contact lens intolerance and aggravation or induction of keratoconjunctivitis sicca in some patients. Recently, it has been shown that these drugs in large dosages or with chronic therapy can produce facial dyskinesia. Many of these cases started with unilateral or bilateral blepharospasm. Lack of pupillary responses, visual hallucinations, and nystagmus usually only occur in toxic states. Most of the ocular side effects in this group are attributed to diphenhydramine, which is the most commonly used drug.

Interactions with Other Drugs:

A. Effect of Antihistamines on Activity of Other Drugs
   1. Alcohol ↑
   2. Anticholinergics ↑
   3. Sedatives and hypnotics ↑
   4. Sympathomimetics ↑
   5. Adrenergic blockers ↓
   6. Barbiturates ↓
   7. Corticosteroids ↓
   8. Phenylbutazone ↓
B. Effect of Other Drugs on Activity of Antihistamines
   1. Monoamine oxidase inhibitors ↑
   2. Phenothiazines ↑
   3. Adrenergic blockers ↓
   4. Barbiturates ↓
   5. Phenylbutazone ↓

References:

Delaney, W. V., Jr.: Explained unexplained anisocoria. JAMA *244*:1475, 1980.
Gilman, A. G., Goodman, L. S., and Gilman, A. (Eds.): The Pharmacological Basis of Therapeutics. 6th Ed., New York, Macmillan, 1980, pp. 622–629.
Miller, D.: Role of the tear film in contact lens wear. Int. Ophthalmol. Clin. *13*(1): 247, 1973.
Nigro, S. A.: Toxic psychosis due to diphenhydramine hydrochloride. JAMA *203*:301, 1968.

Wyngaarden, V. B., and Seevers, M. H.: Toxic effects of antihistaminic drugs. JAMA 145:277, 1951.

Class: Antiparkinsonism Agents

Generic Name: Amantadine

Proprietary Name: Contenton (Germ.), Mantadix (Fr.), PK-Merz (Germ.), Symmetrel, Virofral (Swed.)

Primary Use: This synthetic antiviral agent is used in the treatment of Parkinson's disease and in the prophylaxis of influenza A_2 (Asian) virus infections.

Ocular Side Effects:

A. Systemic Administration
1. Decreased vision
2. Visual hallucinations
3. Oculogyric crises
4. Eyelids or conjunctiva
   a. Photosensitivity
   b. Purpura
   c. Eczema
   d. Loss of eyelashes or eyebrows (?)
5. Mydriasis — may precipitate narrow-angle glaucoma
6. Cornea
   a. Edema
   b. Punctate keratitis

Clinical Significance: Ocular side effects due to amantadine are rare except for decreased vision, which is transitory and seldom significant. All ocular effects appear to be dose-related and are reversible with discontinued amantadine usage. Visual hallucinations are often lilliputian and colored. In the Registry, there are three separate reports of superficial punctate keratitis which disappeared within 4 to 7 days after discontinuing the drug. One case of corneal edema was associated with edema of the lower limbs, which is also a known adverse effect. One case of sudden bilateral loss of vision in an otherwise normal eye has been reported secondary to amantadine; this sudden loss of vision was reversible after discontinuing the drug for several weeks.

Interactions with Other Drugs:

    A. Effect of Amantadine on Activity of Other Drugs
       1. Anticholinergics ↑

References:

AMA Drug Evaluations. 4th Ed., New York, John Wiley & Sons, 1980, pp. 1374–1375.
American Hospital Formulary Service. Washington, D.C., American Society of Hospital Pharmacists, Vol. I, 8:18, 1978, Vol. II, 92:00, 1977.
Gilman, A. G., Goodman, L. S., and Gilman, A. (Eds.): The Pharmacological Basis of Therapeutics. 6th Ed., New York, Macmillan, 1980, p. 483.
Pearlman, J. T., Kadish, A. H., and Ramseyer, J. C.: Vision loss associated with amantadine hydrochloride use. JAMA 237:1200, 1977.
Postma, J. U., and Van Tilburg, W.: Visual hallucinations and delirium during treatment with amantadine (Symmetrel). J. Am. Geriatr. Soc. 23:212, 1975.
Selby, G.: Treatment of parkinsonism. Drugs 11:61, 1976.
Wade, A. (Ed.): Martindale: The Extra Pharmacopoeia. 27th Ed., London, Pharmaceutical Press, 1977, pp. 854–856.

Generic Name: 1. Benztropine; 2. Biperiden; 3. Chlorphenoxamine; 4. Cycrimine; 5. Procyclidine; 6. Trihexyphenidyl

Proprietary Name: 1. Cogentin, Cogentinol (Germ.); 2. Akineton, Akinophyl (Fr.); 3. Clorevan (G.B.), Phenoxene, Systral (Fr., Germ., Swed.); 4. Pagitane; 5. Kemadrin, Osnervan (Germ.); 6. Anti-Spas (Austral.), Antitrem, Aparkane (Canad.), Artane, Benzhexol (G.B.), Hexyphen, Novohexidyl (Canad.), Pargitan (Germ., Swed.), Peragit (Denm., Norw.), Pipanol, Tremin, Trihexy (Canad.), Trixyl (Canad.)

Primary Use: These anticholinergic agents are used in the management of Parkinson's disease and in the control of extrapyramidal disorders due to central nervous system drugs such as reserpine or the phenothiazines.

Ocular Side Effects:

    A. Systemic Administration
       1. Pupils
          a. Mydriasis — may precipitate narrow-angle glaucoma
          b. Decreased reaction to light
       2. Decreased vision
       3. Decrease or paralysis of accommodation
       4. Visual hallucinations
       5. Retinal pigmentary changes (?)

Clinical Significance: The degree of anticholinergic activity of these drugs which induce ocular side effects varies with each agent. With benztropine, adverse ocular reactions are common; while with biperiden, they are rare. In the younger age groups, decreased accommodation may cause considerable inconveniences which may be partially reversed by topical ocular application of a weak, long-acting anticholinesterase. There are a few cases in the Registry of these drugs precipitating glaucoma in patients on recommended dosages. Hallucinations in patients on these drugs are primarily of people, normal size, and in color, and they disappear if the dosage of the drug is reduced.

Interactions with Other Drugs:

A. Effect of Anticholinergics on Activity of Other Drugs
   1. Barbiturates ↑ (chlorphenoxamine)
B. Effect of Other Drugs on Activity of Anticholinergics
   1. Antihistamines ↑
   2. Monoamine oxidase inhibitors ↑
   3. Phenothiazines ↑
   4. Tricyclic antidepressants ↑

References:

AMA Drug Evaluations. 4th Ed., New York, John Wiley & Sons, 1980, pp. 247–252.
Gilbert, G. J.: Hallucinations from levodopa. JAMA *235*:597, 1976.
Medina, C., Kramer, M. D., and Kurland, A. A.: Biperiden in the treatment of phenothiazine-induced extrapyramidal reactions. JAMA *182*:1127, 1962.
Physicians' Desk Reference. 35th Ed., Oradell, N.J., Medical Economics Co., 1981, pp. 754, 964, 993, 1088, 1172.
Selby, G.: Treatment of parkinsonism. Drugs *11*:61, 1976.
Walsh, F. B., and Hoyt, W. F.: Clinical Neuro-Ophthalmology. 3rd Ed., Baltimore, Williams & Wilkins, Vol. III, 1969, pp. 2618, 2661, 2664.

Generic Name: Caramiphen

Proprietary Name: Caramiphen

Primary Use: This anticholinergic agent is used in the treatment of Parkinson's disease.

Ocular Side Effects:

A. Systemic Administration
   1. Mydriasis — may precipitate narrow-angle glaucoma
   2. Paralysis of accommodation
   3. Retrobulbar neuritis
   4. Scotomas

Clinical Significance: Significant ocular side effects due to caramiphen are very rare. Only one case of retrobulbar neuritis has been reported; however, it was well documented. The retrobulbar neuritis occurred each time caramiphen therapy was restarted.

Interactions with Other Drugs:

  A. Effect of Other Drugs on Activity of Caramiphen
   1. Antihistamines ↑
   2. Monoamine oxidase inhibitors ↑
   3. Phenothiazines ↑
   4. Tricyclic antidepressants ↑

References:

Bruckner, R.: Über pharmakologische Beeinflussung des Augendruckes bei verschie-
  denen Körperlagen. Ophthalmologica *116*:200, 1948.
Grant, W. M.: Toxicology of the Eye. 2nd Ed., Springfield, Charles C Thomas, 1974,
  p. 228.
Hermans, G.: Le système moteur. Bull. Soc. Belge Ophtalmol. *160*:97, 1972.
Leibold, J. E.: Drugs having toxic effect on the optic nerve. Int. Ophthalmol. Clin.
  11(2):137, 1971.
Lubeck, M. J.: Effects of drugs on ocular muscles. Int. Ophthalmol. Clin. *11*(2):
  35, 1971.
Walsh, F. B., and Hoyt, W. F.: Clinical Neuro-Ophthalmology. 3rd Ed., Baltimore,
  Williams & Wilkins, Vol. III, 1969, p. 2664.

Generic Name: Levodopa

Proprietary Name: Bendopa, Berkdopa (G.B.), Bio Dopa, Brocadopa (G.B.), Dopar, Dopastral (Swed.), Emeldopa (S. Afr.), Helfo-dopa (Germ.), Larodopa, Ledopa (Fr.), Levopa (G.B.), Parda, Parkidopa (Swed.), Rio-Dopa, Sobiodopa (Fr.), Speciadopa (Fr.), Syndopa (Austral.), Veldopa (G.B.)

Primary Use: This beta-adrenergic blocking agent is used in the management of Parkinson's disease.

Ocular Side Effects:

  A. Systemic Administration
   1. Pupils
      a. Mydriasis — may precipitate narrow-angle glaucoma
      b. Miosis
   2. Widening of palpebral fissure
   3. Decreased vision
   4. Diplopia

5. Blepharospasm
6. Horner's syndrome
   a. Miosis
   b. Ptosis
7. Paresis of extraocular muscles — especially V cranial nerve
8. Blepharoclonus
9. Visual hallucinations
10. Oculogyric crises
11. Eyelids or conjunctiva
    a. Allergic reactions
    b. Edema
    c. Lupoid syndrome
12. Subconjunctival or retinal hemorrhages secondary to drug-induced anemia
13. Loss of eyelashes or eyebrows (?)
14. Papilledema secondary to pseudotumor cerebri (?)
15. Stimulation of malignant melanoma (?)

Clinical Significance: While numerous ocular side effects due to levodopa are known, they appear to be dose-dependent and reversible. Pupillary side effects are variable. Initially, mydriasis may occur and has been reported to precipitate narrow-angle glaucoma. After a few weeks of levodopa therapy, miosis is not uncommon. Lid responses also appear to be variable. In some patients, levodopa produces ptosis, sometimes unilateral, while blepharospasm is reported in other patients. Visual hallucinations are menacing and primarily of normal size people and in color. These hallucinations can be stopped or decreased in frequency by reducing the drug dosage. Oculogyric crises have been precipitated by levodopa, primarily in patients with a prior history of encephalitis. One case of drug-induced pseudotumor cerebri occurred in a patient on carbidopa and levodopa. Since levodopa is an intermediate in melanin synthesis, there is a question whether it might induce or stimulate the growth of melanomas. Although there are no proved data to support this, alternate forms of antiparkinsonian therapy have been suggested for susceptible patients.

Interactions with Other Drugs:
   A. Effect of Levodopa on Activity of Other Drugs
      1. Sympathomimetics ↓
   B. Effect of Other Drugs on Activity of Levodopa
      1. Anticholinergics ↑
      2. Tricyclic antidepressants ↑
      3. Adrenergic blockers ↓
      4. Phenothiazines ↓

References:

Barone, D. A., and Martin, H. L.: Causes of pseudotumor cerebri and papilledema. Arch. Intern. Med. *139*:830, 1979.

Fermaglich, J., and Delaney, P.: Levodopa and melanoma. JAMA *241*:883, 1979.

Gilbert, G. J.: Hallucinations from levodopa. JAMA *235*:597, 1976.

Karch, F. E.: Drugs affecting autonomic functions or the extrapyramidal system. In Dukes, M. N. G. (Ed.): Side Effects of Drugs Annual 4. Amsterdam, Excerpta Medica, 1980, pp. 97–98.

Spiers, A. S. D.: Mydriatic responses to sympathomimetic amines in patients treated with L-Dopa. Lancet *2*:1301, 1969.

Spiers, A. S. D., Calne, D. B., and Fayers, P. M.: Miosis during L-Dopa therapy. Br. Med. J. *2*:639, 1970.

Yahr, M. D., et al.: Treatment of parkinsonism with levodopa. Arch. Neurol. *21*:343, 1969.

Class: Cholinesterase Reactivators

Generic Name: Pralidoxime

Proprietary Name: Contrathion (Fr.), Protopam

Primary Use: This cholinesterase reactivator is used as an antidote for poisoning due to organophosphate pesticides or other chemicals which have anticholinesterase activity. It is also of value in the control of overdosage by anticholinesterase agents used in the treatment of myasthenia gravis.

Ocular Side Effects:

A. Systemic Administration
 1. Decreased vision
 2. Diplopia
 3. Decreased accommodation
B. Local Ophthalmic Use or Exposure — Subconjunctival Injection
 1. Irritation
  a. Hyperemia
  b. Burning sensation
 2. Subconjunctival hemorrhages
 3. Iritis
 4. Reverses miosis
 5. Reverses accommodative spasms

Clinical Significance: Pralidoxime commonly causes adverse ocular reactions after systemic administration. These effects are of rapid onset, last from a few minutes to a few hours, and are completely reversible. In one series, up to 60 percent of patients using the agent complained of misty vision, heaviness of the eye, blurred near vision, or decreased accommodation, especially after sudden head movement. Ocular side effects from subconjunctival injection are also transitory and reversible.

Interactions with Other Drugs:

A. Effect of Pralidoxime on Activity of Other Drugs
    1. Anticholinesterases ↓
B. Contraindications
    1. Analgesics
    2. Phenothiazines
    3. Succinylcholine

References:

AMA Drug Evaluations. 4th Ed., New York, John Wiley & Sons, 1980, pp. 1455–1456.

Byron, H. M., and Posner, H.: Clinical evaluation of Protopam. Am. J. Ophthalmol. 57:409, 1964.

Dekking, H. M.: Stopping the action of strong miotics. Ophthalmologica *148*:428, 1964.

Holland, P., and Parkes, D. C.: Plasma concentrations of the oxime pralidoxime mesylate (P2S) after repeated oral and intramuscular administration. Br. J. Ind. Med. 33:43, 1976.

Jager, B. V., and Stagg, G. N.: Toxicity of diacetyl monoxime and of pyridine-2-aldoxime methiodide in man. Bull. Johns Hopkins Hosp. *102*:203, 1958.

Taylor, W. J. R., et al.: Effects of a combination of atropine, metaraminol and pyridine aldoxime methanesulfonate (AMP therapy) on normal human subjects. Can. Med. Assoc. J. *93*:957, 1965.

Class: Muscle Relaxants

Generic Name: Baclofen

Proprietary Name: Lioresal

Primary Use: This chlorophenyl derivative of gamma-aminobutyric acid is useful for alleviation of spasticity symptoms resulting from multiple sclerosis and other disorders of the spinal cord.

Ocular Side Effects:

A. Systemic Administration
1. Decreased vision
2. Decreased accommodation
3. Diplopia
4. Visual hallucinations
5. Pupils
   a. Mydriasis — may precipitate narrow-angle glaucoma
   b. Miosis
   c. Decreased reaction to light
6. Nystagmus
7. Strabismus

Clinical Significance: Ocular side effects from baclofen are rare and transient. Usually, the adverse effects can be abolished by reduction of the dosage of baclofen without loss of benefit. Hallucinations have occurred sometimes with treatment but usually after abrupt withdrawal of this drug. Therefore, except for serious adverse reactions, the dose should be reduced slowly when the drug is discontinued. Accommodation disorders have been reported in overdosage situations.

References:

Hedley, D. W., Maroun, J. A., and Espir, M. L. E.: Evaluation of baclofen (Lioresal) for spasticity in multiple sclerosis. Postgrad. Med. J. *51*:615, 1975.
Paulson, G. W.: Overdose of Lioresal. Neurology *26*:1105, 1976.
Physicians' Desk Reference. 35th Ed., Oradell, N. J., Medical Economics Co., 1981, p. 905.
Skausig, O. B., and Korsgaard, S.: Hallucinations and baclofen. Lancet *1*:1258, 1977.
Stein, R.: Hallucinations after sudden withdrawal of baclofen. Lancet *2*:44, 1977.

Generic Name: Dantrolene

Proprietary Name: Dantrium

Primary Use: This skeletal muscle relaxant is effective in controlling the manifestations of clinical spasticity resulting from serious chronic disorders, such as spinal cord injury, stroke, cerebral palsy, or multiple sclerosis.

Ocular Side Effects:

A. Systemic Administration
1. Decreased vision
2. Eyelids or conjunctiva

   a. Photosensitivity
   b. Urticaria
3. Diplopia
4. Lacrimation
5. Visual hallucinations

Clinical Significance: Ocular side effects due to dantrolene are transient and seldom of clinical significance. Decreased vision, diplopia, and excessive lacrimation are the most common adverse ocular effects. Visual hallucinations associated with the use of this drug usually subside upon drug withdrawal; however, several days may be required.

References:

American Hospital Formulary Service. Washington, D.C., American Society of Hospital Pharmacists, Vol. I, *12*:20, 1975.
Andrews, L. G., Muzumdar, A. S., and Pinkerton, A. C.: Hallucinations associated with dantrolene sodium therapy. Can. Med. Assoc. J. *112*:148, 1975.
Physicians' Desk Reference. 35th Ed., Oradell, N.J., Medical Economics Co., 1981, p. 1273.
Silverman, H. I., and Harvie, R. J.: Adverse effects of commonly used systemic drugs on the human eye — Part III. Am J. Optom. Physiol. Optics *52*:275, 1975.
Wade, A. (Ed.): Martindale: The Extra Pharmacopoeia. 27th Ed., London, Pharmaceutical Press, 1977, pp. 939–940.

Generic Name: 1. Mephenesin; 2. Methocarbamol

Proprietary Name: 1. Decontractyl (Fr., Germ.), Mervaldin, Myanesin, Oranixon, Rhex (Germ.), Tolserol (Canad.); 2. Delaxin, Lumirelax (Fr.), Metho-500, Methocabal (Jap.), Parabaxin, Robaxin, Romethocarb, SK-Methocarbamal, Tresortil (Denm.)

Primary Use: These centrally acting muscle relaxants are used in the treatment of acute musculoskeletal disorders. Mephenesin has also been used as an adjunct to anesthesia and in the treatment of Parkinson's disease and tetanus.

Ocular Side Effects:

A. Systemic Administration
   1. Decreased vision
   2. Nystagmus — horizontal, vertical, or rotatory
   3. Diplopia
   4. Ptosis (mephenesin)
   5. Ciliary hyperemia (mephenesin)
   6. Decreased intraocular pressure (mephenesin)

7. Paresis of extraocular muscles (mephenesin)
8. Conjunctivitis — nonspecific (methocarbamol)

Clinical Significance: Ocular side effects due to these muscle relaxants are much more common after intravenous administration than when given orally. Adverse ocular reactions are transitory and usually of little consequence. Ptosis, ciliary hyperemia, decreased intraocular pressure, and paresis of extraocular muscles are only seen with mephenesin, while nonspecific conjunctivitis has only been reported with methocarbamol.

Interactions with Other Drugs:

A. Effect of Muscle Relaxants on Activity of Other Drugs
    1. Barbiturates ↑
    2. Phenothiazines ↑
    3. Sedatives and hypnotics ↑

References:

Gilman, A. G., Goodman, L. S., and Gilman, A. (Eds.): The Pharmacological Basis of Therapeutics. 6th Ed., New York, Macmillan, 1980, pp. 488–489.
Grant, W. M.: Toxicology of the Eye. 2nd Ed., Springfield, Charles C Thomas, 1974, pp. 646, 677.
Schlesinger, E. B., Drew, A. L., and Wood, B.: Clinical studies in the use of Myanesin. Am. J. Med. 4:365, 1948.
Stephen, C. R., and Chandy, J.: Clinical and experimental studies with Myanesin. Can. Med. Assoc. J. 57:463, 1947.
Walsh, F. B., and Hoyt, W. F.: Clinical Neuro-Ophthalmology. 3rd Ed., Baltimore, Williams & Wilkins, Vol. III, 1969, p. 2648.

Generic Name: Orphenadrine

Proprietary Name: Disipal, Flexon, Flexor, Mephenamin (Germ.), Norflex, Orpadrex (S. Afr.)

Primary Use: This antihistaminic agent is used in the treatment of skeletal muscle spasm and the associated pain of parkinsonism.

Ocular Side Effects:

A. Systemic Administration
    1. Pupils
        a. Mydriasis — may precipitate narrow-angle glaucoma
        b. Absence of reaction to light
    2. Decreased vision

3. Decrease or paralysis of accommodation
4. Diplopia
5. Subconjunctival or retinal hemorrhages secondary to drug-induced anemia
6. Decreased tolerance to contact lenses (?)

Clinical Significance: Ocular side effects due to orphenadrine are transient and probably the result of its weak anticholinergic effect. These are seldom a significant clinical problem, although narrow-angle glaucoma has been precipitated secondary to drug-induced mydriasis. Nonreactive dilated pupils are only seen in overdose situations.

Interactions with Other Drugs:

A. Effect of Orphenadrine on Activity of Other Drugs
   1. Anticholinergics ↑
   2. Phenothiazines ↑
   3. Phenylbutazone ↓
B. Effect of Other Drugs on Activity of Orphenadrine
   1. Antihistamines ↑
   2. Monoamine oxidase inhibitors ↑
   3. Phenothiazines ↑
   4. Tricyclic antidepressants ↑

References:

AMA Drug Evaluations. 4th Ed., New York, John Wiley & Sons, 1980, pp. 275–276.
Bennett, N. B., and Kohn, J.: Case report: Orphenadrine overdose. Cerebral manifestations treated with physostigmine. Anaesth. Intensive Care 4:67, 1976.
Curry, A. S.: Twenty-one uncommon cases of poisoning. Br. Med. J. 1:687, 1962.
Davidson, S. I.: Reports of ocular adverse reactions. Trans. Ophthalmol. Soc. U. K. 93:495–510, 1973.
Gilman, A. G., Goodman, L. S., and Gilman, A. (Eds.): The Pharmacological Basis of Therepeutics. 6th Ed., New York, Macmillan, 1980, pp. 485–487.
Heinonen, J., et al.: Orphenadrine poisoning. A case report supplemented with animal experiments. Arch. Toxikol. 23:264, 1968.
Physicians' Desk Reference. 35th Ed., Oradell, N.J., Medical Economics Co., 1981, p. 1459.
Selby, G.: Treatment of parkinsonism. Drugs 11:61, 1976.
Stoddart, J. C., Parkin, J. M., and Wynne, N. A.: Orphenadrine poisoning. A case report. Br. J. Anaesth. 40:789, 1968.

XI

Oncolytic Agents

Class: Antineoplastic Agents

Generic Name: 1. Bleomycin; 2. Cactinomycin; 3. Dactinomycin; 4. Daunorubicin; 5. Doxorubicin; 6. Mitomycin

Proprietary Name: 1. Blenoxane; 2. Cactinomycin; 3. Cosmegen; 4. Cerubidin (G.B.), Cerubidine, Daunoblastin (Germ.), Daunoblastina (Ital.), Ondena (Germ.); 5. Adriacin (Jap.), Adriamycin; 6. Ametycine (Fr.), Mutamycin

Primary Use: *Systemic:* These antibiotics are used in a variety of malignant conditions. Bleomycin is a polypeptide antibiotic used in the management of squamous cell carcinomas, lymphomas, and testicular carcinomas. Cactinomycin and dactinomycin are antibiotics used in the management of choriocarcinoma, rhabdomyosarcoma, Wilms' tumor, testicular neoplasms, and carcinoid syndrome. Daunorubicin is used in the treatment of acute leukemia, and doxorubicin is used in sarcomas, lymphomas, and leukemia. Mitomycin is useful in the therapy of disseminated adenocarcinoma of the stomach or pancreas. *Ophthalmic:* Mitomycin is used topically after a pterygium operation in an attempt to prevent recurrence.

Ocular Side Effects:

A. Systemic Administration
    1. Eyelids or conjunctiva
        a. Allergic reactions
        b. Erythema
        c. Conjunctivitis — nonspecific (doxorubicin)
        d. Edema
        e. Hyperpigmentation
        f. Angioneurotic edema (daunorubicin)
        g. Urticaria

2. Decreased vision (mitomycin)
3. Subconjunctival or retinal hemorrhages secondary to drug-induced anemia
4. Lacrimation (doxorubicin)
5. Loss of eyelashes or eyebrows
6. Ocular teratogenic effects (?)

B. Local Ophthalmic Use or Exposure — Mitomycin
   1. Blepharoconjunctivitis
   2. Uveitis
   3. Scleral degeneration
   4. Increased intraocular pressure
   5. Iris prolapse

Clinical Significance: Ocular side effects are generally reversible and transitory, except for their teratogenic effects. Lacrimation has been seen due to doxorubicin. Although red discoloration of the tears has not been reported, doxorubicin can turn the urine red. Adverse effects following topical ophthalmic applications of mitomycin usually develop about a week later, but several cases have developed as late as 16 months. Many of these drugs have a direct irritant effect on the skin, eyes, mucous membranes, and other tissues, and, therefore, inadvertent ocular exposure should be avoided.

References:

Apt, L., and Gaffney, W. L.: Congenital eye abnormalities from drugs during pregnancy. In Leopold, I. H. (Ed.): Symposium on Ocular Therapy. St. Louis, C. V. Mosby, Vol. VII, 1974, pp. 1–22.
Cancer chemotherapy. Med. Lett. Drugs Ther. 22:101, 1980.
Grant, W. M.: Toxicology of the Eye. 2nd Ed., Springfield, Charles C Thomas, 1974, pp. 93, 718.
Knowles, R. S., and Virden, J. E.: Handling of injectable antineoplastic agents. Br. Med. J. 2:589, 1980.
Manalo, F. B., Marks, A., and Davis, H. L., Jr.: Doxorubicin toxicity. Onycholysis, plantar callus formation, and epidermolysis. JAMA 233:56, 1975.
Van Dyk, J. J., et al.: Adriamycin in the treatment of cancer. S. Afr. Med. J. 50:61, 1976.

Generic Name: 1. Busulfan; 2. Carmustine, BCNU; 3. Chlorambucil; 4. Cyclophosphamide; 5. Dacarbazine, DIC; 6. Lomustine, CCNU; 7. Mechlorethamine; 8. Melphalan; 9. Semustine; 10. Triethylenemelamine (Tretamine); 11. Uracil Mustard (Uramustine)

Proprietary Name: 1. Busulphan (G.B.), Misulban (Fr.), Myleran; 2. BiCNU; 3. Chloraminophene (Fr.), Leukeran; 4. Cytoxan, Endoxan (Austral., Fr., Germ., S. Afr.), Endoxana (G.B.), Enduxan (Braz.),

Genoxal (Span.), Procytox (Canad.), Sendoxan (Norw., Swed.); 5. DTIC-Dome; 6. CeeNU; 7. Caryolysine (Fr.), Mustargen, Mustine (G.B.); 8. Alkeran; 9. Methyl-CCNU; 10. TEM; 11. Uracil Mustard

Primary Use: These alkylating agents are used in the treatment of Hodgkin's disease, lymphomas, multiple myeloma, leukemia, neuroblastoma, and retinoblastoma. Chlorambucil, cyclophosphamide, mechlorethamine, melphalan, and uracil mustard are nitrogen mustards, and carmustine, lomustine, and semustine are nitrosureas. Busulfan is an alkyl sulfonate, dacarbazine is a triazene, and triethylenemelamine is an ethylenimine derivative.

Ocular Side Effects:

A. Systemic Administration
   1. Eyelids or conjunctiva
       a. Allergic reactions
       b. Hyperemia (carmustine)
       c. Erythema
       d. Blepharoconjunctivitis — nonspecific (cyclophosphamide, melphalan)
       e. Hyperpigmentation (busulfan, chlorambucil, cyclophosphamide, uracil mustard)
       f. Photosensitivity (cyclophosphamide, dacarbazine)
       g. Urticaria (busulfan, dacarbazine)
       h. Exfoliative dermatitis (chlorambucil)
   2. Decreased vision
   3. Subconjunctival or retinal hemorrhages secondary to drug-induced anemia
   4. Nonspecific ocular irritation (cyclophosphamide)
       a. Lacrimation
       b. Hyperemia
       c. Ocular pain
       d. Edema
       e. Burning sensation
   5. Cataracts (busulfan)
   6. Keratoconjunctivitis sicca (busulfan, chlorambucil)
   7. Corneal edema (melphalan)
   8. Loss of eyelashes or eyebrows
   9. Precipitation of herpes zoster
   10. Ocular teratogenic effects (?)

Clinical Significance: In general, ocular side effects due to these alkylating agents are uncommon, transitory, and seldom of major significance. However, with long-term use, busulfan has caused cataracts and keratoconjunctivitis sicca. Hyperpigmentation of the skin and mucous membranes seen with some of these agents is an indication for discontinued drug use and is reversible. Loss of eyelashes or eyebrows is almost always seen only with severe drug-induced alopecia. One case of possible melphalan-aggravated Fuchs' dystrophy causing acute corneal hydration has been reported. Herpes zoster, which occurs commonly in patients with lymphomas, may be precipitated by the drug's immunosuppressive effects. Ocular teratogenic effects seen with busulfan include microphthalmia and atypical tapetoretinal degeneration. Inadvertent topical ocular exposure with these agents has caused severe conjunctival irritation and has been suspected of causing corneal opacities.

References:

American Hospital Formulary Service. Washington, D.C., American Society of Hospital Pharmacists, Vol. I, *10*:00, 1977.
Apt, L., and Gaffney, W. L.: Congenital eye abnormalities from drugs during pregnancy. In Leopold, I. H. (Ed.): Symposium on Ocular Therapy. St. Louis, C. V. Mosby Co., 1974, Vol. VII, pp. 1–22.
Green, A. A., and Naiman, J. L.: Chlorambucil poisoning. Am. J. Dis. Child. *116*:190, 1968.
Johnson, D. R., and Burns, R. P.: Blepharoconjunctivitis associated with cancer chemotherapy. Trans. Pac. Coast Oto-Ophthalmol. Soc. *46*:43, 1965.
Kapur, T. R.: Systemic photosensitivity towards cyclophosphamide (Endoxan). Indian J. Dermatol. *42*:5, 1976.
Richardson, R. B., et al.: An unusual ocular complication after anesthesia. Anesthesiology *43*:357, 1975.
Rosell Costa, R., et al.: Catarata por busulfan. Med. Clin. *63*:417, 1974.
Rugh, R., and Skaredoff, L.: Radiation and radiomimetic chlorambucil and the fetal retina. Arch. Ophthalmol. *74*:382, 1965.
Saraux, H., and Lefrancois, A.: Degenerative Netzhauterkrankungen nach Behandlung der Mutter mit Busulfan wahrend der Schwangerschaft. Klin. Monatsbl. Augenheilkd. *170*:818, 1977.
Sidi, Y., Douer, D., and Pinkhas, J.: Sicca syndrome in a patient with toxic reaction to busulfan. JAMA *238*:1951, 1977.

Generic Name: Cytarabine. See under *Class: Antiviral Agents.*

Generic Name: 1. Floxuridine; 2. Fluorouracil

Proprietary Name: *Systemic:* 1. FUDR; 2. Adrucil, 5 FU *Topical:* 2. Efudex, Fluoroplex

Primary Use: These fluorinated pyrimidine antimetabolites are used in the management of carcinoma of the colon, rectum, breast, stomach, and pancreas. Fluorouracil is also used topically for actinic keratoses and intradermally for skin cancer.

Ocular Side Effects:

A. Systemic Administration
   1. Nonspecific ocular irritation
      a. Lacrimation
      b. Hyperemia
      c. Photophobia
      d. Ocular pain
      e. Edema
      f. Burning sensation
   2. Decreased vision
   3. Scarring with occlusion of lacrimal canaliculi or punctum
   4. Eyelids or conjunctiva
      a. Cicatricial ectropion
      b. Erythema
      c. Edema
      d. Hyperpigmentation
      e. Photosensitivity
      f. Ulceration
      g. Loss of eyelashes or eyebrows
   5. Nystagmus
   6. Decreased convergence or divergence
   7. Diplopia
   8. Decreased accommodation
   9. Ocular teratogenic effects (?)
B. Topical Administration — Fluorouracil
   1. Irritation
      a. Lacrimation
      b. Ocular pain
      c. Edema
      d. Burning sensation
   2. Eyelids or conjunctiva
      a. Allergic reactions
      b. Hyperpigmentation
      c. Photosensitivity
      d. Subconjunctival hemorrhages
   3. Periorbital edema
C. Local Ophthalmic Use or Exposure — Intradermal Eyelid Injection (Fluorouracil)
   1. Cicatricial ectropion
   2. Eyelids or conjunctiva — hyperpigmentation

Clinical Significance: Fluorouracil is one of the most commonly used cytotoxic drugs in the palliative treatment of solid tumors. Since its therapeutic dose is often close to its toxic level, between 25 to 35 percent of patients on systemic therapy have some ocular side effects. The most common adverse ocular effects are a low-grade blepharitis and conjunctival irritation with symptoms well out of proportion to the clinical findings. These reactions occur within the first few weeks of therapy and are only transitory, but discontinuation of the drug may be required in some patients. Neurotoxicity which possibly affects the brain stem and causes oculomotor disturbances can occur. On long-term therapy, the drug has been found in tears, which possibly causes a local irritation resulting in a cicatricial reaction in the conjunctiva, punctum, canaliculi, and lacrimal sac. If recognized early, some cases have been reversed; however, in most cases, the scarring is irreversible with epiphora resulting. In addition, cicatricial ectropion secondary to long-term systemic fluorouracil has developed. As with the lacrimal outflow system, this is reversible early, but most require surgical correction. Ointments containing fluorouracil used in the treatment of skin lesions near the eye have caused significant ocular irritation requiring discontinuation of this form of therapy. Ocular side effects due to local therapy are usually reversible, if the eye had only limited exposure. Direct injection of fluorouracil into the eyelids for the treatment of basal cell carcinoma can also cause cicatricial ectropion; hyperpigmentation may also occur, but this is usually reversible.

References:

Bixenman, W. W., Nicholls, J. V. V., and Warwick, O. H.: Oculomotor disturbances associated with 5-fluorouracil chemotherapy. Am. J. Ophthalmol. 83:789, 1977.
Christophidis, N., et al.: Lacrimation and 5-fluorouracil. Ann. Intern. Med. 89:574, 1978.
Christophidis, N., et al.: Ocular side effects with 5-fluorouracil. Aust. NZ J. Med. 9: 143, 1979.
Fraunfelder, F. T.: Interim report: National Registry of Possible Ocular Side Effects. Ophthalmology 87:87, 1980.
Haidak, D. J., Hurwitz, B. S., and Yeung, K. Y.: Tear-duct fibrosis (dacryostenosis) due to 5-fluorouracil. Ann. Intern. Med. 88:657, 1978.
Hamersley, J., et al.: Excessive lacrimation from fluorouracil treatment. JAMA 225: 747, 1973.
Physicians' Desk Reference. 35th Ed., Oradell, N.J., Medical Economics Co., 1981, pp. 565, 1500.
Straus, D. J., et al.: Cicatricial ectropion secondary to 5 fluorouracil therapy. Med. Pediatr. Oncol. 3:15, 1977.

Generic Name: Hydroxyurea

Proprietary Name: Hydrea, Litalir (Germ.)

Primary Use: This substituted urea preparation is used in the management of chronic granulocytic leukemia, carcinoma of the ovary, and malignant melanoma.

Ocular Side Effects:

A. Systemic Administration
  1. Subconjunctival or retinal hemorrhages secondary to drug-induced anemia
  2. Eyelids or conjunctiva
     a. Erythema
     b. Hyperpigmentation
     c. Atrophy
     d. Scaling
     e. Loss of eyelashes or eyebrows (?)
  3. Visual hallucinations
  4. Ocular teratogenic effects (?)

Clinical Significance: Adverse ocular reactions due to hydroxyurea are quite rare. Ocular side effects other than teratogenic effects are reversible and transitory after the drug is discontinued.

References:

Apt, L., and Gaffney, W. L.: Congenital eye abnormalities from drugs during pregnancy. In Leopold, I. II. (Ed.): Symposium on Ocular Therapy. St. Louis, C. V. Mosby, Vol. VII, 1974, pp. 1–22.
Gilman, A. G., Goodman, L. S., and Gilman, A. (Eds.): The Pharmacological Basis of Therapeutics. 6th Ed., New York, Macmillan, 1980, p. 1299.
Kennedy, B. J., Smith, L. R., and Goltz, R. W.: Skin changes secondary to hydroxyurea therapy. Arch. Dermatol. *111*:183, 1975.
Physicians' Desk Reference. 35th Ed., Oradell, N.J., Medical Economics Co., 1981, p. 1708.

Generic Name: 1. Mercaptopurine; 2. Thioguanine

Proprietary Name: 1. Purinethol; 2. Lanvis (G.B.)

Primary Use: These purine analogs are used in the treatment of acute and some forms of chronic leukemias.

Ocular Side Effects:

A. Systemic Administration
  1. Eyelids or conjunctiva
     a. Hyperpigmentation
     b. Icterus

2. Subconjunctival or retinal hemorrhages secondary to drug-induced anemia
3. Ocular teratogenic effects (?)

Clinical Significance: Ocular side effects due to these antimetabolites are seldom of clinical importance. Between 10 and 40 percent of patients with acute leukemia receiving mercaptopurine may develop conjunctival icterus.

Interactions with Other Drugs:

A. Effect of Other Drugs on Activity of Purine Analogs
   1. Salicylates ↑
   2. Sulfonamides ↑

References:

American Hospital Formulary Service. Washington, D.C., American Society of Hospital Pharmacists, Vol. I, 10:00, 1978, 1981.
Apt, L., and Gaffney, W. L.: Congenital eye abnormalities from drugs during pregnancy. In Leopold, I. H. (Ed.): Symposium on Ocular Therapy. St. Louis, C. V. Mosby, Vol. VII, 1974, pp. 1–22.
Dukes, M. N. G. (Ed.): Meyler's Side Effects of Drugs. Amsterdam, Excerpta Medica, Vol. VIII, 1975, p. 964.
Gilman, A. G., Goodman, L. S., and Gilman, A. (Eds.): The Pharmacological Basis of Therapeutics. 6th Ed., New York, Macmillan, 1980, pp. 1285–1287.

Generic Name: Methotrexate

Proprietary Name: Ledertrexate (Fr.), Mexate

Primary Use: This folic acid antagonist is effective in the treatment of certain neoplastic diseases and in the management of psoriasis.

Ocular Side Effects:

A. Systemic Administration
   1. Eyelids or conjunctiva
      a. Allergic reactions
      b. Erythema
      c. Blepharoconjunctivitis
      d. Depigmentation
      e. Hyperpigmentation
      f. Photosensitivity
      g. Urticaria
      h. Lyell's syndrome

2. Decreased vision
3. Nonspecific ocular irritation
   a. Lacrimation
   b. Hyperemia
   c. Photophobia
   d. Ocular pain
   e. Burning sensation
4. Periorbital edema
5. Subconjunctival or retinal hemorrhages secondary to drug-induced anemia
6. Keratitis
7. Loss of eyelashes or eyebrows
8. Ocular teratogenic effects (?)

Clinical Significance: Both systemic and ocular side effects due to methotrexate are common. In the opinion of some oncologists, about 25 percent of patients on this drug will develop periorbital edema, blepharitis, conjunctival hyperemia, increased lacrimation, or photophobia. In spite of minimal blepharoconjunctivitis, occasional patients have marked subjective complaints.

Interactions with Other Drugs:

A. Effect of Other Drugs on Activity of Methotrexate
   1. Analgesics ↑
   2. Salicylates ↑
   3. Sulfonamides ↑

References:

American Hospital Formulary Service. Washington, D. C., American Society of Hospital Pharmacists, Vol. I, 10:00, 1973.
Bonadonna, G., et al.: Combination chemotherapy as an adjuvant treatment in operable breast cancer. N. Engl. J. Med. 294:405, 1976.
Fraunfelder, F. T.: Interim report: National Registry of Drug-Induced Ocular Side Effects. Ophthalmology 87:87, 1980.
Havener, W. H.: Ocular Pharmacology. 4th Ed., St. Louis, C. V. Mosby, 1978, pp. 199–200.
Johnson, D. R., and Burns, R. P.: Blepharoconjunctivitis associated with cancer chemotherapy. Trans. Pac. Coast Oto-Ophthalmol. Soc. 46:43, 1965.
Lischka, G.: Auffallend rasche Wirkung des Methotrexats bei Psoriasis eines 82 jahrigen Patienten mit gleichzeitigen Nebenwirkungen am Auge. Hautarzt. 19:473, 1968.
Margileth, D. A., et al.: Blindness during remission in two patients with acute lymphoblastic leukemia. A possible complication of multimodality therapy. Cancer 39:58, 1977.

Generic Name: Mithramycin

Proprietary Name: Mithracin

Primary Use: This cytostatic antibiotic is used primarily in the treatment of testicular neoplasms.

Ocular Side Effects:

A. Systemic Administration
   1. Subconjunctival or retinal hemorrhages
   2. Periorbital pallor
   3. Ocular teratogenic effects (?)

Clinical Significance: The main adverse reaction to mithramycin is severe thrombocytopenia which causes a bleeding diathesis which may also affect the eye. A striking periorbital pallor may occur in patients taking this drug. No reports of other drugs causing this unusual reaction have been made.

References:

AMA Drug Evaluations. 4th Ed., New York, John Wiley & Sons, 1980, pp. 906, 1185.
Dukes, M. N. G. (Ed.): Meyler's Side Effects of Drugs. Amsterdam, Excerpta Medica, Vol. IX, p. 742.
Wade, A. (Ed.): Martindale: The Extra Pharmacopoeia. 27th Ed., London, Pharmaceutical Press, 1977, pp. 161–162.

Generic Name: Mitotane

Proprietary Name: Lysodren

Primary Use: This adrenal cytotoxic agent is used in the treatment of inoperable adrenocortical carcinoma.

Ocular Side Effects:

A. Systemic Administration
   1. Decreased vision
   2. Diplopia
   3. Cataracts
   4. Retinal pigmentary changes
   5. Papilledema
   6. Retinal hemorrhages
   7. Ocular teratogenic effects (?)

Clinical Significance: While systemic side effects due to mitotane occur commonly, adverse ocular reactions occur infrequently. Significant ocular side effects do occur, but seldom require discontinued drug use because of the seriousness of the underlying disease.

References:

AMA Drug Evaluations. 4th Ed., New York, John Wiley & Sons, 1980, pp. 1180–1181.
Apt, L., and Gaffney, W. L.: Congenital eye abnormalities from drugs during pregnancy. In Leopold, I. H. (Ed.): Symposium on Ocular Therapy. St. Louis, C. V. Mosby, Vol. VII, 1974, pp. 1–22.
Gilman, A. G., Goodman, L. S., and Gilman, A. (Eds.): The Pharmacological Basis of Therapeutics. 6th Ed., New York, Macmillan, 1980, pp. 1300–1301.
Physicians' Desk Reference. 35th Ed., Oradell, N.J., Medical Economics Co., 1981, p. 714.

Generic Name: Procarbazine

Proprietary Name: Matulane, Natulan (G.B.), Natulanar (Swed.)

Primary Use: This methylhydrazine derivative is used in the management of generalized Hodgkin's disease.

Ocular Side Effects:

A. Systemic Administration
  1. Subconjunctival or retinal hemorrhages secondary to drug-induced anemia
  2. Eyelids or conjunctiva
     a. Erythema
     b. Hyperpigmentation
     c. Photosensitivity
     d. Purpura
     e. Exfoliative dermatitis
     f. Lyell's syndrome
  3. Nystagmus
  4. Photophobia
  5. Diplopia
  6. Decreased accommodation
  7. Papilledema
  8. Loss of eyelashes or eyebrows (?)
  9. Ocular teratogenic effects (?)

Clinical Significance: Numerous adverse ocular reactions have been caused by procarbazine with the most frequent secondary to drug-induced hematologic disorders. Most ocular side effects are transitory and reversible with discontinued drug use, and seldom are of major clinical significance.

Interactions with Other Drugs:

A. Synergistic Activity
   1. Analgesics
   2. Antihistamines
   3. Barbiturates
   4. Phenothiazines
B. Contraindications
   1. Local anesthetics
   2. Sympathomimetics
   3. Tricyclic antidepressants

References:

AMA Drug Evaluations. 4th Ed., New York, John Wiley & Sons, 1980, pp. 1181–1182.
Apt, L. and Gaffney, W. L.: Congenital eye abnormalities from drugs during pregnancy. In Leopold, I. H. (Ed.): Symposium of Ocular Therapy. St. Louis, C. V. Mosby Co., Vol. VII, 1974, pp. 1–22.
Dukes, M. N. G., (Ed.): Meyler's Side Effects of Drugs. Amsterdam, Excerpta Medica, Vol. VIII, 1975, pp. 947, 978.
Gilman, A. G., Goodman, L. S., and Gilman, A. (Eds.): The Pharmacological Basis of Therapeutics. 6th Ed., New York, Macmillan, 1980, pp. 1299–1300.
Physicians' Desk Reference. 35th Ed., Oradell, N.J., Medical Economics Co., 1981, p. 1513.

Generic Name: Tamoxifen

Proprietary Name: Nolvadex

Primary Use: This antiestrogen is used primarily in the palliative treatment of advanced breast carcinoma in postmenopausal women.

Ocular Side Effects:

A. Systemic Administration
   1. Decreased vision
   2. Corneal opacities
   3. Retinopathy
   4. Macular edema
   5. Ocular teratogenic effects (?)

Clinical Significance: Recently in the literature and confirmed by cases in the Registry, this drug has been implicated to cause corneal opacities, decreased visual acuity, and retinopathy. These patients are generally on higher than usual drug dosage, and the visual symptoms are seldom seen prior to 12 to 18 months. The corneal opacities seen with this agent are whorl-like subepithelial corneal deposits, not unlike those seen with chloroquine. Retinal findings are quite striking in these patients, since they appear as superficial refractile deposits in the posterior pole, primarily in the perimacular area. The abnormalities seem to lie superficial to the retinal blood vessels. Macular edema has been seen with this entity as well.

References:

Beck, M., and Mills, P. V.: Ocular assessment of patients treated with tamoxifen. Cancer Treat. Rep. 63:1833, 1979.

Fraunfelder, F. T.: Interim report: National Registry of Possible Drug-Induced Ocular Side Effects. Ophthalmology 87:87, 1980.

Kaiser-Kupfer, M. I.: Role of the ophthalmologist in the therapy of breast carcinoma. Trans. Ophthalmol. Soc. U.K. 98:184, 1978.

Kaiser-Kupfer, M. I., and Lippman, M. E.: Tamoxifen retinopathy. Cancer Treat. Rep. 62:315, 1978.

Physicians' Desk Reference. 35th Ed., Oradell, N.J., Medical Economics Co., 1981, p. 1760.

Generic Name: Thiotepa

Proprietary Name: Thio-Tepa (G.B.), Tifosyl (Swed.)

Primary Use: *Systemic:* This ethylenimine derivative is used in the management of carcinomas of the breast and ovary, lymphomas, Hodgkin's disease, and various sarcomas. *Ophthalmic:* This topical agent is used to inhibit pterygium recurrence and possibly to prevent corneal neovascularization after chemical injuries.

Ocular Side Effects:

A. Systemic Administration
  1. Eyelids or conjunctiva
     a. Erythema
     b. Urticaria
     c. Loss of eyelashes or eyebrows
  2. Subconjunctival or retinal hemorrhages secondary to drug-induced anemia
  3. Acute fibrinous uveitis (?)
  4. Ocular teratogenic effects (?)
B. Local Ophthalmic Use or Exposure
  1. Irritation

2. Eyelids or conjunctiva
   a. Allergic reactions
   b. Depigmentation
   c. Poliosis
3. Delayed corneal wound healing
4. Keratitis
5. Corneal edema
6. Occlusion of lacrimal punctum
7. Corneal ulceration (?)
8. Ocular teratogenic effects (?)

Clinical Significance: Ocular side effects due to topical ophthalmic thiotepa application are rare. While ocular irritation and allergic reactions are the most common, depigmentation of the eyelids may be the most disturbing ocular reaction. Eyelid depigmentation has been reported to occur 6 years after topical ocular use of thiotepa, and, in some instances, it has been permanent. This depigmentation due to thiotepa is probably enhanced by excessive exposure to sunlight. Use of thiotepa for many months in dosages of 4 to 6 times daily has caused significant keratitis and conjunctivitis. The Registry has received one report of unilateral punctal occlusion possibly due to topical ocular use of this drug. Corneal ulcerations have been attributed to thiotepa when it was used in alkaline injuries; however, this is difficult to substantiate due to the coexisting alkaline damage.

References:

Asregadoo, E. R.: Surgery, thio-tepa, and corticosteroid in the treatment of pterygium. Am. J. Ophthalmol. 74:960, 1972.
Berkow, J. W., Gills, J. P., and Wise, J. B.: Depigmentation of eyelids after topically administered thiotepa. Arch. Ophthalmol. 82:415, 1969.
Cassady, J. R.: The inhibition of pterygium recurrence by Thiotepa. Am. J. Ophthalmol. 61:886, 1966.
Greenspan, E. M., Jaffrey, I., and Bruckner, H.: Thiotepa, cutaneous reactions, and efficacy. JAMA 237:2288, 1977.
Hornblass, A., et al.: A delayed side effect of topical thiotepa. Ann. Ophthalmol. 6: 1155, 1974.
Howitt, D., and Karp, E. J.: Side-effect of topical thio-tepa. Am. J. Ophthalmol. 68: 473, 1969.
Olander, K., Haik, K. G., and Haik, G. M.: Management of pterygia. Should thiotepa be used? Ann. Ophthalmol. 10:853, 1978.

Generic Name: Urethan

Proprietary Name: Urethan

Primary Use: This carbamic acid ester is used in the management of multiple myeloma and leukemia.

Ocular Side Effects:

  A. Systemic Administration
1. Subconjunctival or retinal hemorrhages secondary to drug-induced anemia
2. Decreased vision
3. Nystagmus
4. Pupils
    a. Mydriasis
    b. Absence of reaction to light
5. Ocular teratogenic effects (?)

Clinical Significance: Adverse ocular reactions due to urethan are rare and seldom of major significance. Nystagmus and pupillary changes have only been seen in extreme toxic states and are probably central in origin. While corneal crystals, iritis, ciliary body cysts, and corneal foreign body sensations have been attributed to urethan, these are more likely due to multiple myeloma and not the drug.

References:

Aronson, S. B., and Shaw, R.: Corneal crystals in multiple myeloma. Arch. Ophthalmol. *61*:541, 1959.

Ashton, N.: Cystic changes and urethane (Correspondence). Arch. Ophthalmol. 78: 416, 1967.

Grant, W. M.: Toxicology of the Eye. 2nd Ed., Springfield, Charles C Thomas, 1974, pp. 1074–1076.

Handley, G. J., and Arney, G. K.: Plasma cell myeloma and associated amino acid disorder: Case with crystalline deposition in the cornea and lens. Arch. Intern. Med. *120*:353, 1967.

Wade, A. (Ed.): Martindale: The Extra Pharmacopoeia. 27th Ed., London, Pharmaceutical Press, 1977, pp. 171–172.

Generic Name: 1. Vinblastine; 2. Vincristine

Proprietary Name: 1. Velban, Velbe (G.B.); 2. Oncovin

Primary Use: These vinca alkaloids are often used in conjunction with other antineoplastic agents. Vinblastine is primarily used in inoperable malignant neoplasms of the breast, the female genital tract, the lung, the testis, and the gastrointestinal tract. Vincristine is primarily used in Hodgkin's disease, lymphosarcoma, reticulum cell sarcoma, rhabdomyosarcoma, neuroblastoma, and Wilms' tumor.

Ocular Side Effects:

A. Systemic Administration
   1. Ptosis
   2. Paresis or paralysis of extraocular muscles
   3. Diplopia
   4. Eyelids
      a. Photosensitivity
      b. Loss of eyelashes or eyebrows
   5. Subconjunctival or retinal hemorrhages secondary to drug-induced anemia
   6. Optic atrophy
   7. Ocular signs of gout (?)
   8. Ocular teratogenic effects (?)
B. Inadvertent Ocular Exposure — Vinblastine
   1. Irritation
      a. Lacrimation
      b. Hyperemia
      c. Photophobia
      d. Edema
   2. Cornea
      a. Keratitis
      b. Superficial gray opacities
   3. Blepharospasm
   4. Decreased vision
   5. Astigmatism
   6. Keratoconjunctivitis sicca (?)

Clinical Significance: Vincristine more commonly causes extraocular muscle paresis and ptosis than vinblastine. These ocular side effects are dose-related and most patients obtain full recovery after these agents are discontinued. The onset of extraocular muscle paresis or paralysis may be seen as early as 2 weeks after commencing therapy. Recent data, published and unpublished, suggest vincristine may cause optic atrophy. Even if this is true, it is a rare event and will be difficult to prove, since most of these patients are on multiple drugs. The ocular signs of gout which may occur include conjunctival hyperemia, uveitis, scleritis, and corneal deposits or ulcerations. An accidental splashing of vinblastine on a patient's eye caused corneal clouding, with vision reduced to seeing hand movements. Vision returned to near normal after a number of weeks with astigmatic correcting lens.

References:

Albert, D. M., Wong, V. G., and Henderson, E. S.: Ocular complications of vincristine therapy. Arch. Ophthalmol. 78:709, 1967.

Bradley, W. G., et al.: The neuromyopathy of vincristine in man. Clinical, electro-physiological and pathological studies. J. Neurol. Sci. *10*:107, 1970.

Fishman, M. L., Bean, S. C., and Cogan, D. G.: Optic atrophy following prophylactic chemotherapy and cranial radiation for acute lymphocytic leukemia. Am. J. Ophthalmol. *82*:571, 1976.

Green, W. R.: Retinal and optic nerve atrophy induced by intravitreous vincristine in the primate. Trans. Am. Ophthalmol. Soc. *73*:389, 1975.

McLendon, B. F., and Bron, A. J.: Corneal toxicity from vinblastine solution. Br. J. Ophthalmol. *62*:97, 1978.

Mosci, L.: Astigmatismo contro regola in un caso di causticazione corneale da vincaleucoblastina. Ann. Ottal. *93*:94, 1967.

Sanderson, P. A., Kuwabara, T., and Cogan, D. G.: Optic neuropathy presumably caused by vincristine therapy. Am. J. Ophthalmol. *81*:146, 1976.

XII

Heavy Metal Antagonists and Miscellaneous Agents

Class: Agents Used to Treat Alcoholism

Generic Name: Disulfiram

Proprietary Name: Antabuse, Esperal (Fr.)

Primary Use: This thiuram derivative is used as an aid in the management of chronic alcoholism.

Ocular Side Effects:

A. Systemic Administration
1. Decreased vision
2. Retrobulbar or optic neuritis
3. Scotomas — central or centrocecal
4. Problems with color vision — dyschromatopsia
5. Eyelids or conjunctiva
   a. Allergic reactions
   b. Erythema
   c. Urticaria
   d. Ptosis (?)
6. Visual hallucinations
7. Extraocular muscles
   a. Paresis or paralysis
   b. Nystagmus
8. Anisocoria
9. Toxic amblyopia

Clinical Significance: Adverse ocular side effects due to disulfiram are uncommon. Retrobulbar neuritis has been well documented by numerous authors, since each time the drug was restarted the optic neuritis, often bilateral, would recur. In most cases, the vision lost during retro-bulbar or optic neuritis returned within a few weeks after the drug therapy was discontinued. This ocular side effect may be more common in higher dosages, in the elderly, or in patients with impaired hepatic function. Other ocular side effects are reversible and seldom of importance.

Interactions with Other Drugs:

   A. Effect of Disulfiram on Activity of Other Drugs
      1. Barbiturates ↑
      2. Sedatives and hypnotics ↑
      3. Alcohol ↓

References:

Debrousse, J. Y.: L'examen systematique du fond d'oeil dans le traitement de l'alco-olisme par le disulfure de tetra-ethyl-thiourane. Sem. Hop. Paris 26:4132, 1950.
Humblet, M.: Nevrite retrobulbaire chronique par Antabuse. Bull. Soc. Belge Oph-talmol. 104:297, 1953.
Norton, A. L., and Walsh, F. B.: Disulfiram-induced optic neuritis. Trans. Am. Acad. Ophthalmol. Otolaryngol. 76:1263, 1972.
Perdriel, G., and Chevaleraud, J.: A propos d'un nouveau cas de névrite optique due au disulfirame. Bull. Soc. Ophtalmol. Fr. 66:159, 1966.
Rainey, J. M., Jr.: Disulfiram toxicity and carbon disulfide poisoning. Am. J. Psychia-try 134:371, 1977.
Wade, A. (Ed.): Martindale: The Extra Pharmacopoeia. 27th Ed., London, Phar-maceutical Press, 1977, pp. 538–539.
Walsh, F. B., and Hoyt, W. F.: Clinical Neuro-Ophthalmology. 3rd Ed. Baltimore, Williams & Wilkins, Vol. III, 1969, p. 2597.

Class: Chelating Agents

Generic Name: Deferoxamine

Proprietary Name: *Systemic:* Desferal, Desferrioxamine (G.B.) *Oph-thalmic:* Desferrioxamine (G.B.)

Primary Use: *Systemic:* This chelating agent is used in the treatment of iron-storage diseases and acute iron poisoning. *Ophthalmic:* This topical agent is used in the treatment of ocular siderosis and hematogenous pigmentation of the cornea.

Ocular Side Effects:

A. Systemic Administration
1. Eyelids or conjunctiva
a. Allergic reactions
b. Erythema
c. Urticaria
2. Decreased vision
3. Cataracts
4. Subconjunctival or retinal hemorrhages secondary to drug-induced anemia (?)
B. Local Ophthalmic Use or Exposure
1. Eyelids or conjunctiva
a. Allergic reactions
b. Hyperemia

Clinical Significance: Adverse ocular side effects due to deferoxamine are rare and seldom significant. Cataracts have been observed in 3 patients who received this drug over prolonged periods in the treatment of chronic iron-storage diseases.

References:

Ciba Pharmaceutical Company. Official literature on new drugs: Deferoxamine mesylate (desferal mesylate). A specific iron-chelating agent for treating acute iron intoxication. Clin. Pharmacol. Ther. *10*:595, 1969.
Davidson, S. I.: Report of ocular adverse reactions. Trans. Ophthalmol. Soc. U. K. *93*:495, 1973.
Gilman, A. G., Goodman, L. S., and Gilman, A. (Eds.): The Pharmacological Basis of Therapeutics. 6th Ed., New York, Macmillan, 1980, pp. 1633–1634.
Grant, W. M.: Toxicology of the Eye. 2nd Ed., Springfield, Charles C Thomas, 1974, pp. 351–352.
Jacobs, J., Greene, H., and Gendel, B. R.: Acute iron intoxication. N. Engl. J. Med. *273*:1124, 1965.
Physicians' Desk Reference. 35th Ed., Oradell, N.J., Medical Economics Co., 1981, p. 794.
Valvo, A.: Desferrioxamine B in ophthalmology. Am. J. Ophthalmol. *63*:98, 1967.

Generic Name: Dimercaprol

Proprietary Name: BAL (British Anti-Lewisite)

Primary Use: This chelating agent is effective in the treatment of arsenic, gold, or mercury poisonings.

Ocular Side Effects:

A. Systemic Administration
1. Nonspecific ocular irritation

        a. Lacrimation
        b. Edema
        c. Burning sensation
    2. Eyelids or conjunctiva
        a. Allergic reactions
        b. Conjunctivitis — nonspecific
        c. Blepharospasm
  B. Inadvertent Ocular Exposure
    1. Irritation
        a. Lacrimation
        b. Photophobia
        c. Burning sensation
    2. Blepharospasm

Clinical Significance: Approximately 50 percent of patients receiving intramuscular injections of dimercaprol experience a burning sensation around their eyes within 15 to 20 minutes. This persists for 1 to 2 hours and is completely reversible. Other ocular manifestations to systemic dimercaprol are also of little consequence, transitory, and reversible. Direct ocular contact with this drug causes significant local irritation which lasts for a few hours but without apparent ocular damage.

References:

Dimercaprol. Council on pharmacy and chemistry. "Bal" (British anti-lewisite) in the treatment of arsenic and mercury poisoning. JAMA *131*:824, 1946.
Grant, W. M.: Toxicology of the Eye. 2nd Ed., Springfield, Charles C Thomas, 1974, pp. 398–399.
Peters, R. A., Stocken, L. A., and Thompson, R. H. S.: British anti-lewisite (BAL). Nature *156*:616, 1945.
Scherling, S. S., and Blondis, R. R.: The effect of chemical warfare agents on the human eye. Milit. Surg. *96*:70, 1945.
Wade, A. (Ed.): Martindale: The Extra Pharmacopoeia. 27th Ed., London, Pharmaceutical Press, 1977, pp. 331–332.

Generic Name: Penicillamine

Proprietary Name: Cuprenil (Pol.), Cuprimine, Depamine (G.B.), Depen, Distamine (G.B.), D-Penamine (Austral.), Metalcaptase (Germ.), Trolovol (Germ.)

Primary Use: This amino acid derivative of penicillin is a potent chelating agent effective in the management of Wilson's disease, cystinuria, and copper, iron, lead, or mercury poisonings.

Ocular Side Effects:

A. Systemic Administration
  1. Myasthenic neuromuscular blocking effect
    a. Paresis or paralysis of extraocular muscles
    b. Ptosis
  2. Visual changes
    a. Myopia
    b. Hypermetropia
  3. Diplopia
  4. Nonspecific ocular irritation
    a. Lacrimation
    b. Hyperemia
    c. Photophobia
    d. Edema
  5. Retina
    a. Pigmentary changes
    b. Hemorrhages
  6. Eyelids or conjunctiva
    a. Blepharoconjunctivitis
    b. Lupoid syndrome
    c. Lyell's syndrome
    d. Pemphigoid lesion
    e. Loss of eyelashes or eyebrows (?)
    f. Yellowing and wrinkling
  7. Cornea
    a. Delayed wound healing (?)
    b. Punctate keratitis (?)
  8. Retrobulbar or optic neuritis
  9. Papilledema
  10. Problems with color vision — dyschromatopsia
  11. Subconjunctival or retinal hemorrhages secondary to drug-induced anemia
  12. Cataracts (?)

Clinical Significance: Adverse ocular reactions to the three isomers of penicillamine (D, DL, and L) are rare. Probably most side effects are due to penicillamine-pyridoxine antagonism. This is most common with the DL or L isomers, and only rarely with the D form. Unfortunately, most of the literature does not differentiate which isomer was prescribed, although now only the D form is used. To date, myopia and papilledema have not been reported with the D isomer form of penicillamine. Myasthenia gravis symptoms associated with penicillamine therapy are not uncommon. It appears that this drug can cause antistriational and antiacetylcholine receptor antibodies. Not infrequently, the first signs of this drug-related myasthenia involve the eyes, with ptosis or extraocular muscle paresis. This drug is now also associated with a number of skin disorders with ocular related abnormalities. It has been implicated in delayed wound healing and proliferation of connective tissue. Retinal changes, such as retinal pigment epithelial defects, have been reported in the literature, and possible retinitis pigmentosa with bone corpuscle-shaped pigment deposits have been reported to the Registry. Penicillamine-induced zinc deficiency may be the cause of keratitis, blepharitis, and loss of eyelashes, but this is unproven to date.

Interactions with Other Drugs:

   A. Cross Sensitivity
       1. Penicillins

References:

Bigger, J. F.: Retinal hemorrhages during penicillamine therapy of cystinuria. Am. J. Ophthalmol. *66*:954, 1968.
Dingle, J., and Havener, W. H.: Ophthalmoscopic changes in a patient with Wilson's disease during long-term penicillamine therapy. Ann. Ophthalmol. *10*:1227, 1978.
Fraunfelder, F. T.: Interim report: National Registry of Possible Drug-Induced Ocular Side Effects. Ophthalmology *87*:87, 1980.
Greer, K. E., Askew, F. C., and Richardson, D. R.: Skin lesions induced by penicillamine. Occurrence in a patient with hepatolenticular degeneration (Wilson disease). Arch. Dermatol. *112*:1267, 1976.
Klingberg, W. G., Prasad, A. S., and Oberleas, D.: Zinc deficiency following penicillamine therapy. In Prasad, A. S., and Oberleas, D. (Eds.): Trace Elements in Human Health and Disease. New York, Academic Press, 1976, p. 51.
Masters, C. L., et al.: Penicillamine-associated myasthenia gravis, antiacetylcholine receptor and antistriational antibodies. Am. J. Med. *63*:689, 1977.
Penicillamine for rheumatoid arthritis. Med. Lett. Drugs Ther. *20*:73, 1978.
Reeback, J., et al.: Penicillamine-induced neuromyotonia. Br. Med. J. *1*:1464, 1979.

Class: Dermatologic Agents

Generic Name: Chrysarobin

Proprietary Name: Chrysarobin

Primary Use: This keratolytic agent is effective in the treatment of psoriasis and parasitic skin infections.

Ocular Side Effects:

A. Systemic Absorption from Topical Application to the Skin
1. Nonspecific ocular irritation
2. Eyelids or conjunctiva
   a. Hyperemia
   b. Brown-violet discoloration
3. Keratoconjunctivitis
4. Punctate keratitis
5. Gray corneal opacities
B. Inadvertent Ocular Exposure
1. Irritation
   a. Lacrimation
   b. Hyperemia
   c. Photophobia
2. Eyelids or conjunctiva
   a. Allergic reactions
   b. Conjunctivitis — nonspecific
   c. Edema
   d. Brown-violet discoloration
3. Keratitis

Clinical Significance: Systemic absorption of chrysarobin through the skin has caused aggravating ocular symptoms. Irritation may be extensive and often takes the form of a keratoconjunctivitis which, in rare instances, may last for weeks. Chrysarobin is highly irritating as well if it comes into direct contact with the eye; however, rarely is permanent damage done. In general, ocular irritation secondary to direct ocular contact or systemic absorption usually subsides 8 to 10 days from the time of last exposure.

References:

Duke-Elder, S.: System of Ophthalmology. St. Louis, C. V. Mosby, Vol. XIV, Part 2, 1972, p. 1189.
Dukes, M. N. G. (Ed.): Meyler's Side Effects of Drugs. Amsterdam, Excerpta Medica, Vol. VII, 1975, p. 345.
Grant, W. M.: Toxicology of the Eye. 2nd Ed., Springfield, Charles C Thomas, 1974, pp. 152, 291.
Wade, A. (Ed.): Martindale: The Extra Pharmacopoeia. 27th Ed., London, Pharmaceutical Press, 1977, p. 442.
Willetts, G. S.: Ocular side-effects of drugs. Br. J. Ophthalmol. 53:252, 1969.

Generic Name: Hexachlorophene

Proprietary Name: Derl, Dermohex (Canad.), E-Z Scrub (G.B.), G-11, Gamophen, Gill Liquid (S. Afr.), Hexachlorone (Canad.), Hexachlorophane (G.B.), Hexacreme (S. Afr.), Hexaklen (S. Afr.), Hexaphenyl (Canad.), Kalacide (S. Afr.), Orahex (Austral.), pHisoHex, Sapoderm (Austral., Canad.), Skrub Kreme, Steridermis (G.B.), Ster-Zac (G.B.), Surgiderm (Canad.), Zalpon (G.B.)

Primary Use: This chlorinated biphenol is a topical germicide with high bacteriostatic activity which is commonly used to degerm the skin.

Ocular Side Effects:

A. Systemic Administration — Inadvertent Oral Ingestion
   1. Decreased vision
   2. Pupils
     a. Miosis
     b. Absence of reaction to light
   3. Optic atrophy
   4. Toxic amblyopia
   5. Ocular teratogenic effects (?)
B. Systemic Absorption from Topical Application to the Skin
   1. Eyelids
     a. Erythema
     b. Photosensitivity
   2. Diplopia
C. Local Ophthalmic Use or Exposure — Inadvertent Ocular Exposure
   1. Irritation
     a. Conjunctivitis
     b. Lacrimation
     c. Hyperemia
     d. Photophobia
     e. Burning sensation
   2. Decreased vision
   3. Cornea
     a. Keratitis
     b. Edema

Clinical Significance: Hexachlorophene is toxic by the oral route. Case reports, both published and unpublished, confirm a predilection of the toxic effect on the optic nerve. Systemic toxicity can also occur from chronic dermatologic use of the drug in underweight, premature infants, in infants with excoriated skin, or in adults if applied several times a day to the skin or vagina. Inadvertent ocular exposure of this agent can produce a severe keratitis involving all layers of the human cornea. A marked reduction of visual acuity has been reported to occur initially, but seldom are these changes irreversible.

References:

Browning, C. W., and Lippas, J.: pHisoHex keratitis. Arch. Ophthalmol. 53:817, 1955.
Gilman, A. G., Goodman, L. S., and Gilman, A. (Eds.): The Pharmacological Basis of Therapeutics. 6th Ed., New York, Macmillan, 1980, pp. 968–969.
Martinez, A. J., Boehm, R., and Hadfield, M. G.: Acute hexachlorophene encephalopathy: Clinico-neuropathological correlation. Acta Neuropathol. 28:93, 1974.
Photosensitivity from drugs, perfumes, and cosmetics. Med. Lett. Drugs Ther. 22:64, 1980.
Slamovits, T. L., Burde, R. M., and Klingele, T. G.: Bilateral optic atrophy caused by chronic oral ingestion and topical application of hexachlorophene. Am. J. Ophthalmol. 89:676, 1980.

Generic Name: 1. Methoxsalen; 2. Trioxsalen

Proprietary Name: 1. Oxsoralen, Soloxsalen (Canad.); 2. Trisoralen

Primary Use: These psoralens are administered topically for the treatment of vitiliginous lesions. The drugs are applied to the affected area and then exposed to long-wave (320 to 400 nm) ultraviolet light source.

Ocular Side Effects:

A. Systemic Absorption from Topical Application to the Skin
    1. Eyelids or conjunctiva
        a. Hyperpigmentation
        b. Erythema
        c. Photosensitivity
        d. Increased incidence of skin cancers
    2. Lens changes
        a. Yellowing (?)
        b. Cataracts (?)
    3. Pigmentary glaucoma

Clinical Significance: A marked increase in clinical interest from the ophthalmic viewpoint has been generated by this group of drugs. Photochemotherapy (PUVA), using 8-methoxypsoralen (8-MOP) plus long-wave ultraviolet light, is now commonplace in the treatment of psoriasis. While it has been shown that free 8-MOP can be detected in human lenses for at least 12 hours following oral ingestion, to date, few cataracts have been reported to the Registry or in the literature. However, lens changes have been produced in animals. These drugs are strong photosensitizers; therefore, a photochemical reaction is possible. For this reason, it is recommended that the lens of the eye be protected from any light source by means of special lenses for a minimum of 12 to 24 hours after drug exposure. To date, no retinal changes have been found. There are, however, clear data that PUVA increases the incidence of skin cancers.

References:

Andersen, K. E., and Maibach, H. I.: Allergic reaction to drugs used topically. Clin. Toxicol. *16*:415, 1980.
Cyrlin, M. N., Pedvis-Leftick, A., and Sugar, J.: Cataract formation in association with ultraviolet photosensitivity. Ann. Ophthalmol. *12*:786, 1980.
Glew, W. B.: Determination of 8-methoxypsoralen in serum, aqueous, and lens: Relation to long-wave ultraviolet phototoxicity in experimental and clinical photochemotherapy. Trans. Am. Ophthalmol. Soc. *77*:464, 1979.
Helland, S., and Bang, G.: Nevus spilus-like hyperpigmentation in psoriatic lesions during PUVA therapy. Acta Derm. Venereol. *60*:81, 1979.
Lerman, S., Megaw, J., and Willis, I.: Potential ocular complications from PUVA therapy and their prevention. J. Invest. Dermatol. *74*:197, 1980.
Lerman, S., Megaw, J., and Willis, I.: The photoreactions of 8-methoxypsoralen with tryptophan and lens proteins. Photochem. Photobiol. *31*:235, 1980.

Class: Diagnostic Aids

Generic Name: Diatrizoate Meglumine and/or Sodium

Proprietary Name: Cardiografin, Cystografin, Gastrografin, Hypaque Meglumine, Radioselectan (Fr.), Renografin, Reno-M, Renovist, Sinografin, Urografin (C.B.), Uropolinum (Pol.), Urovist (Germ.)

Primary Use: This organic iodide is used in excretion urography, aortography, pediatric angiocardiography, and peripheral arteriography.

Ocular Side Effects:

  A. Systemic Administration
   1. Decreased vision
   2. Eyelids or conjunctiva
       a. Allergic reactions
       b. Hyperemia
       c. Conjunctivitis — follicular
       d. Edema
       e. Angioneurotic edema
       f. Urticaria
   3. Nonspecific ocular irritation
       a. Lacrimation

      b. Photophobia
      c. Ocular pain
      d. Burning sensation
   4. Corneal infiltrates
   5. Visual fields
      a. Scotoma
      b. Hemianopsia
   6. Retinal vascular disorders
      a. Hemorrhages
      b. Thrombosis

Clinical Significance: Ocular complications associated with the intravenous administration of radiopaque dyes have been well documented. These complications usually result either from the toxic, irritative, or hypersensitivity responses on the vessel or the production of emboli. A number of hypersensitivity responses have occurred with these agents, especially perilimbal corneal infiltrates not unlike that seen with staphylococcal hypersensitivity reactions. These infiltrates clear on topical ocular steroids without complication. This drug has also been reported to layer out in the anterior chamber—like a hypopyon—in a 2-week postoperative cataract patient. In the absence of pathologic confirmation, retinal or cerebral emboli with resultant secondary complications have been variously interpreted as cholesterol crystals, fat, air, dislodged atheromatous plaques, and the injected contrast media.

References:

Baum, J. L., and Bierstock, S. R.: Peripheral corneal infiltrates following intravenous injection of diatrizoate meglumine. Am. J. Ophthalmol. 85:613, 1978.

Browne, J. S., and Andy, O. J.: Complications from Hypaque cerebral arteriography. Surg. Forum 9:732, 1958.

Guerry, D., III, and Wiesinger, H.: Ocular complications of carotid arteriography. Am. J. Ophthalmol. 55:241, 1963.

Haney, W. P., and Preston, R. E.: Ocular complications of carotid arteriography in carotid occlusive disease. Arch. Ophthalmol. 67:127, 1962.

Levine, R. A., and Henry, M. D.: Ischemic infarction of the retina. Am. J. Ophthalmol. 55:365, 1963.

Priluck, I. A., Buettner, H., and Robertson, D. M.: Acute macular neuroretinopathy. Am. J. Ophthalmol. 86:775, 1978.

Class: Immunosuppressants

Generic Name: Azathioprine

Proprietary Name: Imuran, Imurek (Germ.), Imurel (Aust., Fr., Swed.)

Primary Use: This imidazolyl derivative of mercaptopurine is used as an adjunct to help prevent rejection in homograft transplantation and to treat various possible autoimmune diseases.

Ocular Side Effects:

A. Systemic Administration
1. Decreased resistance to infection
2. Delayed corneal wound healing
3. Retinal pigmentary changes
4. Subconjunctival or retinal hemorrhages secondary to drug-induced anemia
5. Loss of eyelashes or eyebrows (?)
6. Ocular teratogenic effects (?)
7. Cataracts (?)

Clinical Significance: Ocular side effects due to azathioprine are uncommon and, except for possible teratogenic effects, are usually reversible upon drug withdrawal. However, there are data that this agent can decrease resistance to infection or even activate some virus infections, such as vaccinia, cytomegalic inclusion disease, and possibly herpes. Inadvertent ocular exposure of the drug will cause irritation.

References:

AMA Drug Evaluations. 4th Ed., New York, John Wiley & Sons, 1980, pp. 1127–1128.
Ellis, P. P.: Ocular Therapeutics and Pharmacology. 5th Ed., St. Louis, C. V. Mosby, 1977, pp. 166–167, 228.
Havener, W. H.: Ocular Pharmacology. 4th Ed., St. Louis, C. V. Mosby, 1978, p. 198.
Knowles, R. S., and Virden, J. E.: Handling of injectable antineoplastic agents. Br. Med. J. 2:589, 1980.
Koch, H. R., and Hockwin, O.: Iatrogenic cataract. Ther. Ggw. *114*:1450, 1975.
Physicians' Desk Reference. 35th Ed., Oradell, N.J., Medical Economics Co., 1981, p. 753.
Wade, A. (Ed.): Martindale: The Extra Pharmacopoeia. 27th Ed., London, Pharmaceutical Press, 1977, pp. 123–127.

Class: Solvents

Generic Name: Dimethyl Sulfoxide, DMSO

Proprietary Name: Domoso, Rimso-50

Primary Use: This is an exceptional solvent with controversial medical therapeutic indications. It is possibly effective in the treatment of musculoskeletal pain, as a solvent for antivirals (IDU) or anticancer drugs, and as an anti-inflammatory agent.

Ocular Side Effects:

A. Systemic or Topical Administration
1. Potentiates the adverse effects of any drug it is combined with
B. Local Ophthalmic Use or Exposure
1. Irritation
a. Burning sensation
2. Eyelids
a. Erythema
b. Photosensitivity

Clinical Significance: DMSO may enhance the ocular side effects of other drugs by increasing the speed and volume of systemic absorption. No cases of any lens changes in man have been reported due to systemic or local ocular exposure. To date, lens and retinal toxicity have been poorly investigated partly because the drug has such a characteristic odor it cannot be used in double-blind studies. There is one study in primates which suggests this agent may cause nuclear sclerosis of the lens. Topical ocular DMSO in high concentrations commonly causes ocular irritation. Topical ocular use is associated with foul oyster type breath; this is because the DMSO drains down the nasolacrimal ducts directly into the oral cavity.

References:

Barnett, K. C., and Noel, P. R. B.: Dimethyl sulphoxide and lens changes in primates. Nature 214:1115, 1967.

Gordon, D. M.: Dimethyl sulfoxide in ophthalmology, with special reference to possible toxic effects. Ann. N. Y. Acad. Sci. 141:392, 1967.

Gordon, D. M., and Kleberger, K. E.: The effect of dimethylsulfoxide (DMSO) on animal and human eyes. Arch. Ophthalmol. 79:423, 1968.

Hanna, C., Fraunfelder, F. T., and Meyer, S. M.: Effects of dimethylsulfoxide on ocular inflammation. Ann. Ophthalmol. 9:61, 1977.

Hull, F. W., Wood, D. C., and Brobyn, R. D.: Eye effects of DMSO. Report of negative results. Northwest. Med. 68:39, 1969.

Kleberger, K. E.: An ophthalmological evaluation of DMSO. Ann. N. Y. Acad. Sci. 141:381, 1967.

Wade, A. (Ed.): Martindale: The Extra Pharmacopoeia. 27th Ed., London, Pharmaceutical Press, 1977, pp. 1461–1463.

Generic Name: Methyl Alcohol

Proprietary Name: Methanol, Rubbing Alcohol, Wood Alcohol

Primary Use: This agent is widely employed industrially as a solvent. It is also used as an adulterant to "denature" the ethyl alcohol that is used for cleaning purposes, paint removal, and a variety of other uses.

Ocular Side Effects:

A. Systemic Administration
1. Decreased vision
2. Pupils
   a. Mydriasis
   b. Decreased reaction to light
3. Horizontal nystagmus
4. Paresis of extraocular muscles
5. Problems with color vision — dyschromatopsia, red-green or blue-yellow defect
6. Visual fields
   a. Scotomas — central, centrocecal, or paracentral
   b. Constriction
7. Retinal vascular disorders
   a. Edema
   b. Hemorrhages
8. Optic atrophy
9. Toxic amblyopia

Clinical Significance: Methyl alcohol is highly poisonous, and consumption in some individuals leads to a rapid loss of vision. Ophthalmoscopically, the first sign of toxicity is hyperemia of discs, followed by peripapillary retinal edema and engorgement of the retinal veins. The more severe the retinal edema, the more likely permanent visual loss will follow. Pupillary dilatation and horizontal nystagmus are common. The earliest changes in the visual fields are due to loss of sensitivity to color. Initially, this occurs for green, followed by red, yellow, and finally blue. Prompt treatment is essential if the toxic effects of methyl alcohol are to be minimized.

References:

Birch, J., et al.: Acquired color vision defects. In Pokorny, J., et al. (Eds.): Congenital and Acquired Color Vision Defects. New York, Grune & Stratton, 1979, pp. 243–348.

Carroll, F. D.: Toxicology of the optic nerve. In Srinivasan, B.D. (Ed.): Ocular Therapeutics. New York, Masson, 1980, pp. 139–144.

Dethlefs, R., and Naraqi, S.: Ocular manifestations and complications of acute methyl alcohol intoxication. Med. J. Aust. 2:483, 1978.

Havener, W. H.: Ocular Pharmacology. 4th Ed., St. Louis, C. V. Mosby, 1978, pp. 406–409.

Walsh, F. B., and Hoyt, W. F.: Clinical Neuro-Ophthalmology. 3rd Ed., Baltimore, Williams & Wilkins, Vol. III, 1969, pp. 2582–2583.

Class: Vaccines

Generic Name: Diphtheria and Tetanus Toxoids and Pertussis (DPT) Vaccine Adsorbed

Proprietary Name: Di-Te-Tuss (Germ.), DT Coq Adsorbe (Fr.), DT Perthydral (Fr.), Tri-Immunol, Triogen, Triple Antigen, Tri-Solgen, Trivax (G.B.), Vaccin Ipad DTC (Fr.)

Primary Use: This combination of diphtheria and tetanus toxoids with pertussis vaccine is the recommended preparation for routine primary immunization and recall injections in children under 7 years of age.

Ocular Side Effects:

A. Systemic Administration
1. Paresis or paralysis of extraocular muscles
2. Eyelids or conjunctiva
   a. Allergic reactions
   b. Urticaria
3. Decreased vision
4. Uveitis
5. Papilledema secondary to pseudotumor cerebri
6. Optic neuritis

Clinical Significance: Adverse ocular reactions secondary to this preparation are rare and transitory. Generalized urticarial reactions have been reported to occur immediately or several hours after injection. Allergic reactions due to preservatives or contaminants of the antigens are seen, although rarely. Neurologic complications, including papilledema, optic neuritis, and decreased vision, have been reported as transient adverse effects, sometimes accompanying encephalitis.

References:

Dolinova, L.: Bilateral uveoretinoneuritis after vaccination with Ditepe (diphtheria, tetanus, and pertussis vaccine). Cs. Oftal. *30*:114, 1974.
Dukes, M. N. G. (Ed.): Meyler's Side Effects of Drugs. Amsterdam, Excerpta Medica, Vol. IX, 1980, pp. 547–550.

McReynolds, W. U., Havener, W. H., and Petrohelos, M. A.: Bilateral optic neuritis following smallpox vaccination and diphtheria-tetanus toxoid. Am. J. Dis. Child. 86:601, 1953.

Walsh, F. B., and Hoyt, W. F.: Clinical Neuro-Ophthalmology. 3rd Ed., Baltimore, Williams & Wilkins, Vol. III, 1969, pp. 2709–2710.

Generic Name: 1. Influenza Virus Vaccine; 2. Measles Virus Vaccine Live; 3. Poliovirus Vaccine; 4. Rabies Immune Globulin and Vaccine; 5. Rubella Virus Vaccine Live

Proprietary Name: 1. Admune (G.B.), Alorbat (Germ., S. Afr.), Fluax, Flu-Imune, Fluogen, Fluzone, Gripovax (Belg.), Influvac (G.B.), Influvaxin (S. Afr.), Mutagrip (Fr.), Nasoflu (G.B.), Vaxigrip (Fr.), Zonomune; 2. Attenuvax, Koplivac (S. Afr.), Lirugen (Austral., Canad., S. Afr.), Mevilin-L (G.B.), M-Vac, Rouvax (Fr.); 3. Diplovax, Oral-Virelon (Germ.), Orimune, Virelon (Germ.); 4. Hyperab; 5. Almevax (G.B.), Cendevax (G.B.), Ervevax (Fr.), Meruvax, Rudivax (Fr.)

Primary Use: These viral vaccines, both live attenuated and inactivated, are used for active immunization against specific viruses.

Ocular Side Effects:

A. Systemic Administration
1. Decreased vision
2. Eyelids or conjunctiva
    a. Erythema
    b. Blepharoconjunctivitis
    c. Edema (poliovirus vaccine)
    d. Urticaria
    e. Purpura (rubella virus vaccine live)
3. Extraocular muscles
    a. Paresis
    b. Diplopia
    c. Nystagmus
    d. Strabismus (measles virus vaccine live)
4. Anterior and posterior uveitis
5. Decreased accommodation (rubella virus vaccine live)
6. Photophobia (rabies vaccine)
7. Toxic amblyopia (influenza virus vaccine)
8. Exophthalmos (poliovirus vaccine)
9. Optic neuritis

Clinical Significance: Adverse ocular reactions due to these viral vaccines are rare and generally transitory. The extraocular muscle abnormalities and uveitis usually occur 2 to 8 days following the vaccination and last for 1 to 7 days. Rarely, an optic neuritis may appear 7 to 10 days following administration. One case of direct ocular exposure to live measles virus vaccine resulted in a keratoconjunctivitis, which resolved within 2 weeks. It has been suggested that patients who have had a demyelinating disease should not receive vaccines.

References:

Behan, P. O.: Diffuse myelitis associated with rubella vaccination. Br. Med. J. *1*: 166, 1977.
Bienfang, D. C., et al.: Ocular abnormalities after influenza immunization. Arch. Ophthalmol. *95*:1649, 1977.
Chan, C. C., Sogg, R. L., and Steinman, L.: Isolated oculomotor palsy after measles immunization. Am. J. Ophthalmol. *89*:446, 1980.
Cormack, H. S., and Anderson, L. A. P.: Bilateral papillitis following antirabic inoculation: Recovery. Br. J. Ophthalmol. *18*:167, 1934.
Hasselbacher, P.: Neuropathy after influenza vaccination. Lancet *1*:551, 1977.
Kirkham, T. H., and MacLellan, A. V.: Strabismus following measles vaccination. Br. Orthop. J. *27*:108, 1970.
Perry, H. D., et al.: Reversible blindness in optic neuritis associated with influenza vaccination. Ann. Ophthalmol. *11*:545, 1979.
Rabin, J.: Hazard of influenza vaccine in neurologic patients. JAMA *225*:63, 1973.
Wade, A. (Ed.): Martindale: The Extra Pharmacopoeia. 27th Ed., London, Pharmaceutical Press, 1977, pp. 1616–1620, 1623–1628.

Generic Name: Smallpox Vaccine

Proprietary Name: Bague-Variole (Fr.), Dryvax

Primary Use: This vaccine is used to provide active immunity against smallpox.

Ocular Side Effects:

A. Systemic Administration
  1. Eyelids or conjunctiva
    a. Erythema
    b. Blepharoconjunctivitis
    c. Edema
    d. Photosensitivity
    e. Urticaria
    f. Purpura
    g. Erythema multiforme
    h. Stevens-Johnson syndrome
    i. Eczema
  2. Cornea

      a. Superficial punctate keratitis
      b. Scarring
  3. Uveitis
  4. Optic neuritis
  5. Decreased vision
  6. Precipitation of herpes virus infections

Clinical Significance: Ocular adverse effects secondary to smallpox vaccine are rare and usually transitory. Vaccinial lesions on the eyelids and the conjunctiva have been seen as secondary inoculations with vaccinia virus from another site. From these lesions, a keratitis may develop which sometimes extends to deeper layers of the cornea with concomitant uveitis. Accidental infection (autoinoculation) of the eye may result in decreased vision. Herpes virus infections have been observed following smallpox vaccination. Allergic reactions are much less common after revaccination than after primary vaccination. Optic neuritis has been reported after revaccination and primary vaccination.

References:

Ferry, B. J.: Adverse reactions after smallpox vaccination. Med. J. Aust. 2:180, 1977.
McReynolds, W. U., Havener, W. H., and Petrohelos, M. A.: Bilateral optic neuritis following smallpox vaccination and diphtheria-tetanus toxoid. Am. J. Dis. Child. 86:601, 1953.
Mathur, S. P., Makhija, J. M., and Mehta, M. C.: Papillitis with myelitis after revaccination. Indian J. Med. Sci. 21:469, 1967.
Ross, J., and Gorin, M.: Vaccinia infection of the eyelids. Two case reports. Eye Ear Nose Throat Month. 48:363, 1969.

Generic Name: Tetanus Toxoid

Proprietary Name: Tetanol (Germ.), Tetatoxoid (Germ.), Tetavax (Fr.), T-Immun (Germ.)

Primary Use: Tetanus toxoid is used prophylactically for wound management in patients not completely immunized.

Ocular Side Effects:

  A. Systemic Administration
    1. Eyelids
      a. Erythema
      b. Urticaria
    2. Paralysis of accommodation
    3. Nystagmus
    4. Optic neuritis (?)

Clinical Significance: Except for local reactions, such as erythema or urticaria, adverse ocular reactions following tetanus toxoid are rare. Recent publications emphasize that overimmunization may lead to adverse reactions. Nystagmus, accommodative paresis, and possibly optic neuritis have been reported as adverse ocular symptoms following tetanus vaccine.

References:

Harrer, V. G., Melnizky, U., and Wendt, H.: Akkommodationsparese und Schluck-lähmung nach Tetanus-Toxoid-Auffrischungsimpfung. Wien. Med. Wochenschr. *15*:296, 1971.

McReynolds, W. U., Havener, W. H., and Petrohelos, M. A.: Bilateral optic neuritis following smallpox vaccination and diphtheria-tetanus toxoid. Am. J. Dis. Child. *86*:601, 1953.

Schlenska, G. K.: Unusual neurological complications following tetanus toxoid administration. J. Neurol. *215*:299, 1977.

XIII

Drugs Used Primarily in Ophthalmology

Class: Agents Used to Treat Glaucoma

Generic Name: Dipivefrin, DPE

Proprietary Name: Propine

Primary Use: This adrenergic agent is indicated as initial therapy for the control of intraocular pressure in chronic open-angle glaucoma.

Ocular Side Effects:

A. Local Ophthalmic Use or Exposure
   1. Decreased intraocular pressure
   2. Irritation
      a. Lacrimation
      b. Hyperemia
      c. Ocular pain
      d. Burning sensation
   3. Eyelids or conjunctiva
      a. Erythema
      b. Conjunctivitis — follicular
   4. Decreased vision
   5. Mydriasis — may precipitate narrow-angle glaucoma
   6. Cystoid macular edema (?)

Clinical Significance: Dipivefrin is a prodrug, which is biotransformed to epinephrine inside the eye. This drug is better tolerated than standard epinephrine preparations; but at concentrations greater than 0.1 percent, there are increased epinephrine-like side effects: stinging, hyperemia, mydriasis with blurred vision, and intolerance. Dipivefrin has been used without contact lens discoloration. This drug has been released only recently, and it is too early to fully evaluate its potential for adverse reactions. However, to date, it is surprisingly free of major adverse effects. While there have been some cases of maculopathy reported to the Registry, these may be only chance occurrences. However, this potential adverse effect should be especially watched for in aphakics.

References:

Kaback, M. B., et al.: The effects of dipivalyl epinephrine on the eye. Am. J. Ophthalmol. *81*:768, 1976.
Mandell, A. I., and Podos, S. M.: Dipivalyl epinephrine (DPE): A new prodrug in the treatment of glaucoma. In Leopold, I. H., and Burns, R. P. (Eds.): Symposium on Ocular Therapy. New York, John Wiley & Sons, Vol. X, 1977, pp. 109–117.
Newton, M. J., and Nesburn, A. B.: Lack of hydrophilic lens discoloration in patients using dipivalyl epinephrine for glaucoma. Am. J. Ophthalmol. *87*:193, 1979.
Theodore, J., and Leibowitz, H. M.: External ocular toxicity of dipivalyl epinephrine. Am. J. Ophthalmol. *88*:1013, 1979.
Yablonski, M. E., et al.: Dipivefrin use in patients with intolerance to topically applied epinephrine. Arch. Ophthalmol. *95*:2157, 1977.
Zimmerman, T. J., Leader, B., and Kaufman, H. E.: Advances in ocular pharmacology. Annu. Rev. Pharmacol. Toxicol. *20*:415, 1980.

Generic Name: Timolol

Proprietary Name: Blocadren, Timolate, Timoptic, Timoptol

Primary Use: This beta-adrenergic blocker is used to treat glaucoma.

Ocular Side Effects:

A. Local Ophthlamic Use or Exposure
1. Decreased intraocular pressure
2. Irritation
    a. Hyperemia
    b. Ocular pain
    c. Burning sensation
3. Decreased vision
4. Punctate keratitis
5. Eyelids or conjunctiva
    a. Allergic reactions
    b. Erythema
    c. Blepharoconjunctivitis
    d. Urticaria
    e. Purpura
    f. Erythema multiforme

6. Myopia
7. Visual hallucinations
8. Decreased corneal reflex
9. Keratoconjunctivitis sicca
10. Myasthenic neuromuscular blocking effect
    a. Paralysis of extraocular muscles
    b. Ptosis
11. Uveitis (?)
12. Loss of eyelashes or eyebrows (?)
13. Cataracts (?)

Clinical Significance: In the history of ocular pharmacology, never has a drug reached such wide acceptance in as short a period of time as has this agent. While some systemic side effects are of major clinical importance, only occasionally are ocular side effects of major clinical significance. If superficial punctate keratitis is noted, corneal sensitivity should be checked since the cornea may be anesthetized. Keratoconjunctivitis sicca has been aggravated while patients were on this agent. Visual loss may become prominent after starting this drug; two types occur, both of which are reversible after the drug is discontinued. The more common is an increased myopia even up to 3 to 4 diopters. The second type is a decrease in vision, occasionally 20/60 to 20/80, which is unexplained. Some have postulated this is due to a vascular effect—decreased perfusion—but, to date, the cause is unknown. Visual hallucinations and even vivid often frightening dreams occur on topical ocular timolol, but this is probably on a systemic absorption basis. To the Registry's knowledge, nearly all ocular side effects attributed to timolol are reversible once the drug is discontinued. While a number of unilateral cataracts have been reported to the Registry following unilateral timolol application, unilateral glaucoma with its various topical antiglaucoma medications can have a higher frequency of cataracts in its own right.

Interactions with Other Drugs:

A. Synergistic Activity
    1. Adrenergic blockers
    2. Carbonic anhydrase inhibitors
    3. Miotics
    4. Sympathomimetics
B. Contraindications
    1. Patients with preexisting asthmatic conditions
    2. Patients with cardiopulmonary problems

References:

Fraunfelder, F. T.: Interim report: National Registry of Possible Drug-Induced Ocular Side Effects. Ophthalmology 87:87, 1980.
Kaufman, H. E.: 1. Timolol maleate. Ophthalmology 87:164, 1980.
Nielsen, N. V., and Eriksen, J. S.: Timolol transitory manifestations of dry eyes in long term treatment. Acta Ophthalmol. 57:418, 1979.
Shaivitz, S. A.: Timolol and myasthenia gravis. JAMA 242:1611, 1979.
Van Buskirk, E. M.: Adverse reactions from timolol administration. Ophthalmology 87:447, 1980.
Wilson, R. P., Spaeth, G. L., and Poryzees, E.: The place of timolol in the practice of ophthalmology. Ophthalmology 87:451, 1980.
Yates, D.: Syncope and visual hallucinations, apparently from timolol. JAMA 244: 768, 1980.

Class: Antibacterial Agents

Generic Name: 1. Colloidal Silver; 2. Silver Nitrate (Argentum Nitrate); 3. Silver Protein (Argentum Protein)

Proprietary Name: 1. Colloidal Silver; 2. Mova Nitrat (Germ.); 3. Argincolor (Fr.), Argyrol, Protargol, Stillargol (Fr.), Veraseptyl (Ital.)

Primary Use: These topical ocular antibacterial agents are effective in the treatment of conjunctivitis and in the prophylaxis of ophthalmia neonatorum.

Ocular Side Effects:

A. Local Ophthalmic Use or Exposure
  1. Silver deposits
     a. Cornea
     b. Conjunctiva
     c. Eyelids
     d. Lens
     e. Lacrimal sac
  2. Irritation
     a. Hyperemia
     b. Photophobia
     c. Ocular pain
     d. Edema
  3. Eyelids or conjunctiva
     a. Allergic reactions

   b. Conjunctivitis — nonspecific
   c. Edema
   d. Symblepharon
4. Scarring or opacities of any ocular structure (silver nitrate — when exposed to caustic concentrations)
5. Decreased vision
6. Problems with color vision — objects have yellow tinge

Clinical Significance: The overall use of silver-containing medication has been decreasing; however, in some countries it is still commonly prescribed. Ocular side effects other than with silver nitrate in caustic concentrations seldom cause serious adverse reactions. Silver nitrate sticks or concentrated solutions have been known to cause severe corneal and conjunctival damage. Conjunctivitis is probably the most common side effect but rarely requires discontinuation of the medication. Topical ocular silver application for even a few months may cause conjunctival silver deposition. Long-term dosage may cause corneal, lens, eyelid, or lacrimal sac silver deposition. Silver deposits in the cornea or lens rarely interfere with vision. Ocular and periocular silver deposits over many years are absorbed, if the drug is discontinued.

References:

Bartlett, R. E.: Generalized argyrosis with lens involvement. Am. J. Ophthalmol. 38:402, 1954.
Friedman, B., and Rotth, A.: Argyrosis corneae. Am. J. Ophthalmol. 13:1050, 1930.
Goldstein, J. H.: Effects of drugs on cornea, conjunctiva, and lids. Int. Ophthalmol. Clin. 11(2):13, 1971.
Grayson, M., and Pieroni, D.: Severe silver nitrate injury to the eye. Am. J. Ophthalmol. 70:227, 1970.
Hanna, C., Fraunfelder, F. T., and Sanchez, J.: Ultrastructural study of argyrosis of the cornea and conjunctiva. Arch. Ophthalmol. 92:18, 1974.
Hornblass, A.: Severe silver nitrate ocular damage in newborn nursery. NY State J. Med. 76:1875, 1976.
Rosen, E.: Argyrolentis. Am. J. Ophthalmol. 33:797, 1950.

Class: Antiviral Agents

Generic Name: Cytarabine

Proprietary Name: Alexan (Belg., Germ.), Aracytine (Fr.), Cytosar

Primary Use: *Systemic:* This antimetabolite is effective in the management of acute granulocytic leukemia, polycythemia vera, and malignant neoplasms. *Ophthalmic:* This topical pyrimidine nucleoside is used in the treatment of herpes simplex keratitis.

Ocular Side Effects:

A. Systemic Administration
   1. Eyelids or conjunctiva
      a. Allergic reactions
      b. Conjunctivitis — nonspecific
      c. Hyperpigmentation
      d. Purpura
   2. Subconjunctival or retinal hemorrhages secondary to drug-induced anemia
   3. Keratitis
   4. Corneal deposits (?)
   5. Loss of eyelashes or eyebrows (?)
   6. Ocular teratogenic effects (?)
B. Local Ophthalmic Use or Exposure
   1. Ocular pain
   2. Iritis
   3. Corneal opacities
   4. Corneal ulceration

Clinical Significance: Ocular side effects due to systemic cytarabine are uncommon and seldom of major clinical significance. Other than the drug's possible teratogenic effects, all adverse ocular reactions are transitory and reversible with discontinued drug use. Because topical cytarabine causes significant corneal toxicity, it has been replaced by equally effective and less toxic antiviral agents. The Registry has received a case report of corneal crystalline deposits following high intravenous dosages, which resolved after the drug was discontinued.

References:

Apt, L., and Gaffney, W. L.: Congenital eye abnormalities from drugs during pregnancy. In Leopold, I. H. (Ed.): Symposium on Ocular Therapy. St. Louis, C. V. Mosby, Vol. VII, 1974, pp. 1–22.

Elliott, G. A., and Schut, A. L.: Studies with cytarabine HCl (CA) in normal eyes of man, monkey and rabbit. Am. J. Ophthalmol. 60:1074, 1965.

Grant, W. M.: Toxicology of the Eye. 2nd Ed., Springfield, Ill., Charles C Thomas, 1974, pp. 346–347.

Havener, W. H.: Ocular Pharmacology. 4th Ed., St. Louis, C. V. Mosby, 1978, pp. 211–213.

Kaufman, H. E., et al.: Corneal toxicity of cytosine arabinoside. Arch. Ophthalmol. 72:535, 1964.

Wade, A. (Ed.): Martindale: The Extra Pharmacopoeia. 27th Ed., London, Pharmaceutical Press, 1977, pp. 141–143.

Generic Name: 1. Idoxuridine, IDU; 2. Trifluridine, F_3T; 3. Vidarabine

Proprietary Name: 1. Dendrid, Herpid (G.B.), Herpidu (S. Afr.), Herplex, Iduridin (Germ., Swed.), Iduviran (Fr.), Kerecid (G.B.), Ophthalmadine (G.B.), Stoxil, Synmiol (Germ.), Virunguent (Germ.); 2. Viroptic; 3. Vira-A

Primary Use: These topical ocular antiviral agents are used in the treatment of herpes simplex keratitis.

Ocular Side Effects:

A. Local Ophthalmic Use or Exposure
   1. Irritation
      a. Lacrimation
      b. Hyperemia
      c. Photophobia
      d. Ocular pain
      e. Edema
   2. Cornea
      a. Superficial punctate keratitis
      b. Filaments
      c. Delayed wound healing
      d. Erosions or indolent ulceration
      e. Stromal opacities
      f. Superficial vascularization (late)
   3. Eyelids or conjunctiva
      a. Allergic reactions
      b. Hyperemia
      c. Conjunctivitis – follicular
      d. Edema
      e. Perilimbal filaments
      f. Conjunctival punctate staining
      g. Conjunctival scarring
   4. Narrowing or occlusion of lacrimal punctum
   5. Ptosis

Clinical Significance: Adverse ocular reactions to these agents are often missed and frequently assumed to be worsening of the clinical disease. Ocular side effects seem to occur most frequently in eyes with decreased tear production. The occasional appearance of corneal clouding, stippling, and small punctate defects in the corneal epithelium is not uncommon. These corneal changes can be painful but will disappear after the drug has been discontinued. However, not all signs and symptoms are reversible after discontinuing use of these drugs, since in some cases ptosis and occlusion of the lacrimal punctum have been permanent. Idoxuridine seems to have the highest degree of local irritation and toxicity, followed by vidarabine and trifluridine. There is evidence of cross reactivity with other pyrimidine analogues, not only ocular but cutaneous as well. Dimethyl sulfoxide and idoxuridine are occasionally combined to enhance the solubility and penetration of the antiviral drug. In one case, a cutaneous herpes simplex lesion treated with this combination developed premalignant epidermal changes. When these agents were discontinued, the epidermis returned to normal. Simultaneous administration of boric acid may increase ocular irritation. In animals, idoxuridine may have ocular teratogenic toxicity, but the Registry is unaware of any such cases in humans, to date.

Interactions with Other Drugs:

A. Contraindications
   1. Boric acid

References:

Amon, R. B., Lis, A. W., and Hanifin, J. M.: Allergic contact dermatitis caused by idoxuridine. Patterns of cross reactivity with other pyrimidine analogues. Arch. Dermatol. *111*:1581, 1975.
Itoi, M., et al.: Teratogenicities of ophthalmic drugs. I. Antiviral ophthalmic drugs. Arch. Ophthalmol. *93*:46, 1975.
Laibson, P. R.: Current therapy of herpes simplex virus infection of the cornea. Int. Ophthalmol. Clin. *13*(4):39, 1973.
McGill, J., et al.: Reassessment of idoxuridine therapy of herpetic keratitis. Trans. Ophthalmol. Soc. U. K. *94*:542, 1974.
McGill, J., Fraunfelder, F. T., and Jones, B. R.: Current and proposed management of ocular herpes simplex. Surv. Ophthalmol. *20*:358, 1976.
Thomson, J., and O'Neill, S. M.: Iodoxuridine in dimethyl sulfoxide: Is it carcinogenic in man? J. Cutan. Pathol. *3*:269, 1976.

Class: Carbonic Anhydrase Inhibitors

Generic Name: 1. Acetazolamide; 2. Dichlorphenamide; 3. Ethoxzolamide; 4. Methazolamide

Proprietary Name: 1. Defiltran (Fr.), Diamox, Diazol (S. Afr.), Didoc (Jap.), Diuramid (Pol.), Glaucomide (Austral.), Glaupax (Swed.), Hydrazol; 2. Daranide, Oralcon (Swed.), Oratrol; 3. Cardrase, Ethamide; 4. Neptazane

Primary Use: These enzyme inhibitors are effective in the treatment of all types of glaucomas. Acetazolamide is also effective in edema due to congestive heart failure, drug-induced edema, and centrencephalic epilepsies.

Ocular Side Effects:

A. Systemic Administration
   1. Decreased intraocular pressure
   2. Decreased vision
   3. Myopia
   4. Decreased accommodation
   5. Forward displacement of lens
   6. Eyelids or conjunctiva
       a. Allergic reactions
       b. Urticaria
       c. Purpura
       d. Lyell's syndrome
   7. Retinal or macular edema
   8. Iritis
   9. Ocular signs of gout
   10. Globus hystericus
   11. Subconjunctival or retinal hemorrhages secondary to drug-induced anemia
   12. Problems with color vision (methazolamide)
       a. Dyschromatopsia
       b. Objects have yellow tinge

Clinical Significance: Ocular side effects due to carbonic anhydrase inhibitors are usually transient and insignificant. Myopia is a common adverse ocular reaction; but since most patients are already receiving miotics, these drugs are incriminated. Cases of gout have been induced by carbonic anhydrase inhibitors since they elevate serum uric acid. The ocular signs of gout include conjunctival hyperemia, uveitis, scleritis, and corneal deposits or ulcerations. There are an increasing number of reports of adverse systemic responses to this group of agents. Possibly, these drugs as much as any others prescribed by ophthalmologists inconvenience or decrease the quality of life of patients. Also, there have been reports of pharmacists inadvertently substituting acetohexamide for acetazolamide.

Interactions with Other Drugs:

A. Effect of Carbonic Anhydrase Inhibitors on Activity of Other Drugs
   1. Diuretics ↑

   2. Erythromycin ↑
   3. Phenothiazines ↑
   4. Tricyclic antidepressants ↑
   5. Urea ↑
   6. Salicylates ↑↓
   7. Sympathomimetics ↑↓
 B. Effect of Other Drugs on Activity of Carbonic Anhydrase Inhibitors
   1. Adrenergic blockers ↑
   2. Diuretics ↑
   3. Monoamine oxidase inhibitors ↑
   4. Sympathomimetics ↑
   5. Tricyclic antidepressants ↑
   6. Urea ↑

References:

Back, M.: Transient myopia after use of acetazoleamide (Diamox). Arch. Ophthalmol. *55*:546, 1956.

Beasley, F. J.: Transient myopia and retinal edema during ethoxzolamide (Cardrase) therapy. Arch. Ophthalmol. *68*:490, 1962.

Galin, M. A., Baras, I., and Zweifach, P.: Diamox-induced myopia. Am. J. Ophthalmol. *54*:237, 1962.

Halpern, A. E., and Kulvin, M. M.: Transient myopia during treatment with carbonic anhydrase inhibitors. Am. J. Ophthalmol. *48*:534, 1959.

Hargett, N. A., et al.: Inadvertent substitution of acetohexamide for acetazolamide. Am. J. Ophthalmol. *84*:580, 1977.

Class: Decongestants

Generic Name: Naphazoline

Proprietary Name: *Nasal:* Imidazyl (Ital.), Privine, Turbine *Ophthalmic:* Ak-Con, Albalon, Allerest, Clear Eyes, Degest, Naphcon, Opticon, Vasoclear

Primary Use: This topical sympathomimetic amine is effective in the symptomatic relief of both nasal and ophthalmic congestion of allergic or inflammatory origin.

Ocular Side Effects:

 A. Local Ophthalmic Use or Exposure
   1. Conjunctival vasoconstriction

2. Irritation
   a. Lacrimation
   b. Reactive hyperemia
3. Mydriasis — may precipitate narrow-angle glaucoma
4. Decreased vision
5. Punctate keratitis
6. Eyelids or conjunctiva
   a. Allergic reactions
   b. Conjunctivitis — nonspecific
7. Increased pigment granules in anterior chamber
8. Retinal vascular occlusion (?)

Clinical Significance: No ocular side effects due to naphazoline are seen except with topical ocular application. Adverse ocular reactions are seldom significant except with frequent or long-term usage. The conjunctival vasculature may fail to respond to the vasoconstrictive properties of naphazoline if it is used excessively or for prolonged periods. The Registry has received reports from ophthalmologists describing a possible association of topical ocular naphazoline with an acute episode of central retinal artery occlusion.

Interactions with Other Drugs:

A. Effect of Naphazoline on Activity of Other Drugs
   1. Tricyclic antidepressants ↑
   2. Analgesics ↓
   3. Anticholinesterases ↓
B. Effect of Other Drugs on Activity of Naphazoline
   1. Alcohol ↑
   2. Anticholinergics ↑
   3. Antihistamines ↑
   4. Tricyclic antidepressants ↑
   5. Phenothiazines ↑↓
   6. Anticholinesterases ↓
C. Contraindications
   1. Monoamine oxidase inhibitors

References:

AMA Drug Evaluations. 4th Ed., New York, John Wiley & Sons, 1980, pp. 453–456.
Gilman, A. G., Goodman, L. S., and Gilman, A. (Eds.) The Pharmacological Basis of Therapeutics. 6th Ed., New York, Macmillan, 1980, p. 168.
Grant, W. M.: Toxicology of the Eye. 2nd Ed., Springfield, Charles C Thomas, 1974, p. 733.
Komi, T., et al.: Inhibitory effect of sodium chondroitin sulfate on epithelial keratitis induced by naphazoline. Am. J. Ophthalmol. 58:892, 1964.

Physicians' Desk Reference. 35th Ed., Oradell, N.J., Medical Economics Co., 1981, p. 509.

———————

Generic Name: Tetrahydrozoline

Proprietary Name: *Nasal:* Tyzanol (Swed.), Tyzine, Yxin (Germ.) *Ophthalmic:* Murine Plus, Soothe, Tetracon, Visine

Primary Use: This topical sympathomimetic amine is effective in the symptomatic relief of both nasal and ophthalmic congestion of allergic or inflammatory origin.

Ocular Side Effects:

A. Local Ophthalmic Use or Exposure
   1. Conjunctival vasoconstriction
   2. Irritation
      a. Lacrimation
      b. Reactive hyperemia
      c. Burning sensation
   3. Mydriasis — may precipitate narrow-angle glaucoma
   4. Decreased intraocular pressure
   5. Punctate keratitis
   6. Decreased vision
   7. Orbital or periorbital pain
   8. Eyelids or conjunctiva
      a. Allergic reactions
      b. Blepharoconjunctivitis — nonspecific
   9. Increased pigment granules in anterior chamber (?)

Clinical Significance: No ocular side effects due to tetrahydrozoline are seen except with topical ocular application. In the drug concentrations available in commercial ophthalmic preparations, ocular side effects are quite rare and usually of little consequence. The Registry received a case report of contact dermatitis and keratitis, which were slow to resolve even months later. However, adverse ocular reactions are almost always reversible with discontinuation of the use of the drug.

Interactions with Other Drugs:

A. Contraindications
   1. Monoamine oxidase inhibitors

References:

AMA Drug Evaluations. 4th Ed., New York, John Wiley & Sons, 1980, pp. 453–454, 458.

American Hospital Formulary Service. Washington, D.C., American Society of Hospital Pharmacists, Vol. II, 52:32, 1977.

Physicians' Desk Reference. 35th Ed., Oradell, N.J., Medical Economics Co., 1981, p. 534.

Physicians' Desk Reference for Ophthalmology. 9th Ed., Oradell, N.J., Medical Economics Co., 1980/81, p. 82.

Class: Miotics

Generic Name: Aceclidine

Proprietary Name: Glaucostat (Fr.)

Primary Use: This topical parasympathomimetic agent is used to lower intraocular pressure in the treatment of open-angle glaucoma.

Ocular Side Effects:

A. Local Ophthalmic Use or Exposure
   1. Miosis
   2. Decreased intraocular pressure
   3. Accommodative spasm
   4. Decreased vision
   5. Irritation
      a. Lacrimation
      b. Hyperemia
      c. Burning sensation
      d. Browache
   6. Problems with color vision — dyschromatopsia
   7. Retinal detachment (?)

Clinical Significance: Although the miotic effect of aceclidine may be slightly greater than that of other miotics in comparable concentrations, the degree of accommodative spasm has been reportedly less. Irritation does not appear to be a common problem with 2 to 4 percent solutions. Aceclidine is not in clinical use in the United States but is available in Europe.

References:

Crandall, D. C., and Leopold, I. H.: The influence of systemic drugs on tear constituents. Ophthalmology 86:115, 1979.

Fechner, P. U., Teichmann, K. D., and Weyrauch, W.: Accommodative effects of aceclidine in the treatment of glaucoma. Am. J. Ophthalmol. 79:104, 1975.

Laroche, J., and Laroche, C.: Nouvelles recherches sur la modification de la vision des couleurs sous l'action des médicaments à dose thérapeutique. Ann. Pharm. Fr. 35:173, 1977.

Lieberman, T. W., and Leopold, I. H.: The use of aceclydine in the treatment of glaucoma. Its effect on intraocular pressure and facility of aqueous humor outflow as compared to that of pilocarpine. Am. J. Ophthalmol. 64:405, 1967.

Romano, J. H.: Double-blind cross-over comparison of aceclidine and pilocarpine in open-angle glaucoma. Br. J. Ophthalmol. 54:510, 1970.

Generic Name: Acetylcholine

Proprietary Name: Acecoline (Canad., Fr.), Covochol (S. Afr.), Miochol

Primary Use: This intraocular quaternary ammonium parasympathomimetic agent is used to produce prompt, short-term miosis.

Ocular Side Effects:

A. Local Ophthalmic Use or Exposure — Subconjunctival or Intracameral Injection
   1. Miosis
   2. Decreased intraocular pressure
   3. Conjunctival hyperemia
   4. Accommodative spasm
   5. Iris atrophy
   6. Blepharoclonus
   7. Lacrimation
   8. Retinal hemorrhages
   9. Paradoxical mydriasis
   10. Decreased anterior chamber depth
   11. Cataract — transient
   12. Corneal edema
   13. Corneal opacities
   14. Retinal detachment (?)

Clinical Significance: Few ocular side effects due to acetylcholine are seen. While miosis is the primary ophthalmic effect, on rare occasions mydriasis may occur. Ocular side effects are rarely of clinical significance; however, a few cases of corneal edema have been reported to the Registry, but it is difficult to distinguish the drug's effects from

13

surgical trauma. Transient lens opacities have been reported, probably on the basis of an osmotic effect. To date, no long-term effect on the lens has been seen due to this drug. If acetylcholine is administered intraocularly, it may cause lacrimation. Bradycardia and hypotension have been seen following irrigation of the anterior chamber with acetylcholine.

Interactions with Other Drugs:

   A. Effect of Other Drugs on Activity of Acetylcholine
      1. Anticholinergics ↓
      2. Sympathomimetics ↓

References:

Babinski, M., Smith, R. B., and Wickerham, E. P.: Hypotension and bradycardia following intraocular acetylcholine injection. Report of a case. Arch. Ophthalmol. 94:675, 1976.

Barraquer, J. I.: Acetylcholine as a miotic agent for use in surgery. Am. J. Ophthalmol. 57:406, 1964.

Catford, G. V., and Millis, E.: Clinical experience in the intraocular use of acetylcholine. Br. J. Ophthalmol. 51:183, 1967.

Fraunfelder, F. T.: Corneal edema after use of carbachol. Arch. Ophthalmol. 97:975, 1979.

Harley, R. D., and Mishler, J. E.: Acetylcholine in cataract surgery. Br. J. Ophthalmol. 50:429, 1966.

Lazar, M., Rosen, N., and Nemet, P.: Miochol-induced transient cataract. Ann. Ophthalmol. 9:1142, 1977.

Rizzuti, A. B.: Acetylcholine in surgery of the lens, iris and cornea. Am. J. Ophthalmol. 63:484, 1967.

Rongey, K. A., and Weisman, H.: Hypotension following intraocular acetylcholine. Anesthesiology 36:412, 1972.

Generic Name: 1. Demecarium; 2. Echothiophate; 3. Isoflurophate, DFP

Proprietary Name: 1. Humorsol, Tosmilen (G.B.); 2. Echodide, Echothiopate (G.B.), Phospholine; 3. Diflupyl (Fr.), Dyflos (G.B.), Floropryl

Primary Use: These topical anticholinesterases are used in the management of open-angle glaucoma, conditions in which movement or constriction of the pupil is desired, and in accommodative esotropia. Demecarium is also used in the early management of ocular myasthenia gravis, and isoflurophate, in periocular louse infestations.

Ocular Side Effects:

   A. Local Ophthalmic Use or Exposure
      1. Miosis

2. Decreased vision
3. Accommodative spasm
4. Irritation
   a. Lacrimation
   b. Hyperemia
   c. Photophobia
   d. Ocular pain
   e. Edema
   f. Burning sensation
5. Cataracts
   a. Anterior or posterior subcapsular
   b. Hydrational changes (?)
   c. Nuclear changes (?)
6. Eyelids or conjunctiva
   a. Allergic reactions
   b. Conjunctivitis — follicular
   c. Edema
   d. Pemphigoid lesion
   e. Depigmentation (isoflurophate)
7. Blepharoclonus
8. Myopia
9. Iris or ciliary body cysts — especially in children
10. Intraocular pressure
    a. Increased — initial
    b. Decreased
11. Iritis
    a. Occasionally fine K.P. (keratitic precipitates)
    b. Activation of latent iritis or uveitis
    c. Formation of anterior or posterior synechiae
12. Decreased scleral rigidity
13. Occlusion of lacrimal canaliculi
14. Decreased anterior chamber depth
15. Hyphema — during surgery
16. Vitreous hemorrhages
17. Decreased size of filtering bleb
18. Corneal deposits (echothiophate)
19. Retinal detachment (?)
20. Atypical band keratopathy (?) (isoflurophate)

Clinical Significance: Ocular side effects are most common with isoflurophate followed by echothiophate and demecarium. Visual complaints with or without accommodative spasm are the most frequent adverse ocular reactions. Drug-induced lens changes are well documented and are primarily seen in the older age group. In shallow anterior chamber angles, these agents are contraindicated since in up to 10 percent of cases they may precipitate narrow-angle glaucoma. This is probably due to peripheral vascular congestion of the iris, which may further aggravate an already compromised angle. Also, these parasympathomimetic agents allow the iris lens diaphragm to come forward and, under certain circumstances, to induce a relative pupillary block. While irritative conjunctival changes are common with long-term usage, allergic reactions are rare. Some retinal surgeons are convinced that these agents cause retinal detachments by exerting traction on the peripheral retina. Cases of irreversible miosis due to long-term therapy have been reported. An atypical band-shaped keratopathy has been said to be due to long-term miotic therapy; however, others suggest this is due to long-term elevation of intraocular pressure and is not drug-induced. There is evidence that a slowly progressive drug-related cicatricial process of the conjunctiva may occur with these drugs, which may be clinically indistinguishable from ocular cicatricial pemphigoid. Patients on topical ocular anticholinesterases and those under treatment for myasthenia may have increased systemic and ocular side effect risks if exposed to organic phosphorous insecticides. Topical demecarium may have the greatest risk, since it has the highest degree of penetrability of the blood-cerebrospinal fluid barrier. This combination has resulted in cardiac arrest, hypotension, gastrointestinal effects, and respiratory failure. In addition, anesthetic deaths have been reported in patients on topical ocular anticholinesterases after receiving succinylcholine. This effect is due to the lowered blood cholinesterase from the topical ocular anticholinesterase agents.

Interactions with Other Drugs:

A. Effect of Anticholinesterases on Activity of Other Drugs
    1. Succinylcholine ↑

References:

Apt, L.: Toxicity of strong miotics in children. In Leopold, I. H. (Ed.): Symposium on Ocular Therapy. St. Louis, C. V. Mosby, 1972, Vol. V, pp. 30–35.
Beasley, H., and Fraunfelder, F. T.: Retinal detachments and topical ocular miotics. Ophthalmology 86:95, 1979.
Grant, W. M.: Toxicology of the Eye. 2nd Ed., Springfield, Charles C Thomas, 1974, pp. 398, 441–442, 706–718.
Havener, W. H.: Ocular Pharmacology. 4th Ed., St. Louis, C. V. Mosby, 1978, pp. 270, 281, 298–314.
Klendshoj, N. C., and Olmsted, E. P.: Observation of dangerous side effect of phospholine iodide in glaucoma therapy. Am. J. Ophthalmol. 56:247, 1963.
Patten, J. T., Cavanagh, H. D., and Allansmith, M. R.: Induced ocular pseudopemphigoid. Am. J. Ophthalmol. 82:272, 1976.
Shaffer, R. N., and Hetherington, J.: Anticholinesterase drugs and cataracts. Am. J. Ophthalmol. 62:613, 1966.

Sugar, H. S.: Pitfalls in glaucoma treatment. Ann. Ophthalmol. *11*:1043, 1979.
Westsmith, R. A., and Abernethy, R. E.: Detachment of retina with use of diisopropyl fluorophosphate (Fluropryl) in treatment of glaucoma. Arch. Ophthalmol. 52:779, 1954.

Generic Name: 1. Neostigmine; 2. Physostigmine

Proprietary Name: 1. Prostigmin; 2. Isopto Eserine

Primary Use: These topical parasympathomimetic agents are used in the management of narrow- and open-angle glaucoma. Neostigmine is also used in the management of ptosis caused by myasthenia gravis.

Ocular Side Effects:

A. Local Ophthalmic Use or Exposure
   1. Miosis
   2. Decreased intraocular pressure
   3. Irritation
      a. Lacrimation
      b. Hyperemia
      c. Photophobia
      d. Ocular pain
   4. Accommodative spasm
   5. Decreased vision
   6. Eyelids or conjunctiva
      a. Allergic reactions
      b. Conjunctivitis — follicular
      c. Blepharoconjunctivitis
      d. Depigmentation
      e. Blepharoclonus
   7. Myopia
   8. Iritis
   9. Iris cysts
   10. Decreased anterior chamber depth
   11. Vitreous hemorrhages
   12. Cataracts
   13. Occlusion of lacrimal punctum
   14. Retinal detachment (?)
   15. Atypical band keratopathy (?) (physostigmine)

Clinical Significance: Ocular side effects due to these anticholinesterases are usually reversible with discontinued drug usage. These agents should be used with caution since peripheral vascular congestion of the iris may precipitate narrow-angle glaucoma. Long-term usage with these drugs is seldom possible, since allergic or irritative conjunctivitis occurs frequently. An allergic blepharitis may cause skin depigmentation. The normal coloration usually returns after discontinuance of the drug. An atypical band keratopathy has been said to be due to long-term miotic therapy; however, others suggest it is due to long-term elevation of intraocular pressure and is not drug-induced. Physostigmine is sensitive to heat and light and becomes discolored. Discolored solutions are irritating and clinically ineffective.

Interactions with Other Drugs:

A. Effect of Anticholinesterases on Activity of Other Drugs
    1. Succinylcholine ↑
    2. Anticholinergics ↓
    3. Local anesthetics ↓
B. Effect of Other Drugs on Activity of Anticholinesterases
    1. Local anesthetics ↓

References:

Crandall, D. C., and Leopold, I. H.: The influence of systemic drugs on tear constituents. Ophthalmology 86:115, 1979.
Cumming, G., Harding, L. K., and Prowse, K.: Treatment and recovery after massive overdose of physostigmine. Lancet 2:147, 1968.
Ellis, P. P.: Ocular Therapeutics and Pharmacology. 5th Ed., St. Louis, C. V. Mosby, 1977, pp. 16, 51.
Grant, W. M.: Toxicology of the Eye. 2nd Ed. Springfield, Ill., Charles C Thomas, 1974, pp. 706–718, 831–832.
Jacklin, H. N.: Depigmentation of the eyelids in eserine allergy. Am. J. Ophthalmol. 59:89, 1965.
Leopold, I. H. (Ed.): Glaucoma Drug Therapy: Monograph I Parasympathetic Agents. Irvine, Calif., Allergan Pharmaceuticals, 1975, pp. 19–21.
Sugar, H. S.: Pitfalls in glaucoma treatment. Ann. Ophthalmol. 11:1043, 1979.

Generic Name: Pilocarpine

Proprietary Name: Adsorbocarpine, Akarpine, Almocarpine, Isopto Carpine, Isopto-Pilocarpine (Fr.), Licarpin (Swed.), Marticarpine (Fr.), Mio-Carpine-SMP (S. Afr.), Mistura P, Nova-Carpine (Canad.), Ocusert, Pilocar, Pilocarpina Lux (Ital.), Pilocel, Pilomiotin, Pilopt (Austral.), Piloptic, PV Carpine, Spersacarpine (S. Afr., Swed.)

Primary Use: This topical ocular parasympathomimetic agent is used in the management of glaucoma and in conditions in which constriction of the pupil is desired.

Ocular Side Effects:

A. Local Ophthalmic Use or Exposure
 1. Pupils
    a. Miosis
    b. Mydriasis — rare
 2. Decreased vision
 3. Paralysis or spasm of accommodation
 4. Intraocular pressure
    a. Increased — initial
    b. Decreased
 5. Decreased anterior chamber depth
 6. Eyleids or conjunctiva
    a. Allergic reactions
    b. Hyperemia
    c. Conjunctivitis — follicular
 7. Irritation
    a. Lacrimation
    b. Ocular pain
    c. Burning sensation
 8. Myopia — transient
 9. Retinal detachment
 10. Punctate keratitis
 11. Blepharoclonus
 12. Iris cysts
 13. Increased axial lens diameter
 14. Decreased scleral rigidity
 15. Cataracts
 16. Problems with color vision — dyschromatopsia
 17. Corneal epithelial microcysts (?)
 18. Atypical band keratopathy (?)

Clinical Significance: Probably the most frequent ocular side effect due to pilocarpine is decrease in vision secondary to miosis or accommodative spasms. Follicular conjunctivitis is common after long-term therapy, but it has minimal clinical significance. Iris cysts are quite rare, and drug-induced lens changes are still debatable. An atypical band-shaped keratopathy has been said to be due to long-term miotic therapy; however, others suggest it is due to long-term elevation of intraocular pressure and is not drug-induced. All miotics are now possibly suspect as a cause of retinal detachments; however, this is probably the case only in diseased retinas. As a rare event, impure pilocarpine may contain jaborine, a stereo-isomer of pilocarpine. Jaborine has an atropine-like reaction, and mydriasis and cycloplegia have been seen clinically. Mothers on topical ocular pilocarpine giving birth may have infants with signs mimicking neonatal meningitis — hyperthermia, restlessness, convulsions, and diaphoresis. Pediatricians should be made aware of this syndrome so unnecessary tests and manipulations are avoided.

Interactions with Other Drugs:

A. Effect of Pilocarpine on Activity of Other Drugs
    1. Alcohol ↑
    2. Anticholinesterases ↑
    3. Urea ↑
    4. Anticholinergics ↓
B. Effect of Other Drugs on Activity of Pilocarpine
    1. Antihistamines ↑
    2. Anticholinesterases ↑
    3. Monoamine oxidase inhibitors ↑
    4. Phenothiazines ↑
    5. Tricyclic antidepressants ↑
    6. Urea ↑
    7. Adrenergic blockers ↓

References:

Abraham, S. V.: Miotic iridocyclitis: Its role in the surgical treatment of glaucoma. Am. J. Ophthalmol. *18*:634, 1959.
Abramson, D. H., et al.: Pilocarpine-induced lens changes. Arch. Ophthalmol. *92*: 464, 1974.
Beasley, H., and Fraunfelder, F. T.: Retinal detachments and topical ocular miotics. Ophthalmology *86*:95, 1979.
Drance, S. M.: The use of miotics in the management of intraocular pressure. In Leopold, I. H., and Burns, R. P. (Eds.): Symposium on Ocular Therapy. New York, John Wiley & Sons, 1979, Vol. XI, pp. 1–9.
Forbes, M.: Influence of miotics on visual fields in glaucoma. Invest. Ophthalmol. *5*:139, 1966.
Kennedy, R. E., Roca, P. D., and Landers, P. H.: Atypical band keratopathy in glaucomatous patients. Am. J. Ophthalmol. *72*:917, 1971.
Lebensohn, J. E.: Spectacular adverse reactions from pilocarpine. Am. J. Ophthalmol. *83*:281, 1977.
Levene, R. Z.: Uniocular miotic therapy. Trans. Am. Acad. Ophthalmol. Otolaryngol. *79*:376, 1975.
Mills, P. V.: Atypical band-shaped keratopathy associated with chronic glaucoma or ocular hypertension. Trans. Ophthalmol. Soc. U. K. *94*:450, 1974.

Class: Mydriatics and Cycloplegics

Generic Name: 1. Cyclopentolate; 2. Tropicamide

Proprietary Name: 1. Ak-Pentolate, Ciclolux (Ital.), Cyclogyl, Cyclopen (Austral.), Cyplegin (Jap.), Mydplegic (Canad.), Mydrilate (G.B.), Zyklolat (Germ.); 2. Mydriacyl, Mydriaticum (Germ.), Myriaticum (S. Afr.)

Primary Use: These topical ocular short-acting anticholinergic mydriatic and cycloplegic agents are used in refractions and fundus examination.

Ocular Side Effects:

   A. Local Ophthalmic Use or Exposure
      1. Decreased vision
      2. Mydriasis — may precipitate narrow-angle glaucoma
      3. Irritation
         a. Hyperemia
         b. Photophobia
         c. Ocular pain
         d. Burning sensation
      4. Decrease or paralysis of accommodation
      5. Increased intraocular pressure
      6. Eyelids or conjunctiva
         a. Allergic reactions
         b. Blepharoconjunctivitis
      7. Visual hallucinations
      8. Synechiae
      9. Keratitis

Clinical Significance: Major ocular side effects due to these drugs are quite rare. Both cyclopentolate and tropicamide can elevate intraocular pressure in open-angle glaucoma and precipitate narrow-angle glaucoma; cycloplegics have been shown to decrease the coefficient outflow. Some have suggested the use of these agents may cause an instability of vitreous face, which could aggravate cystoid macular edema. This, however, is debatable. Visual hallucinations or psychotic reactions after topical applications are primarily seen with cyclopentolate. Systemic adverse reactions from these agents are not uncommon, especially in children. Disorientation, somnolence, hyperactivity, vasomotor collapse, tachycardia, and even death have been reported. There have also been cases of addiction to topical ocular application of these drugs, since some patients get a CNS "high" from their use.

Interactions with Other Drugs:

A. Effect of Other Drugs on Activity of Anticholinergics
   1. Antihistamines ↑
   2. Phenothiazines ↑
   3. Tricyclic antidepressants ↑

References:

Awan, K. J.: Adverse systemic reactions of topical cyclopentolate hydrochloride. Ann. Ophthalmol. 8:695, 1976.
Awan, K. J.: Systemic toxicity of cyclopentolate hydrochloride in adults following topical ocular instillation. Ann. Ophthalmol. 8:803, 1976.
Bauer, C. R., Trottier, M. C. T., and Stern, L.: Systemic cyclopentolate (Cyclogyl) toxicity in the newborn infant. J. Pediatr. 82:501, 1973.
Ostler, H. B.: Cycloplegics and mydriatics. Tolerance, habituation, and addiction to topical administration. Arch. Ophthalmol. 93:432, 1975.
Praeger, D. L., and Miller, S. N.: Toxic effects of cyclopentolate (Cyclogel). Am. J. Ophthalmol. 58:1060, 1964.
Simcoe, C. W.: Cyclopentolate (Cyclogyl) toxicity. Arch. Ophthalmol. 67:406, 1962.
Strokes, H. R.: Drug reactions reported in a survey in South Carolina. Ophthalmology 86:161, 1979.
Wahl, J. W.: Systemic reaction to tropicamide. Arch. Ophthalmol. 82:320, 1969.
Yamaji, R.: Study of pseudomyopia. Acta Soc. Ophthalmol. Jap. 72:2083, 1968.

Class: Ophthalmic Dyes

Generic Name: 1. Alcian Blue; 2. Fluorescein; 3. Rose Bengal; 4. Trypan Blue

Proprietary Name: *Systemic:* 2. Ak-Fluor, Fluorescite, Funduscein *Ophthalmic:* 1. Alcian Blue; 2. Fluor-Amps (G.B.), Fluoreseptic, Fluorets (G.B.), Fluor-I-Strip, Fluoro-I-Strip (G.B.), Ful-Glo; 3. Rose Bengal; 4. Trypan Blue

Primary Use: *Systemic:* Fluorescein is used to study the aqueous secretion of the ciliary body and to aid in the diagnosis of internal carotid artery insufficiency. *Ophthalmic:* These topical dyes are used in various ocular diagnostic tests.

Ocular Side Effects:

A. Systemic Administration (Fluorescein)
   1. Stains ocular fluids and tissues yellow-green

2. Eyelids or conjunctiva
   a. Allergic reactions
   b. Hyperemia
   c. Yellow-orange discoloration
   d. Angioneurotic edema
   e. Urticaria
B. Local Ophthalmic Use or Exposure
   1. Stains mucus and connective tissue blue (alcian blue)
   2. Stains ocular fluids and tissues yellow-green (fluorescein)
   3. Stains degenerated epithelial cells and mucus red (rose bengal)
   4. Stains degenerated epithelial cells and mucus blue (trypan blue)
   5. Irritation
      a. Ocular pain
      b. Burning sensation
   6. Eyelids or conjunctiva
      a. Blue discoloration (alcian blue, trypan blue)
      b. Yellow-orange discoloration (fluorescein)
      c. Red discoloration (rose bengal)
   7. Problems with color vision (fluorescein)
      a. Objects have yellow tinge

Clinical Significance: Ocular side effects due to these ophthalmic dyes are rare and transient. Solutions of fluorescein can readily become contaminated with Pseudomonas because fluorescein inactivates the preservatives found in most ophthalmic solutions. Rose bengal, especially in concentrations above 1 percent, may cause significant ocular irritation after topical ocular instillation. If the corneal epithelium is not intact, the topical application of alcian blue may cause long-term or even permanent stromal deposits of the dye.

References:

Grant, W. M.: Toxicology of the Eye. 2nd Ed. Springfield, Charles C Thomas, 1974, pp. 430–435, 495, 888, 1068–1069.
Havener, W. H.: Ocular Pharmacology. 4th Ed., St. Louis, C. V. Mosby, 1978, pp. 421–423.
Norn, M. S.: Vital staining of cornea and conjunctiva. Acta Ophthalmol. (Suppl.) 113:7, 1972.
Paterson, C. A.: Effects of drugs on the lens. Int. Ophthalmol. Clin. 11(2):63, 1971.

Class: Ophthalmic Implants

Generic Name: Silicone

Proprietary Name: Silicone

Primary Use: Various silicone polymers of various viscosities or solids are used in ophthalmology as lubricants, implants, and volume expanders.

Ocular Side Effects:

A. Local Ophthalmic Use or Exposure
1. Burning sensation — topical application of liquid silicone
2. Increase postoperative infections — silicone implants
3. Granulomatous reactions — silicone implants
4. Migration within the eye — intraocular liquid silicone
   a. Cataracts
   b. Endothelial damage with corneal edema or vascularization

Clinical Significance: Silicone solutions or solids rarely cause adverse ocular reactions; however, under certain circumstances significant side effects may occur. Like any foreign body buried within tissue, the implant, even if inert, will be encased by some scar tissue or even granulomatous tissue. Postoperative infection rates are also higher if an implant is included in the procedure. As with silicone liquids placed in other areas of the body, the solution within the eye may with time migrate to new locations. Since the usual site of injection is intravitreal, with time the solution may come in contact with the lens or enter the anterior chamber with the possibility of affecting the lens or cornea.

References:

Armaly, M. F.: Ocular tolerance to silicones. Arch. Ophthalmol. 68:390, 1962.
Cibis, P. A., et al.: The use of liquid silicone in retinal detachment surgery. Arch. Ophthalmol. 68:590, 1962.
Lee, P., et al.: Intravitreous injection of silicone. Ann. Ophthalmol. 1:15, 1969.
Martola, E. L., and Dohlman, C. H.: Silicone oil in the anterior chamber of the eye. Acta Ophthalmol. 41:75, 1963.
Morgan, J. F., and Hill, J. C.: Silicone fluid as a lubricant for artificial eyes. Am. J. Ophthalmol. 58:767, 1964.
Okun, E.: The current status of silicone oil. (Analysis of long-term successes). In Irvine, A. R., and O'Malley, C. (Eds.): Advances in Vitreous Surgery. Springfield, C. C Thomas, 1976, pp. 518–522.
Rosengren, B.: Silicone injection into the vitreous in hopeless cases of retinal detachment. Acta Ophthalmol. 47:757, 1969.
Spivey, B. E., Allen, L., and Burns, C. A.: The Iowa enucleation implant; a 10 year evaluation of technique and results. Am. J. Ophthalmol. 67:171, 1969.
Sugar, H. S., and Okamura, I. D.: Ocular findings six years after intravitreal silicone injection. Arch. Ophthalmol. 94:612, 1976.

Class: Ophthalmic Preservatives

Generic Name: Benzalkonium

Proprietary Name: Roccal (G.B.), Zephiran

Primary Use: This topical ocular quaternary ammonium agent is used as a preservative in ophthalmic solutions and as a germicidal cleaning solution for contact lenses.

Ocular Side Effects:

A. Local Ophthalmic Use or Exposure
1. Irritation
   a. Lacrimation
   b. Hyperemia
   c. Photophobia
   d. Edema
2. Punctate keratitis
3. Gray corneal epithelial haze
4. Pseudomembrane formation
5. Decreased corneal epithelial microvilli
6. Delayed corneal wound healing (?)

Clinical Significance: Adverse ocular reactions to benzalkonium are not uncommon, even at exceedingly low concentrations. Concentrations as low as 0.01 percent may cause cell damage by emulsification of the cell wall lipids. Almost all ocular side effects are reversible after use of the drug is discontinued, and most of the damage is fairly superficial. A case report to the Registry showed irreversible corneal damage with vascularization when 1:1000 benzalkonium was inadvertently placed in both eyes and irrigated out 20 minutes later. Benzalkonium may also destroy the corneal epithelial microvilli, and thereby possibly prevent adherence of the mucoid layer of the tear film to the cornea. This drug also allows for an increased penetration of some drugs through the corneal epithelium, and is added to some commercial ophthalmic preparations for this reason. Benzalkonium binds to soft contact lenses, and the use of preservatives has been said to concentrate in this way, possibly causing increased epithelial breakdown. However, this statement has been denied by a number of investigators. This agent is clearly toxic to the corneal endothelium and even in the small amounts used in ophthalmic solutions may cause problems in diseased denuded corneas which receive multiple topical ocular applications daily.

References:

Gasset, A. R.: Benzalkonium chloride toxicity to the human cornea. Am. J. Ophthalmol. *84*:169, 1977.

Green, K., et al.: Rabbit endothelial response to ophthalmic preservatives. Arch. Ophthalmol. *95*:2218, 1977.

Lavine, J. B., Binder, P. S., and Wickham, M. G.: Antimicrobials and the corneal endothelium. Ann. Ophthalmol. *11*:1517, 1979.

Lemp, M. A.: Artificial tear solutions. Int. Ophthalmol. Clin. *13*(1):221, 1973.

Lemp, M. A., and Holly, F. J.: Ophthalmic polymers as ocular wetting agents. Ann. Ophthalmol. *4*:15, 1972.

Leopold, I. H.: Local toxic effect of detergents on ocular structures. Arch. Ophthalmol. *34*:99, 1945.

Pfister, R. R., and Burstein, N.: The effects of ophthalmic drugs, vehicles, and preservatives on corneal epithelium: A scanning electron microscope study. Invest. Ophthalmol. *15*:246, 1976.

Swan, K. C.: Reactivity of the ocular tissues to wetting agents. Am. J. Ophthalmol. *27*:1118, 1944.

Generic Name: 1. Mercuric Oxide (Hydrargyric Oxide Flavum); 2. Nitromersol; 3. Phenylmercuric Acetate; 4. Phenylmercuric Nitrate (Phenylhydrargyric Nitrate); 5. Thimerosal

Proprietary Name: 1. Ophtosept (Germ.), Pagenstecher's Ointment (G.B.), Yellow Mercuric Oxide; 2. Metaphen (Austral., Canad.); 3. Nylmerate; 4. Clean-N-Soak, Phe-Mer-Nite, Vaxoid (Austral.); 5. Merseptyl (Fr.), Mersol, Merthiolate, Thiomersal (G.B.)

Primary Use: These topical ocular organomercurials are used as antiseptics, preservatives, and antibacterial or antifungal agents in ophthalmic solutions and ointments.

Ocular Side Effects:

A. Local Ophthalmic Use or Exposure
1. Eyelids or conjunctiva
   a. Allergic reactions
   b. Hyperemia
   c. Erythema
   d. Blepharoconjunctivitis
   e. Edema
2. Bluish-gray mercury deposits
   a. Eyelids
   b. Conjunctiva
   c. Cornea (mercuric oxide)
   d. Lens (mercuric oxide and phenylmercuric acetate or nitrate)

Clinical Significance: Adverse ocular side effects due to these organo-mercurials are rare and seldom of significance. The most striking side effect is mercurial deposits in various ocular and periocular tissues. This is an apparently harmless side effect since it is asymptomatic, and no visual impairments due to it have been found. Conjunctival mercurial deposits are seen around blood vessels near the cornea, corneal deposits are in the peripheral Descemet's membrane, and lens deposits are mainly in the pupillary area. Thimerosal is now a commonly used preservative in many ophthalmic contact lens solutions. Mercurialentis has not been seen with thimerosal at concentrations of 0.005 percent, the concentration used as a preservative in some ophthalmic solutions. Unfortunately, in antifungal therapeutic concentrations, these mercurials are too toxic for ocular use. There are a surprisingly large number of people allergic to thimerosal. In fact, one Japanese series claimed that with time up to 50 percent of eye patients became hypersensitive. In the United States, one author claimed a 10-percent hypersensitivity reaction rate. To evaluate this agent as a factor for ocular intolerance, one can perform thimerosal skin testing.

References:

Abrams, J. D.: Iatrogenic mercurialentis. Trans. Ophthalmol. Soc. U. K. 83:263, 1963.

Abrams, J. D., and Majzoub, V.: Mercury content of the human lens. Br. J. Ophthalmol. 54:59, 1970.

Fraunfelder, F. T.: Interim report: National Registry of Possible Drug-Induced Ocular Side Effects. Ophthalmology 87:87, 1980.

Suzuki, H.: Allergic conjunctivitis and blepharoconjunctivitis caused by thimerosal (preservative). Jpn. J. Clin. Ophthalmol. 26:7, 1972.

Theodore, F. H.: Drug sensitivities and irritations of the conjunctiva. JAMA 151:25, 1953.

Wade, A. (Ed.): Martindale: The Extra Pharmacopoeia. 27th Ed., London, Pharmaceutical Press, 1977, pp. 526, 536, 906, 1281–1283.

Willetts, G. S.: Ocular side-effects of drugs. Br. J. Ophthalmol. 53:252, 1969.

Class: Proteolytic Enzymes

Generic Name: Chymotrypsin

Proprietary Name: Alpha Chymar, Alphacutanee (Fr.), Aphlozyme (Fr.), Catarase, Chymar (G.B.), Chymar-Zon (G.B.), Enzeon, Kimopsin (Austral., Jap.), Quimotrase (Canad.), Zolyse, Zonulyn (Canad.), Zonulysin (G.B.)

Primary Use: This intraocular proteolytic enzyme is effective in lysing zonular fibers in intracapsular lens extraction.

Ocular Side Effects:

A. Local Ophthalmic Use or Exposure
1. Lyses zonular fibers
2. Forward displacement of lens
3. Increased intraocular pressure
4. Uveitis
5. Induce or aggravate scleritis
6. Corneal edema
7. Increased striate keratopathy (?)
8. Delayed corneal wound healing (?)
9. Retinal detachment (?)
10. Iridoplegia (?)
11. Keratitis (?)

Clinical Significance: Surprisingly few ocular side effects are seen with this potent enzyme when it is used in the concentrations recommended. The most common adverse ocular reaction is transient glaucoma, which usually appears 2 to 5 days after cataract surgery and spontaneously subsides within a week. This agent can affect the retina; however, clinically it would probably have to be injected into the vitreous to reach toxic retinal levels. There are a number of case reports in the Registry of corneal edema after injection into the anterior segment of the eye, but it is difficult to know if this is secondary to glaucoma, surgical trauma, or a drug effect.

References:

Havener, W. H.: Ocular Pharmacology. 4th Ed., St. Louis, C. V. Mosby, 1978, pp. 46–67.

Kirsch, R. E.: Glaucoma following cataract extraction associated with use of alpha-chymotrypsin. Arch. Ophthalmol. 72:612, 1964.

Maumenee, A. E.: Effects of alpha-chymotrypsin on the retina. Trans. Am. Acad. Ophthalmol. Otolaryngol. 64:33, 1960.

Menezo, J. L., Suarez, R., and Menezo, V.: Verbleibende Irislähmung und Keratitis filiformis: Seltene Komplikationen nach Kataraktoperationen. Klin. Monatsbl. Augenheilkd. 166:523, 1975.

Rains, D. E., Rains, K. P., and Coker, H. G.: Enzymatic zonulolysis in cataract surgery: Historical review and present use. Ann. Ophthalmol. 6:511, 1974.

Troutman, R. C.: National survey on the facility of cataract extraction, operative and immediate postoperative complications. Trans. Am. Acad. Ophthalmol. Otolaryngol. 64:37, 1960.

Watson, P. G.: Treatment of scleritis and episcleritis. Trans. Ophthalmol. Soc. U. K. 94:76, 1974.

Generic Name: Urokinase

Proprietary Name: Abbokinase, Breokinase, Win-Kinase

Primary Use: This proteolytic enzyme is injected into the anterior chamber or vitreous to possibly aid in the removal of blood.

Ocular Side Effects:

A. Local Ophthalmic Use or Exposure
   1. Hypopyon
   2. Uveitis
   3. Intraocular pressure
      a. Increased
      b. Decreased
   4. Bleeding (?)

Clinical Significance: After intravitreal injections of urokinase, as high as a 50-percent incidence of sterile hypopyon has occurred. This is thought to be cellular debris in the anterior chamber which usually absorbs within 5 days. Uveitis usually is mild although severe cases have been seen.

References:

Cleary, P. E., et al.: Intravitreal urokinase in the treatment of vitreous haemorrhage. Trans. Ophthalmol. Soc. U. K. *94*:587, 1974.
Dugmore, W. N., and Raichand, M.: Intravitreal urokinase in the treatment of vitreous hemorrhage. Am. J. Ophthalmol. 75:779, 1973.
Forrester, J. V., and Williamson, J.: Lytic therapy in vitreous hemorrhage. Trans. Ophthalmol. Soc. U. K. *94*:583, 1974.
Pierse, D.: The use of urokinase in the anterior chamber. Trans. Ophthalmol. Soc. U. K. *84*:271, 1964.
Sellors, P. J. H., Kanski, J. J., and Watson, D. M.: Intravitreal urokinase in the management of vitreous haemorrhage. Trans. Ophthalmol. Soc. U. K. *94*:591, 1974.

Class: Topical Local Anesthetics

Generic Name: 1. Benoxinate; 2. Butacaine; 3. Cocaine; 4. Dibucaine (Cinchocaine); 5. Dyclonine; 6. Phenacaine; 7. Piperocaine; 8. Proparacaine (Proxymetacaine); 9. Tetracaine

Proprietary Name: *Injection:* 4. Nupercaine; 7. Metycaine; 9. Amethocaine (G.B.), Contralgin (Germ.), Decicain (Austral.), Pantocain

(Germ.), Pontocaine *Ophthalmic:* 1. Conjuncain (Germ.), Dorsacaine, Novesine (Austral., Germ., S. Afr.); 2. Butacaine; 3. Cocaine; 4. Dibucaine; 5. Dyclonine; 6. Phenacaine; 7. Piperocaine; 8. Ak-Taine, Alcaine, Ophthaine, Ophthetic; 9. Amethocaine (G.B.), Anacel, Pontocaine

Street Name: *Nasal, Oral:* 3. Bernice, Bernies, C, Coke, Flake, Girl, Gold Dust, Happy Dust, Heaven Dust, Snow

Primary Use: *Injection:* Dibucaine, piperocaine, and tetracaine are effective in infiltrative nerve block, peridural, caudal, and spinal anesthesia. *Nasal, Oral:* Cocaine is a potent central nervous system stimulant which is commonly available on the illicit drug market. *Ophthalmic:* These topical local anesthetics are used in diagnostic and surgical procedures.

Ocular Side Effects:

A. Systemic Administration — Injection
1. Decreased vision
2. Miosis
3. Paralysis of extraocular muscles
4. Diplopia
5. Blepharoclonus
6. Photosensitivity (dibucaine)

B. Systemic Administration — Nasal or Oral (Cocaine)
1. Decreased vision
2. Visual hallucinations
3. Photosensitivity
4. Pupils
   a. Mydriasis
   b. Absence of reaction to light — toxic states
5. Paralysis of accommodation
6. Exophthalmos

C. Local Ophthalmic Use or Exposure
1. Corneal epithelium
   a. Punctate keratitis
   b. Gray, ground glass appearance
   c. Edema
   d. Softening, erosions, and sloughing
   e. Filaments
   f. Ulceration
2. Corneal stroma
   a. Yellow-white opacities
   b. Vascularization
   c. Scarring
3. Iritis

4. Irritation
   a. Lacrimation
   b. Hyperemia
   c. Ocular pain
   d. Burning sensation
5. Delayed corneal wound healing
6. Eyelids or conjunctiva
   a. Allergic reactions
   b. Blepharoconjunctivitis
7. Decreased stability of corneal tear film
8. Subconjunctival hemorrhages
9. Decreased blink reflex
10. Hypopyon
11. Inhibits bacterial growth
12. Inhibits fluorescence of fluorescein
13. Decreased vision
14. Conjunctival vasoconstriction (cocaine)
15. Mydriasis — may precipitate narrow-angle glaucoma (cocaine)
16. Paralysis of accommodation (cocaine)
17. Visual hallucinations — especially Lilliputian (cocaine)
18. Ptosis (?) (cocaine)

Clinical Significance: Few significant ocular side effects are seen with these agents if they are given topically for short periods of time; however, prolonged use will inevitably cause severe and permanent corneal damage and visual loss. Local anesthetics inhibit the rate of corneal epithelial cell migration by disruption of cytoplasmic action in filaments which may be important in the epithelial cell migration to close corneal wounds. Chronic use of local anesthetics has been shown recently to cause dense yellow-white rings within the corneal stroma. This may occur as early as the sixth or as late as the sixtieth day after initial use. The ring resembles a Wessely ring and often resolves once the local anesthetic is discontinued. Transient superficial corneal irregularities and edema may interfere with biomicroscopy or fundus examinations even after a single application. Recent data suggest that topical local anesthetics adversely affect superficial corneal epithelial microvilli. This may be the reason the stability of the tear film is adversely affected by these agents. Currently, proparacaine is probably the most commonly used topical local anesthetic since it causes the least irritation. Tetracaine may cause ocular irritation long after its local anesthetic effect wears off. Proparacaine has been reported to be one of the three more common topical ocular drugs causing allergic dermatitis. The other two drugs are atropine and neomycin. While most of these agents decrease the fluorescence of fluorescein, benoxinate decreases it the least. One case of an inadvertent anterior chamber injection of tetracaine has been reported, wherein wrinkling of Descemet's membrane, semidilated nonreactive pupils, and bullous keratopathy which did not respond to therapy occurred. A report of bilateral blindness secondary to topical cocaine drug abuse has been reported. Cocaine can potentiate sympathomimetic drugs, such as epinephrine, so that they should not be mixed or used conjointly, if possible. Numerous systemic reactions from topical ocular applications of local anesthetics have been reported. Many of these occur in part from the fear of the impending procedure or possibly an oculocardiac reflex. Side effects reported to the Registry include syncope, convulsions, and possible anaphylactic shock.

Interactions with Other Drugs:

A. Effect of Topical Local Anesthetics on Activity of Other Drugs
   1. Succinylcholine ↑
   2. Sympathomimetics ↑
   3. Adrenergic blockers ↓
   4. Sulfonamides ↓

References:

Bellows, J. G.: Surface anesthesia in ophthalmology; comparison of some drugs used. Arch. Ophthalmol. *12*:824, 1934.

Burns, R. P., et al.: Chronic toxicity of local anesthetics on the cornea. In Leopold, I. H., and Burns, R. P. (Eds.): Symposium on Drug Therapy. New York, John Wiley & Sons, 1977, Vol. X, pp. 31–44.

Burns, R. P., and Gipson, I.: Toxic effects of local anesthetics. JAMA *240*:347, 1978.

Cocaine. Med. Lett. Drugs Ther. *21*:18, 1979.

Eerden, A. A. J. J. v. d.: Changes in corneal epithelium due to local anesthetics. Ophthalmologica *143*:154, 1962.

Epstein, D. L., and Paton, D.: Keratitis from misuse of corneal anesthetics. N. Engl. J. Med. *279*:396, 1968.

Fraunfelder, F. T., Sharp, J. D., and Silver, B. E.: Possible adverse effects from topical ocular anesthetics. Doc. Ophthalmol. *18*:341, 1979.

Knapp, H.: On cocaine and its use in ophthalmic and general surgery. Arch. Ophthalmol. *68*:31, 1962.

Ravin, J. G., and Ravin, L. C.: Blindness due to illicit use of topical cocaine. Ann. Ophthalmol. *11*:863, 1979.

Siegel, R. K.: Cocaine hallucinations. Am. J. Psychiatry *135*:309, 1978.

Class: Topical Osmotic Agents

Generic Name: Sodium Chloride

Proprietary Name: Adsorbonac, Hyperopto, Hypersal, Muro-128, Ocean, Ocurins

Primary Use: This topical ocular hypertonic salt solution is used to reduce corneal edema.

Ocular Side Effects:

A. Local Ophthalmic Use or Exposure — Topical Application
   1. Irritation
      a. Hyperemia
      b. Ocular pain
      c. Burning sensation
   2. Corneal dehydration
   3. Subconjunctival hemorrhages
B. Local Ophthalmic Use or Exposure — Subconjunctival Injection
   1. Conjunctival hyperemia
   2. Increased intraocular pressure

Clinical Significance: Few significant adverse ocular reactions are seen with commercial topical sodium chloride solutions. The most frequent ocular side effects are irritation and discomfort, which are primarily related to the frequency of application. At suggested dosages all ocular side effects are reversible and transient.

References:

Grant, W. M.: Toxicology of the Eye. 2nd Ed., Springfield, Charles C Thomas, 1974, p. 929.
Maurice, D. M.: Influence on corneal permeability of bathing with solutions of differing reaction and tonicity. Br. J. Ophthalmol. 39:463, 1955.
Physicians' Desk Reference for Ophthalmology. 9th Ed., Oradell, N.J., Medical Economics Co., 1980/81, pp. 102, 108.
Walsh, F. B., and Hoyt, W. F.: Clinical Neuro-Ophthalmology. 3rd Ed., Baltimore, Williams & Wilkins, Vol. III, 1969, p. 2710.

Index of Side Effects

Lists of drugs causing the following side effects appear on page 389 and following pages.

Abnormal Conjugate Deviations
Abnormal ERG or EOG
Abnormal Visual Sensations
Absence of Foveal Reflex. See *Decreased or Absent Foveal Reflex*
Absence of Pupillary Reaction to Light. See *Decreased or Absent Pupillary Reaction to Light*
Accommodative Spasm
Anisocoria
Blepharitis. See also *Blepharoconjunctivitis*
Blepharoclonus
Blepharoconjunctivitis. See also *Blepharitis; Conjunctivitis—Follicular; Conjunctivitis — Nonspecific*
Blepharospasm
Cataracts
Colored Haloes around Lights
Conjunctival Deposits. See *Eyelids or Conjunctiva — Deposits*
Conjunctival Edema. See *Eyelids or Conjunctiva — Edema*
Conjunctival Hyperemia
Conjunctivitis. See also *Blepharoconjunctivitis*
  Follicular
  Nonspecific
Constriction of Visual Fields. See *Visual Field Defects*
Corneal Deposits
Corneal Discoloration
Corneal Edema
Corneal Opacities
Corneal Scarring
Corneal Ulceration

Corneal Vascularization
Cortical Blindness
Decreased Accommodation. See *Decreased or Paralysis of Accommodation*
Decreased Anterior Chamber Depth
Decreased Convergence
Decreased Corneal Reflex
Decreased Dark Adaptation
Decreased Dark Perception
Decreased Foveal Reflex. See *Decreased or Absent Foveal Reflex*
Decreased Intraocular Pressure
Decreased Lacrimation
Decreased or Absent Foveal Reflex
Decreased or Absent Pupillary Reaction to Light
Decreased or Paralysis of Accommodation
Decreased Resistance to Infection
Decreased Spontaneous Eye Movements
Decreased Tear Lysozymes
Decreased Tolerance to Contact Lenses
Decreased Vision
Delayed Corneal Wound Healing
Diplopia
Dyschromatopsia
Enlarged Blind Spot. See *Visual Field Defects*
Exophthalmos
Eyelids — Depigmentation. See *Eyelids or Conjunctiva — Depigmentation*

Abnormal ERG or EOG (Cont'd)
Thiethylperazine
Thiopental
Thiopropazate
Thioproperazine
Thioridazine
Trifluoperazine
Triflupromazine
Trimeprazine
Vinbarbital

Abnormal Visual Sensations
Acetyldigitoxin
Amodiaquine
Aspirin
Bromide
Capreomycin
Chloroquine
Clomiphene
Clonidine (?)
Cycloserine
Deslanoside
Digitalis
Digitoxin
Digoxin
Ergot (?)
Gitalin
Guanethidine
Hashish
Hydralazine
Hydroxychloroquine
Lanatoside C
LSD
Lysergide
Marihuana
Mecamylamine
Mescaline
Nalidixic Acid
Ouabain
Paramethadione
Pentylenetetrazol
Phenytoin
Piperazine
Piperidolate

Propantheline
Psilocybin
Quinine
Sodium Salicylate
Streptomycin
Tetrahydrocannabinol
THC
Thiabendazole
Trimethadione
Tryparsamide

Accommodative Spasm
Aceclidine
Acetylcholine
Carbachol
Demecarium
DFP
Digitalis
Echothiophate
Guanethidine
Isoflurophate
Methylene Blue
Morphine
Neostigmine
Opium
Physostigmine
Pilocarpine

Anisocoria
Alcohol
Antazoline
Bromide
Bromisovalum
Brompheniramine
Carbinoxamine
Carbromal
Chlorpheniramine
Clemastine
Dexbrompheniramine
Dexchlorpheniramine
Diacetylmorphine
Dimethindene
Diphenhydramine
Diphenylpyraline

Disulfiram
Doxylamine
Ethchlorvynol
Hashish
Isocarboxazid
LSD
Lysergide
Marihuana
Mescaline
Methaqualone
Nialamide
Oral Contraceptives
Phenelzine
Pheniramine
Psilocybin
Pyrilamine
Tetrahydrocannabinol
THC
Tranylcypromine
Trichloroethylene
Tripelennamine
Triprolidine

Blepharitis
Aminosalicylate (?)
Aminosalicylic Acid (?)
Isosorbide
Mannitol
Meperidine

Blepharoclonus
Acetylcholine
Allobarbital
Ambenonium
Amobarbital
Amodiaquine
Aprobarbital
Barbital
Bupivacaine
Butabarbital
Butalbital
Butallylonal
Butethal

Carbachol
Chloroprocaine
Chloroquine
Clofibrate
Cyclobarbital
Cyclopentobarbital
Demecarium
DFP
Dibucaine
Echothiophate
Edrophonium
Etidocaine
Heptabarbital
Hexethal
Hexobarbital
Hydroxychloroquine
Isoflurophate
Levodopa
Lidocaine
Mephobarbital
Mepivacaine
Methacholine
Metharbital
Methitural
Methohexital
Neostigmine
Pentobarbital
Phenobarbital
Physostigmine
Pilocarpine
Piperocaine
Prilocaine
Primidone
Probarbital
Procaine
Propoxycaine
Pyridostigmine
Secobarbital
Talbutal
Tetracaine
Thiamylal
Thiopental
Vinbarbital

Blepharoconjunctivitis
Amithiozone
Amoxicillin
Ampicillin
Atropine
Aurothioglucose
Aurothioglycanide
Bacitracin
Benoxinate
Benzathine Penicillin G
Bromide
Butacaine
Carbenicillin
Cloxacillin
Cocaine
Cyclopentolate
Cyclophosphamide
Dibucaine
Dicloxacillin
Dyclonine
Epinephrine
Gold Au[198]
Gold Sodium Thiomalate
Gold Sodium Thiosulfate
Hetacillin
Homatropine
Hydrabamine Penicillin V
Influenza Virus Vaccine
Insulin
Iodine Solution
Measles Virus Vaccine Live
Melphalan
Mercuric Oxide
Methicillin
Methotrexate
Mitomycin
Nafcillin
Neostigmine
Nitromersol
Oxacillin
Penicillamine
Phenacaine
Phenylmercuric Acetate
Phenylmercuric Nitrate

Physostigmine
Piperocaine
Poliovirus Vaccine
Potassium Penicillin G
Potassium Penicillin V
Potassium Phenethicillin
Procaine Penicillin G
Proparacaine
Rabies Immune Globulin and
 Vaccine
Rifampin
Rubella Virus Vaccine Live
Smallpox Vaccine
Tetracaine
Tetrahydrozoline
Thimerosal
Timolol
Tropicamide

Blepharospasm
Amitriptyline
Amodiaquine
Amoxapine (?)
Amphetamine (?)
Antazoline
Brompheniramine
Carbinoxamine
Chloroquine
Chlorpheniramine
Clemastine
Clomipramine
Desipramine
Dexbrompheniramine
Dexchlorpheniramine
Dextroamphetamine (?)
Dimercaprol
Dimethindene
Diphenhydramine
Diphenylpyraline
Doxepin
Doxylamine
Emetine
Hashish
Hydroxychloroquine

Imipramine
Levodopa
Marihuana
Methamphetamine (?)
Nortriptyline
Pentylenetetrazol
Pheniramine
Phenmetrazine (?)
Protriptyline
Pyrilamine
Tetrahydrocannabinol
THC
Trimipramine
Tripelennamine
Tripolidine
Vinblastine

Cataracts
Acetophenazine
Acetylcholine
Adrenal Cortex Injection
Alcohol
Aldosterone
Allopurinol (?)
Amodiaquine
Azathioprine (?)
Betamethasone
Busulfan
Butaperazine
Calcitriol (?)
Carbamazepine (?)
Carbromal (?)
Carphenazine
Chloroquine
Chlorpromazine
Chlorprothixene
Cholecalciferol (?)
Clomiphene (?)
Cobalt
Colchicine (?)
Cortisone
Deferoxamine
Demecarium
Desoxycorticosterone

Dexamethasone
Dextrothyroxine (?)
DFP
Diazoxide
Diethazine
Droperidol (?)
Echothiophate
Edrophonium
Ergocalciferol (?)
Ergonovine (?)
Ergot (?)
Ergotamine (?)
Ethopropazine
Ethotoin (?)
Fludrocortisone
Fluorometholone
Fluphenazine
Fluprednisolone
Haloperidol (?)
Hydrocortisone
Hydroxychloroquine
Ibuprofen (?)
Isoflurophate
Medrysone
Mephenytoin (?)
Meprednisone
Mesoridazine
Methdilazine
Methotrimeprazine
Methoxsalen (?)
Methylergonovine (?)
Methylprednisolone
Methysergide (?)
Mitotane
Naproxen (?)
Neostigmine
Paramethasone
Penicillamine (?)
Perazine
Periciazine
Perphenazine
Phenmetrazine
Physostigmine
Pilocarpine

Cataracts (Cont'd)
Piperacetazine
Piperazine (?)
Prednisolone
Prednisone
Prochlorperazine
Promazine
Promethazine
Propiomazine
Silicone
Thiethylperazine
Thiopropazate
Thioproperazine
Thioridazine
Thiothixene
Timolol (?)
Triamcinolone
Trifluoperazine
Trifluperidol (?)
Triflupromazine
Trimeprazine
Trioxsalen (?)
Vitamin A (?)
Vitamin D₂ (?)
Vitamin D₃ (?)

Colored Haloes Around Lights
Acetophenazine
Acetyldigitoxin
Amiodarone
Amodiaquine
Amyl Nitrite
Betamethasone
Butaperazine
Carphenazine
Chloroquine
Chlorpromazine
Cortisone
Deslanoside
Dexamethasone
Diethazine
Digitalis
Digitoxin
Digoxin

Ethopropazine
Fluorometholone
Fluphenazine
Gitalin
Hydrocortisone
Hydroxychloroquine
Lanatoside C
Medrysone
Mesoridazine
Methdilazine
Methotrimeprazine
Nitroglycerin
Oral Contraceptives
Ouabain
Paramethadione
Perazine
Periciazine
Perphenazine
Piperacetazine
Prednisolone
Prochlorperazine
Promazine
Promethazine
Propiomazine
Quinacrine
Thiethylperazine
Thiopropazate
Thioproperazine
Thioridazine
Trifluoperazine
Triflupromazine
Trimeprazine
Trimethadione

Conjunctival Hyperemia
Acetohexamide
Acetylcholine
Adrenal Cortex Injection
Aldosterone
Alseroxylon
Amithiozone
Aurothioglucose
Aurothioglycanide
BCNU

Betamethasone
Bupivacaine
Carbachol
Carmustine
Chloral Hydrate
Chloroprocaine
Chlorpropamide
Chrysarobin
Cimetidine
Clindamycin
Colchicine
Cortisone
Deferoxamine
Deserpidine
Desoxycorticosterone
Dexamethasone
Dextrothyroxine
Diacetylmorphine
Diatrizoate Meglumine and
   Sodium
Erythromycin
Ether
Etidocaine
Fludrocortisone
Fluorescein
Fluprednisolone
F_3T
Gold Au^{198}
Gold Sodium Thiomalate
Gold Sodium Thiosulfate
Griseofulvin
Hydrocortisone
Idoxuridine
IDU
Iodide and Iodine Solutions and
   Compounds
Levothyroxine
Lidocaine
Lincomycin
Liothyronine
Liotrix
Mepivacaine
Meprednisone
Mercuric Oxide

Methacholine
Methyldopa
Methylprednisolone
Metoprolol
Nitromersol
Norepinephrine
Oxprenolol
Oxyphenbutazone
Paramethasone
Phenoxybenzamine
Phenylbutazone
Phenylmercuric Acetate
Phenylmercuric Nitrate
Pilocarpine
Practolol
Prednisolone
Prednisone
Prilocaine
Procaine
Propoxycaine
Propranolol
Radioactive Iodides
Rauwolfia Serpentina
Rescinnamine
Reserpine
Rifampin
Sodium Chloride
Syrosingopine
Thiabendazole
Thimerosal
Thyroglobulin
Thyroid
Tolazamide
Tolazoline
Tolbutamide
Triamcinolone
Trifluridine
Vancomycin
Vidarabine

Conjunctivitis—Follicular
   Amphotericin B
   Carbachol
   Demecarium

Conjunctivitis—Follicular (Cont'd)
DFP
Diatrizoate Meglumine and
   Sodium
Dipivefrin
DPE
Echothiophate
Framycetin
F₃T
Gentamicin
Hyaluronidase
Idoxuridine
IDU
Isoflurophate
Neomycin
Neostigmine
Physostigmine
Pilocarpine
Scopolamine
Sulfacetamide
Sulfamethizole
Sulfisoxazole
Trifluridine
Vidarabine

Conjunctivitis—Nonspecific
Acenocoumarol
Acetaminophen
Acetanilid
Acetohexamide
Allobarbital
Amobarbital
Anisindione
Antipyrine
Aprobarbital
Aspirin
Barbital
Butabarbital
Butalbital
Butallylonal
Butethal
Carbamazepine
Carbimazole
Chlordiazepoxide

Chlorpropamide
Chrysarobin
Clofibrate
Clonazepam
Clorazepate
Colloidal Silver
Cyclobarbital
Cyclopentobarbital
Cytarabine
Dextran
Diazepam
Dicumarol
Diethylcarbamazine
Dimercaprol
Diphenadione
Disopyramide
Doxorubicin
Edrophonium
Emetine
Ephedrine
Ethotoin
Ethyl Biscoumacetate
Flurazepam
Heparin
Heptabarbital
Hexethal
Hexobarbital
Hydralazine
Iodide and Iodine Solutions and
   Compounds
Ketoprofen
Lorazepam
Meperidine
Mephenytoin
Mephobarbital
Metharbital
Methimazole
Methitural
Methocarbamol
Methohexital
Methyldopa
Methylthiouracil
Metoprolol
Morphine

Naphazoline
Naproxen
Nitrazepam
Opium
Oxazepam
Oxprenolol
Oxyphenbutazone
Oxyphenonium
Pentobarbital
Phenacetin
Phenindione
Phenobarbital
Phenprocoumon
Phenylbutazone
Prazepam
Primidone
Probarbital
Propranolol
Propylthiouracil
Radioactive Iodides
Secobarbital
Silver Nitrate
Silver Protein
Sodium Salicylate
Streptomycin
Sulfacetamide
Sulfachlorpyridazine
Sulfacytine
Sulfadiazine
Sulfadimethoxine
Sulfamerazine
Sulfameter
Sulfamethazine
Sulfamethizole
Sulfamethoxazole
Sulfamethoxypyridazine
Sulfanilamide
Sulfaphenazole
Sulfapyridine
Sulfasalazine
Sulfathiazole
Sulfisoxazole
Talbutal
Thiamylal

Thiopental
Tolazamide
Tolbutamide
Vinbarbital
Warfarin

Corneal Deposits
Acetophenazine
Acid Bismuth Sodium Tartrate
Alcohol
Amiodarone
Amodiaquine
Aurothioglucose
Aurothioglycanide
Bismuth Oxychloride
Bismuth Sodium Tartrate
Bismuth Sodium Thioglycollate
Bismuth Sodium Triglycollamate
Bismuth Subcarbonate
Bismuth Subsalicylate
Butaperazine
Calcitriol
Carphenazine
Chloroquine
Chlorpromazine
Chlorprothixene
Cholecalciferol
Colloidal Silver
Cytarabine (?)
Diethazine
Echothiophate
Epinephrine
Ergocalciferol
Ethopropazine
Ferrocholinate
Ferrous Fumarate
Ferrous Gluconate
Ferrous Succinate
Ferrous Sulfate
Fluphenazine
Gold Au[198]
Gold Sodium Thiomalate
Gold Sodium Thiosulfate
Hydroxychloroquine

14

Corneal Deposits (Cont'd)
Indomethacin
Iron Dextran
Iron Sorbitex
Meperidine (?)
Mercuric Oxide
Mesoridazine
Methdilazine
Methotrimeprazine
Perazine
Periciazine
Perphenazine
Piperacetazine
Polysaccharide-Iron Complex
Prochlorperazine
Promazine
Promethazine
Propiomazine
Quinacrine
Silver Nitrate
Silver Protein
Thiethylperazine
Thiopropazate
Thioproperazine
Thioridazine
Thiothixene
Trifluoperazine
Triflupromazine
Trimeprazine
Vitamin D_2
Vitamin D_3

Corneal Discoloration
Antimony Lithium Thiomalate
Antimony Potassium Tartrate
Antimony Sodium Tartrate
Antimony Sodium Thioglycollate
Chlortetracycline
Ferrocholinate
Ferrous Fumarate
Ferrous Gluconate
Ferrous Succinate
Ferrous Sulfate
Iodine Solution

Iron Dextran
Iron Sorbitex
Methylene Blue
Polysaccharide-Iron Complex
Quinacrine
Sodium Antimonylgluconate
Stibocaptate
Stibogluconate
Stibophen
Tetracycline

Corneal Edema
Acetophenazine
Acetylcholine
Amantadine
Amodiaquine
Amphotericin B
Bacitracin
Benoxinate
Benzathine Penicillin G
Butacaine
Butaperazine
Carbachol
Carphenazine
Chloramphenicol
Chloroquine
Chlorpromazine
Chlortetracycline
Chymotrypsin
Cocaine
Colistin
Dibucaine
Diethazine
Dyclonine
Epinephrine
Erythromycin
Ethopropazine
Fluphenazine
Hexachlorophene
Hydrabamine Penicillin V
Hydroxychloroquine
Melphalan
Mesoridazine
Methdilazine

Methicillin
Methotrimeprazine
Neomycin
Perazine
Periciazine
Perphenazine
Phenacaine
Phenylephrine
Piperacetazine
Piperocaine
Polymyxin B
Potassium Penicillin G
Potassium Penicillin V
Potassium Phenethicillin
Procaine Penicillin G
Prochlorperazine
Promazine
Promethazine
Proparacaine
Propiomazine
Quinacrine
Streptomycin
Tetracaine
Tetracycline
Thiethylperazine
Thiopropazate
Thioproperazine
Thioridazine
Thiotepa
Trifluoperazine
Triflupromazine
Trimeprazine

Corneal Opacities
Acetylcholine
Alcohol
Benoxinate
Broxyquinoline (?)
Butacaine
Chlorambucil (?)
Chloroform
Chrysarobin
Clofazimine
Cloxacillin

Cocaine
Cytarabine
Dibucaine
Dyclonine
Emetine
Ether
Ethotoin (?)
F₃T
Ibuprofen (?)
Idoxuridine
IDU
Iodochlorhydroxyquin (?)
Iodoquinol (?)
Mephenytoin (?)
Oxyphenbutazone
Phenacaine
Phenylbutazone
Piperocaine
Practolol
Proparacaine
Protriptyline
Silver Nitrate
Tamoxifen
Tetracaine
Trichloroethylene
Trifluridine
Vidarabine
Vinblastine

Corneal Scarring
Benoxinate
Butacaine
Cocaine
Dibucaine
Dyclonine
Iodine Solution
Oxyphenbutazone
Phenacaine
Phenylbutazone
Piperocaine
Proparacaine
Silver Nitrate
Smallpox Vaccine
Tetracaine

Corneal Ulceration
Alcohol
Amiodarone
Aspirin
Aurothioglucose
Aurothioglycanide
Benoxinate
Butacaine
Chloroform
Cocaine
Cytarabine
Dibucaine
Dyclonine
Emetine
Ferrocholinate
Ferrous Fumarate
Ferrous Gluconate
Ferrous Succinate
Ferrous Sulfate
F_3T
Gold Au^{198}
Gold Sodium Thiomalate
Gold Sodium Thiosulfate
Idoxuridine
IDU
Iron Dextran
Iron Sorbitex
Oxyphenbutazone
Phenacaine
Phenylbutazone
Piperocaine
Polysaccharide-Iron Complex
Practolol
Proparacaine
Sodium Salicylate
Sulindac (?)
Tetracaine
Thiotepa (?)
Trichloroethylene
Trifluridine
Vidarabine

Corneal Vascularization
Benoxinate
Butacaine

Cocaine
Dibucaine
Dyclonine
F_3T
Ibuprofen
Idoxuridine
IDU
Iodine Solution
Oxyphenbutazone
Phenacaine
Phenylbutazone
Piperocaine
Proparacaine
Tetracaine
Trifluridine
Vidarabine

Cortical Blindness
Bendroflumethiazide (?)
Benzthiazide (?)
Chloroform (?)
Chlorothiazide (?)
Chlorthalidone (?)
Cyclothiazide (?)
Ether (?)
Hydrochlorothiazide (?)
Hydroflumethiazide (?)
Methadone (?)
Methyclothiazide (?)
Methylergonovine (?)
Metolazone (?)
Nitrous Oxide (?)
Polythiazide (?)
Quinethazone (?)
Sulfacetamide
Sulfachlorpyridazine
Sulfacytine
Sulfadiazine
Sulfadimethoxine
Sulfamerazine
Sulfameter
Sulfamethazine
Sulfamethizole
Sulfamethoxazole
Sulfamethoxypyridazine

Sulfanilamide
Sulfaphenazole
Sulfapyridine
Sulfasalazine
Sulfathiazole
Sulfisoxazole
Thiopental (?)
Trichlormethiazide (?)

Decreased Anterior Chamber Depth
Acetylcholine
Demecarium
DFP
Echothiophate
Edrophonium
Isoflurophate
Neostigmine
Physostigmine
Pilocarpine
Sulfacetamide
Sulfachlorpyridazine
Sulfadiazine
Sulfadimethoxine
Sulfamerazine
Sulfameter
Sulfamethazine
Sulfamethizole
Sulfamethoxazole
Sulfamethoxypyridazine
Sulfanilamide
Sulfaphenazole
Sulfapyridine
Sulfasalazine
Sulfathiazole
Sulfisoxazole

Decreased Convergence
Alcohol
Allobarbital
Amobarbital
Amphetamine
Aprobarbital
Barbital
Bromide
Bromisovalum

Butabarbital
Butalbital
Butallylonal
Butethal
Carbon Dioxide
Chloral Hydrate
Cyclobarbital
Cyclopentobarbital
Dextroamphetamine
Floxuridine
Fluorouracil
Heptabarbital
Hexethal
Hexobarbital
Mephobarbital
Methamphetamine
Metharbital
Methitural
Methohexital
Metocurine Iodide
Morphine
Opium
Pentobarbital
Phenmetrazine
Phenobarbital
Phenytoin
Primidone
Probarbital
Secobarbital
Talbutal
Thiamylal
Thiopental
Tubocurarine
Vinbarbital

Decreased Corneal Reflex
Amitriptyline
Amodiaquine
Bromide
Carbon Dioxide
Carisoprodol
Chloroquine
Clorazepate
Desipramine
Diazepam

Decreased Corneal Reflex (Cont'd)
  Glutethimide
  Hydroxychloroquine
  Imipramine
  Meprobamate
  Methyprylon
  Nortriptyline
  Paraldehyde
  Phencyclidine
  Propranolol
  Protriptyline
  Timolol
  Trichloroethylene

Decreased Dark Adaptation
  Alcohol
  Amodiaquine
  Carbon Dioxide
  Chloroquine
  Hashish
  Hydroxychloroquine
  Indomethacin (?)
  LSD
  Lysergide
  Marihuana
  Mescaline
  Psilocybin
  Tetrahydrocannabinol
  THC

Decreased Depth Perception
  Alcohol
  Chlordiazepoxide
  Clonazepam
  Clorazepate
  Diazepam
  Flurazepam
  Lorazepam
  Nitrazepam
  Oxazepam
  Prazepam
  Sulfacetamide
  Sulfachlorpyridazine
  Sulfacytine

Sulfadiazine
Sulfadimethoxine
Sulfamerazine
Sulfameter
Sulfamethazine
Sulfamethizole
Sulfamethoxazole
Sulfamethoxypyridazine
Sulfanilamide
Sulfaphenazole
Sulfapyridine
Sulfasalazine
Sulfathiazole
Sulfisoxazole

Decreased Intraocular Pressure
  Aceclidine
  Acetazolamide
  Acetylcholine
  Acetyldigitoxin
  Alcohol
  Allobarbital
  Alseroxylon
  Amobarbital
  Amyl Nitrite
  Aprobarbital
  Aspirin
  Barbital
  Bendroflumethiazide
  Benzthiazide
  Betamethasone
  Bupivacaine
  Butabarbital
  Butalbital
  Butallylonal
  Butethal
  Carbachol
  Carisoprodol (?)
  Chloroform
  Chlorothiazide
  Chlorthalidone
  Clofibrate (?)
  Clonidine
  Cortisone

Decreased Intraocular Pressure
(Cont'd)
Quinethazone
Rauwolfia Serpentina
Rescinnamine
Reserpine
Secobarbital
Sodium Salicylate
Spironolactone
Succinylcholine
Syrosingopine
Talbutal
Tetraethylammonium
Tetrahydrocannabinol
Tetrahydrozoline
THC
Thiamylal
Thiopental
Timolol
Tolazoline
Trichlormethiazide
Trichloroethylcne
Trifluperidol
Trimethaphan
Trimethidinium
Trolnitrate
Tubocurarine
Urea
Urokinase
Vinbarbital
Vitamin A

Decreased Lacrimation
Acetophenazine
Amitriptyline
Antazoline
Atropine
Azatadine
Belladonna
Brompheniramine
Butaperazine
Carbinoxamine
Carphenazine
Chlorisondamine

Chlorpheniramine
Chlorpromazine
Clemastine
Cyproheptadine
Desipramine
Dexbrompheniramine
Dexchlorpheniramine
Diethazine
Dimethindene
Diphenhydramine
Diphenylpyraline
Doxylamine
Ether
Ethopropazine
Fluphenazine
Hashish
Hexamethonium
Homatropine
Imipramine
Marihuana
Mesoridazine
Methdilazine
Methotrimeprazine
Methscopolamine
Methyldopa
Methylthiouracil
Metoprolol (?)
Morphine
Nitrous Oxide
Nortriptyline
Opium
Oxprenolol
Perazine
Periciazine
Perphenazine
Pheniramine
Piperacetazine
Practolol
Prochlorperazine
Promazine
Promethazine
Propiomazine
Propranolol (?)
Protriptyline

Pyrilamine
Scopolamine
Tetrahydrocannabinol
THC
Thiethylperazine
Thiopropazate
Thioproperazine
Thioridazine
Trichloroethylene
Trifluoperazine
Triflupromazine
Trimeprazine
Tripelennamine
Triprolidine

Decreased or Absent Foveal Reflex
  Amodiaquine
  Broxyquinoline
  Chloroquine
  Hydroxychloroquine
  Iodochlorhydroxyquin
  Iodoquinol
  Quinine

*Decreased or Absent Pupillary
Reaction to Light*
  Acetaminophen
  Acetanilid
  Acetophenazine
  Alcohol
  Allobarbital
  Amitriptyline
  Amobarbital
  Amoxapine
  Amoxicillin (?)
  Amphetamine
  Ampicillin (?)
  Antazoline
  Antimony Lithium Thiomalate
  Antimony Potassium Tartrate
  Antimony Sodium Tartrate
  Antimony Sodium
    Thioglycollate
  Aprobarbital

Aspirin
Baclofen
Barbital
Benztropine
Biperiden
Bromide
Bromisovalum
Brompheniramine
Butabarbital
Butalbital
Butallylonal
Butaperazine
Butethal
Calcitriol
Carbenicillin (?)
Carbinoxamine
Carbon Dioxide
Carbromal
Carisoprodol
Carphenazine
Chloramphenicol
Chlorcyclizine
Chlordiazepoxide
Chlorpheniramine
Chlorphenoxamine
Chlorpromazine
Chlorprothixene
Cholecalciferol
Clemastine
Clomipramine
Clonazepam
Clonidine
Clorazepate
Cloxacillin (?)
Cocaine
Cyclizine
Cyclobarbital
Cyclopentobarbital
Cycrimine
Desipramine
Dexbrompheniramine
Dexchlorpheniramine
Dextroamphetamine
Diacetylmorphine

Decreased or Absent Pupillary
Reaction to Light (Cont'd)

Diazepam
Dicloxacillin (?)
Diethazine
Dimethindene
Diphenhydramine
Diphenylpyraline
Doxepin
Doxylamine
Emetine
Ergocalciferol
Ergot
Ethopropazine
Fenfluramine
Fluphenazine
Flurazepam
Glutethimide
Heptabarbital
Hetacillin (?)
Hexachlorophene
Hexethal
Hexobarbital
Imipramine
Insulin
Isocarboxazid
Isoniazid
Lorazepam
LSD
Lysergide
Meclizine
Meperidine
Mephobarbital
Meprobamate
Mescaline
Mesoridazine
Methamphetamine
Methaqualone
Metharbital
Methdilazine
Methicillin (?)
Methitural
Methohexital
Methotrimeprazine

Methyl Alcohol
Methyprylon
Nafcillin (?)
Neomycin
Nialamide
Nitrazepam
Nortriptyline
Orphenadrine
Oxacillin (?)
Oxazepam
Pargyline
Pentobarbital
Pentylenetetrazol
Perazine
Periciazine
Perphenazine
Phenacetin
Phencyclidine
Phenelzine
Pheniramine
Phenmetrazine
Phenobarbital
Phenytoin
Piperacetazine
Prazepam
Primidone
Probarbital
Prochlorperazine
Procyclidine
Promazine
Promethazine
Propantheline
Propiomazine
Protriptyline
Psilocybin
Pyrilamine
Quinine
Secobarbital
Sodium Antimonylgluconate
Sodium Salicylate
Stibocaptate
Stibogluconate
Stibophen
Talbutal

Thiamylal
Thiethylperazine
Thiopental
Thiopropazate
Thioproperazine
Thioridazine
Thiothixene
Tranylcypromine
Trichloroethylene
Trifluoperazine
Triflupromazine
Trihexyphenidyl
Trimeprazine
Trimipramine
Tripelennamine
Triprolidine
Urethan
Vinbarbital
Vitamin D_2
Vitamin D_3

*Decreased or Paralysis of
Accommodation*
Acetazolamide
Acetophenazine
Adiphenine
Alcohol
Ambutonium
Aminosalicylate (?)
Aminosalicylic Acid (?)
Amitriptyline
Amodiaquine
Amoxapine
Amphetamine
Anisindione
Anisotropine
Antazoline
Atropine
Baclofen
Belladonna
Bendroflumethiazide
Benzathine Penicillin G
Benzphetamine
Benzthiazide

Benztropine
Betamethasone
Bethanechol
Biperiden
Bromide
Butaperazine
Caramiphen
Carbachol
Carbamazepine
Carbinoxamine
Carbon Dioxide
Carisoprodol
Carphenazine
Chloramphenicol
Chlordiazepoxide
Chloroquine
Chlorothiazide
Chlorphenoxamine
Chlorphentermine
Chlorpromazine
Chlorprothixene
Chlorthalidone
Clemastine
Clidinium
Clomipramine
Clonazepam
Clorazepate
Cocaine
Cortisone
Cyclopentolate
Cycloserine (?)
Cyclothiazide
Cycrimine
Desipramine
Dexamethasone
Dextroamphetamine
Diacetylmorphine
Diazepam
Dibucaine
Dichlorphenamide
Dicyclomine
Diethazine
Diethylpropion
Diphemanil

Decreased or Paralysis of Accommodation (*Cont'd*)

Diphenadione
Diphenhydramine
Diphenylpyraline
Doxepin
Doxylamine
Droperidol
Emetine
Ergot
Ethchlorvynol
Ethopropazine
Ethoxzolamide
Fenfluramine
Floxuridine
Fluorometholone
Fluorouracil
Fluphenazine
Flurazepam
Furosemide (?)
Glutethimide
Glycopyrrolate
Haloperidol
Hashish
Hexamethonium
Hexocyclium
Homatropine
Hydrabamine Penicillin V
Hydrochlorothiazide
Hydrocortisone
Hydroflumethiazide
Hydromorphone
Hydroxyamphetamine
Hydroxychloroquine
Imipramine
Iodide and Iodine Solutions and
   Compounds
Isoniazid
Isopropamide
Ketoprofen
Lorazepam
Loxapine
LSD
Lysergide

Marihuana
Mecamylamine
Medrysone
Mepenzolate
Meprobamate
Mescaline
Mesoridazine
Methacholine
Methamphetamine
Methantheline
Methaqualone (?)
Methazolamide
Methdilazine
Methixene
Methotrimeprazine
Methscopolamine
Methyclothiazide
Methylatropine Nitrate
Methylene Blue
Methyprylon
Methysergide
Metolazone
Morphine
Nalidixic Acid
Naproxen
Nitrazepam
Nortriptyline
Opium
Orphenadrine
Oxazepam
Oxymorphone
Oxyphencyclimine
Oxyphenonium
Pargyline
Pentazocine
Pentolinium
Perazine
Periciazine
Perphenazine
Phendimetrazine
Phenindione
Phenmetrazine
Phentermine
Phenytoin

Pilocarpine
Pipenzolate
Piperacetazine
Piperazine
Piperidolate
Piperocaine
Poldine
Polythiazide
Potassium Penicillin G
Potassium Penicillin V
Potassium Phenethicillin
Pralidoxime
Prazepam
Prednisolone
Procaine Penicillin G
Procarbazine
Prochlorperazine
Procyclidine
Promazine
Promethazine
Propantheline
Propiomazine
Protriptyline
Psilocybin
Pyrilamine
Quinethazone
Radioactive Iodides
Rubella Virus Vaccine Live
Scopolamine
Streptomycin
Tetanus Toxoid
Tetracaine
Tetraethylammonium
Tetrahydrocannabinol
THC
Thiethylperazine
Thiopropazate
Thioproperazine
Thioridazine
Thiothixene
Trichlormethiazide
Trichloroethylene
Tridihexethyl
Trifluoperazine

Trifluperidol
Triflupromazine
Trihexyphenidyl
Trimeprazine
Trimethaphan
Trimethidinium
Trimipramine
Tripelennamine
Tropicamide

Decreased Resistance to Infection
Adrenal Cortex Injection
Aldosterone
Azathioprine
Betamethasone
Cortisone
Desoxycorticosterone
Dexamethasone
Fludrocortisone
Fluorometholone
Fluprednisolone
Hydrocortisone
Medrysone
Meprednisone
Methylprednisolone
Paramethasone
Prednisolone
Prednisone
Triamcinolone

Decreased Spontaneous Eye Movements
Alcohol
Alseroxylon
Amitriptyline
Bromide
Carbamazepine
Chlordiazepoxide
Clonazepam
Clorazepate
Deserpidine
Desipramine
Diazepam
Flurazepam

Decreased Spontaneous Eye Movements (Cont'd)
Imipramine
Lithium Carbonate
Lorazepam
Nitrazepam
Nortriptyline
Oxazepam
Prazepam
Protriptyline
Rauwolfia Serpentina
Rescinnamine
Reserpine
Syrosingopine

Decreased Tear Lysozymes
Adrenal Cortex Injection
Aldosterone
Betamethasone
Cortisone
Desoxycorticosterone
Dexamethasone
Fludrocortisone
Fluprednisolone
Hydrocortisone
Insulin
Meprednisone
Methylprednisolone
Paramethasone
Practolol
Prednisolone
Prednisone
Triamcinolone

Decreased Tolerance to Contact Lenses
Antazoline
Azatadine
Brompheniramine
Carbinoxamine
Chlorcyclizine
Chlorpheniramine
Clemastine
Clomiphene

Cyclizine
Cyproheptadine
Dexbrompheniramine
Dexchlorpheniramine
Diemethindene
Diphenhydramine
Diphenylpyraline
Doxylamine
Furosemide
Meclizine
Oral Contraceptives
Orphenadrine (?)
Pheniramine
Pyrilamine
Tripelennamine
Triprolidine

Decreased Vision
Aceclidine
Acetaminophen
Acetanilid
Acetazolamide
Acetohexamide
Acetophenazine
Acetyldigitoxin
Acid Bismuth Sodium Tartrate (?)
Adiphenine
Adrenal Cortex Injection
Alcohol
Aldosterone
Alkavervir
Allobarbital
Allopurinol
Alseroxylon
Aluminum Nicotinate
Amantadine
Ambenonium
Ambutonium
Aminosalicylate (?)
Aminosalicylic Acid (?)
Amiodarone
Amithiozone
Amitriptyline

Amobarbital
Amodiaquine
Amoxapine
Amphetamine
Amphotericin B
Amyl Nitrite
Anisindione
Anisotropine
Antazoline
Antimony Lithium Thiomalate
Antimony Potassium Tartrate
Antimony Sodium Tartrate
Antimony Sodium Thioglycollate
Antipyrine
Aprobarbital
Aspirin
Atropine
Azatadine
Bacitracin
Baclofen
Barbital
BCNU
Belladonna
Bendroflumethiazide
Benoxinate
Benzathine Penicillin G
Benzphetamine
Benzthiazide
Benztropine
Betamethasone
Biperiden
Bismuth Oxychloride (?)
Bismuth Sodium Tartrate (?)
Bismuth Sodium
    Thioglycollate (?)
Bismuth Sodium
    Triglycollamate (?)
Bismuth Subcarbonate (?)
Bismuth Subsalicylate (?)
Bromide
Bromisovalum
Brompheniramine
Broxyquinoline
Bupivacaine

Busulfan
Butabarbital
Butacaine
Butalbital
Butallylonal
Butaperazine
Capreomycin
Carbachol
Carbamazepine
Carbinoxamine
Carbon Dioxide
Carbromal
Carisoprodol
Carmustine
Carphenazine
CCNU
Cefazolin (?)
Cephalexin (?)
Cephaloglycin (?)
Cephaloridine (?)
Cephalothin (?)
Cephradine (?)
Chloral Hydrate
Chlorambucil
Chloramphenicol
Chlorcyclizine
Chlordiazepoxide
Chloroform
Chloroprocaine
Chloroquine
Chlorothiazide
Chlorpheniramine
Chlorphenoxamine
Chlorphentermine
Chlorprocaine
Chlorpromazine
Chlorpropamide
Chlorprothixene
Chlortetracycline
Chlorthalidone
Clemastine
Clidinium
Clofibrate
Clomiphene

Decreased Vision (Cont'd)

Clomipramine
Clonazepam
Clonidine
Clorazepate
Cobalt
Cocaine
Codeine
Colchicine
Colloidal Silver
Cortisone
Cryptenamine
Cyclizine
Cyclobarbital
Cyclopentobarbital
Cyclopentolate
Cyclophosphamide
Cycloserine
Cyclothiazide
Cycrimine
Cyproheptadine
Dacarbazine
Dantrolene
Dapsone
Deferoxamine
Demecarium
Demeclocyline
Deserpidine
Desipramine
Deslanoside
Desoxycorticosterone
Dexamethasone
Dexbrompheniramine
Dexchlorpheniramine
Dextroamphetamine
Dextrothyroxine
DFP
Diatrizoate Meglumine and
    Sodium
Diazepam
Diazoxide
Dibucaine
DIC
Dichlorphenamide

Dicumarol
Dicyclomine
Diethazine
Diethylpropion
Digitalis
Digitoxin
Digoxin
Dimethindene
Diphemanil
Diphenadione
Diphenhydramine
Diphenylpyraline
Diphtheria and Tetanus Toxoids
    and Pertussis (DPT) Vaccine
    Adsorbed
Dipivefrin
Disopyramide
Disulfiram
Doxepin
Doxycycline
Doxylamine
DPE
Droperidol
Dyclonine
Echothiophate
Edrophonium
Emetine
Ephedrine
Epinephrine
Ergonovine
Ergot
Ergotamine
Erythrityl Tetranitrate
Ethacrynic Acid
Ethambutol
Ethchlorvynol
Ether
Ethionamide
Ethopropazine
Ethosuximide
Ethoxzolamide
Etidocaine
Fenfluramine
Floxuridine

Decreased Vision (Cont'd)

Metharbital
Methazolamide
Methdilazine
Methitural
Methixene
Methocarbamol
Methohexital
Methotrexate
Methotrimeprazine
Methscopolamine
Methsuximide
Methyclothiazide
Methyl Alcohol
Methylatropine Nitrate
Methyldopa
Methylene Blue
Methylergonovine
Methylphenidate
Methylprednisolone
Methyprylon
Methysergide
Metoclopramide
Metolazone
Metoprolol
Minocycline
Mitomycin
Mitotane
Morphine
Nalidixic Acid
Nalorphine
Naloxone
Naphazoline
Naproxen
Neostigmine
Niacin
Niacinamide
Nialamide
Nicotinyl Alcohol
Nitrazepam
Nitrofurantoin
Nitroglycerin
Nitrous Oxide
Nortriptyline

Nystatin
Opium
Oral Contraceptives
Orphenadrine
Ouabain
Oxazepam
Oxprenolol
Oxygen
Oxymorphone
Oxyphenbutazone
Oxyphencyclimine
Oxyphenonium
Oxytetracycline
Paraldehyde
Paramethasone
Pentaerythritol Tetranitrate
Pentazocine
Pentobarbital
Pentolinium
Perazine
Perhexilene
Periciazine
Perphenazine
Phenacaine
Phenacetin
Phencyclidine
Phendimetrazine
Phenelzine
Phenindione
Pheniramine
Phenmetrazine
Phenobarbital
Phensuximide
Phentermine
Phenylbutazone
Phenylephrine
Phenytoin
Physostigmine
Pilocarpine
Pipenzolate
Piperacetazine
Piperazine
Piperidolate
Piperocaine

Decreased Vision (Cont'd)
Thiopental
Thiopropazate
Thioproperazine
Thioridazine
Thiothixene
Thyroglobulin
Thyroid
Timolol
Tolazamide
Tolbutamide
Tranylcypromine
Triamcinolone
Trichlormethiazide
Trichloroethylene
Tridihexethyl
Triethylenemelamine
Trifluoperazine
Trifluperidol
Triflupromazine
Trihexyphenidyl
Trimeprazine
Trimethaphan
Trimethidinium
Trimipramine
Tripelennamine
Triprolidine
Trolnitrate
Tropicamide
Tryparsamide
Uracil Mustard
Urea
Urethan
Veratrum Viride Alkaloids
Vinbarbital
Vinblastine
Warfarin

Delayed Corneal Wound Healing
Adrenal Cortex Injection
Aldosterone
Azathioprine
Benoxinate
Benzalkonium (?)

Betamethasone
Butacaine
Chymotrypsin (?)
Cocaine
Colchicine
Cortisone
Desoxycorticosterone
Dexamethasone
Dibucaine
Dyclonine
Fludrocortisone
Fluorometholone
Fluprednisolone
F_3T
Hydrocortisone
Idoxuridine
IDU
Iodine Solution
Medrysone
Meprednisone
Methylprednisolone
Paramethasone
Penicillamine (?)
Phenacaine
Piperocaine
Prednisolone
Prednisone
Proparacaine
Sulfacetamide
Sulfamethizole
Sulfisoxazole
Tetracaine
Thiotepa
Triamcinolone
Trifluridine
Vidarabine

Diplopia
Acetohexamide
Acetophenazine
Acetyldigitoxin
Adrenal Cortex Injection
Alcohol
Aldosterone

Allobarbital
Allopurinol (?)
Ambenonium
Amitriptyline
Amobarbital
Amodiaquine
Amoxicillin (?)
Amphotericin B
Ampicillin (?)
Antazoline
Aprobarbital
Aspirin
Aurothioglucose
Aurothioglycanide
Azatadine
Bacitracin
Baclofen
Barbital
Benzathine Penicillin G
Betamethasone
Bromide
Bromisovalum
Brompheniramine
Broxyquinoline
Bupivacaine
Butabarbital
Butalbital
Butallylonal
Butaperazine
Butethal
Carbamazepine
Carbenicillin (?)
Carbinoxamine
Carbon Dioxide
Carbromal
Carisoprodol
Carphenazine
Cephaloridine
Chlorcyclizine
Chlordiazepoxide
Chloroprocaine
Chloroquine
Chlorpheniramine
Chlorpromazine

Chlorpropamide
Chlorprothixene
Clemastine
Clomiphene
Clonazepam
Clonidine (?)
Clorazepate
Cloxacillin (?)
Colchicine
Colistimethate
Colistin
Cortisone
Cyclizine
Cyclobarbital
Cyclopentobarbital
Cyproheptadine
Dantrolene
Desipramine
Deslanoside
Desoxycorticosterone
Dexamethasone
Dexbrompheniramine
Dexchlorpheniramine
Dextrothyroxine
Diazepam
Diazoxide
Dibucaine
Dicloxacillin (?)
Diethazine
Digitalis
Digitoxin
Digoxin
Dimethindene
Diphenhydramine
Diphenylpyraline
Disopyramide (?)
Doxylamine
Edrophonium
Ergot (?)
Ethchlorvynol
Ethionamide
Ethopropazine
Ethosuximide
Ethotoin

Diplopia (Cont'd)
  Etidocaine
  Floxuridine
  Fludrocortisone
  Fluorouracil
  Fluphenazine
  Fluprednisolone
  Flurazepam
  Gitalin
  Glutethimide
  Gold Au[198]
  Gold Sodium Thiomalate
  Gold Sodium Thiosulfate
  Guanethidine
  Hashish
  Heptabarbital
  Hetacillin (?)
  Hexachlorophene
  Hexethal
  Hexobarbital
  Hydrabamine Penicillin V
  Hydrocortisone
  Hydroxychloroquine
  Ibuprofen
  Imipramine
  Indomethacin
  Influenza Virus Vaccine
  Insulin
  Iodochlorhydroxyquin
  Iodoquinol
  Isocarboxazid
  Isoniazid
  Ketamine
  Lanatoside C
  Levodopa
  Levothyroxine
  Lidocaine
  Liothyronine
  Liotrix
  Lorazepam
  Marihuana
  Measles Virus Vaccine Live
  Meclizine
  Mephenesin

Mephenytoin
Mephobarbital
Mepivacaine
Meprednisone
Meprobamate
Mesoridazine
Methaqualone
Metharbital
Methdilazine
Methicillin (?)
Methitural
Methocarbamol
Methohexital
Methotrimeprazine
Methsuximide
Methylene Blue
Methylpentynol
Methylprednisolone
Methyprylon
Metoclopramide
Metocurine Iodide
Minocycline
Mitotane
Morphine
Nafcillin (?)
Nalidixic Acid
Nialamide
Nitrazepam
Nitrofurantoin
Norepinephrine
Nortriptyline
Opium
Oral Contraceptives
Orphenadrine
Ouabain
Oxacillin (?)
Oxazepam
Oxyphenbutazone
Paramethadione
Paramethasone
Penicillamine
Pentazocine
Pentobarbital
Perazine

Periciazine
Perphenazine
Phencyclidine
Phenelzine
Pheniramine
Phenobarbital
Phensuximide
Phenylbutazone
Phenytoin
Piperacetazine
Piperocaine
Poliovirus Vaccine
Polymyxin B
Potassium Penicillin G
Potassium Penicillin V
Potassium Phenethicillin
Pralidoxime
Prazepam
Prednisolone
Prednisone
Prilocaine
Primidone
Probarbital
Procaine
Procaine Penicillin G
Procarbazine
Prochlorperazine
Promazine
Promethazine
Propiomazine
Propoxycaine
Propranolol
Protriptyline
Pyridostigmine
Pyrilamine
Quinidine
Rabies Immune Globulin and
    Vaccine
Rubella Virus Vaccine Live
Secobarbital
Sodium Salicylate
Succinylcholine
Sulindac
Sulthiame

Talbutal
Tetracaine
Tetracycline
Tetrahydrocannabinol
THC
Thiamylal
Thiethylperazine
Thiopental
Thiopropazate
Thioproperazine
Thioridazine
Thiothixene
Thyroglobulin
Thyroid
Tolazamide
Tolbutamide
Tranylcypromine
Triamcinolone
Trichloroethylene
Trifluoperazine
Triflupromazine
Trimeprazine
Trimethadione
Tripelennamine
Triprolidine
Tubocurarine
Valproate Sodium
Valproic Acid
Vinbarbital
Vinblastine
Vincristine
Vitamin A

Dyschromatopsia
Aceclidine
Acenocoumarol
Acetohexamide
Acetophenazine
Acetyldigitoxin
Adrenal Cortex Injection
Alcohol
Aldosterone
Allobarbital
Alseroxylon

Dyschromatopsia (Cont'd)

Amitriptyline (?)
Amobarbital
Amodiaquine
Amyl Nitrite
Aprobarbital
Aspirin
Atropine
Barbital
Belladonna
Betamethasone
Bromide
Broxyquinoline
Butabarbital
Butalbital
Butallylonal
Butaperazine
Butethal
Carbon Dioxide
Carphenazine
Chloramphenicol
Chlordiazepoxide
Chloroquine
Chlorpromazine
Chlorpropamide
Chlortetracycline
Clonazepam
Clorazepate
Cortisone
Cyclobarbital
Cyclopentobarbital
Deserpidine
Desipramine (?)
Deslanoside
Desoxycorticosterone
Dexamethasone
Diazepam
Diethazine
Digitalis
Digitoxin
Digoxin
Disulfiram
Epinephrine
Ergonovine

Ergotamine
Erythromycin
Ethambutol
Ethchlorvynol
Ethionamide
Ethopropazine
Ferrocholinate (?)
Ferrous Fumarate (?)
Ferrous Gluconate (?)
Ferrous Succinate (?)
Ferrous Sulfate (?)
Fludrocortisone
Fluorometholone
Fluphenazine
Fluprednisolone
Flurazepam
Furosemide
Gitalin
Hashish
Heptabarbital
Hetacillin (?)
Hexethal
Hexobarbital
Homatropine
Hydrocortisone
Hydroxychloroquine
Ibuprofen
Imipramine (?)
Indomethacin
Iodide and Iodine Solutions and
    Compounds
Iodochlorhydroxyquin
Iodoquinol
Iron Dextran (?)
Iron Sorbitex (?)
Isocarboxazid
Isoniazid
Lanatoside C
Lidocaine
Lorazepam
LSD
Lysergide
Marihuana
Medrysone

Dyschromatopsia (Cont'd)
  Tetrahydrocannabinol
  THC
  Thiabendazole
  Thiamylal
  Thiethylperazine
  Thiopental
  Thiopropazate
  Thioproperazine
  Thioridazine
  Tolazamide
  Tolbutamide
  Tranylcypromine
  Triamcinolone
  Trichloroethylene
  Trifluoperazine
  Triflupromazine
  Trimeprazine
  Trimethadione
  Vinbarbital

Exophthalmos
  Adrenal Cortex Injection
  Aldosterone
  Betamethasone
  Carbimazole
  Cocaine
  Cortisone
  Desoxycorticosterone
  Dexamethasone
  Dextrothyroxine
  Fludrocortisone
  Fluprednisolone
  Hydrocortisone
  Iodide and Iodine Solutions and
    Compounds
  Levothyroxine
  Liothyronine
  Liotrix
  Lithium Carbonate
  Meprednisone
  Methimazole
  Methylprednisolone
  Methylthiouracil

  Oral Contraceptives
  Paramethasone
  Poliovirus Vaccine
  Prednisolone
  Prednisone
  Propranolol
  Propylthiouracil
  Radioactive Iodides
  Thyroglobulin
  Thyroid
  Triamcinolone
  Vitamin A

Eyelids — Eczema
  Amantadine
  Emetine
  Methyldopa
  Piperazine
  Practolol
  Quinacrine
  Smallpox Vaccine

Eyelids — Erythema
  Allopurinol
  Amitriptyline
  Amoxapine
  Antazoline
  Aurothioglucose
  Aurothioglycanide
  BCNU
  Benzathine Penicillin G
  Benzphetamine
  Betamethasone
  Bleomycin
  Bromide
  Brompheniramine
  Busulfan
  Cactinomycin
  Carbinoxamine
  Carmustine
  CCNU
  Cefazolin
  Cephalexin
  Cephaloglycin

Eyelids — Exfoliative Dermatitis (Cont'd)

Propiomazine
Propoxycaine
Propoxyphene
Propranolol
Propylthiouracil
Quinacrine
Quinidine
Radioactive Iodides
Rifampin
Secobarbital
Sulfacetamide
Sulfachlorpyridazine
Sulfacytine
Sulfadiazine
Sulfadimethoxine
Sulfamerazine
Sulfameter
Sulfamethazine
Sulfamethizole
Sulfamethoxazole
Sulfamethoxypyridazine
Sulfanilamide
Sulfaphenazole
Sulfapyridine
Sulfasalazine
Sulfathiazole
Sulfisoxazole
Talbutal
Thiabendazole
Thiamylal
Thiethylperazine
Thiopental
Thiopropazate
Thioproperazine
Thioridazine
Thiothixene
Tolazamide
Tolbutamide
Tridihexethyl
Trifluoperazine
Trifluperidol
Triflupromazine

Trimeprazine
Trimethadione
Trolnitrate
Vancomycin
Vinbarbital

Eyelids — Urticaria

Acenocoumarol
Acetaminophen
Acetanilid
Acetazolamide
Allobarbital
Allopurinol
Aluminum Nicotinate
Amitriptyline
Amobarbital
Amoxapine
Amoxicillin
Ampicillin
Anisindione
Antazoline
Antimony Lithium Thiomalate
Antimony Potassium Tartrate
Antimony Sodium Tartrate
Antimony Sodium Thioglycollate
Antipyrine
Aprobarbital
Aspirin
Aurothioglucose
Aurothioglycanide
Bacitracin
Barbital
Bendroflumethiazide
Benzathine Penicillin G
Benzphetamine
Benzthiazide
Bleomycin
Brompheniramine
Bupivacaine
Busulfan
Butabarbital
Butalbital
Butallylonal
Cactinomycin

Eyelids — Urticaria (Cont'd)

Hydralazine
Hydrochlorothiazide
Hydroflumethiazide
Hydromorphone
Ibuprofen
Imipramine
Indomethacin
Influenza Virus Vaccine
Insulin
Iodide and Iodine Solutions and
  Compounds
Iron Dextran
Isosorbide
Lidocaine
Lincomycin
Lorazepam
Loxapine
Mannitol
Measles Virus Vaccine Live
Mephobarbital
Mepivacaine
Meprobamate
Methacycline
Methadone
Metharbital
Methazolamide
Methicillin
Methimazole
Methitural
Methohexital
Methotrexate
Methyclothiazide
Methyldopa
Methylphenidate
Methylthiouracil
Methyprylon
Metoclopramide
Metolazone
Metoprolol
Minocycline
Mitomycin
Morphine
Nafcillin

Nalidixic Acid
Naproxen
Neomycin
Niacin
Niacinamide
Nicotinyl Alcohol
Nitrazepam
Nitrofurantoin
Nortriptyline
Opium
Oral Contraceptives
Oxacillin
Oxazepam
Oxymorphone
Oxyphenbutazone
Oxytetracycline
Pentobarbital
Phenacetin
Phendimetrazine
Phenindione
Pheniramine
Phenobarbital
Phenprocoumon
Phentermine
Phenylbutazone
Piperazine
Poliovirus Vaccine
Polythiazide
Potassium Penicillin G
Potassium Penicillin V
Potassium Phenethicillin
Practolol
Prazepam
Prilocaine
Primidone
Probarbital
Procaine
Procaine Penicillin G
Propoxycaine
Propylthiouracil
Protriptyline
Pyrilamine
Quinacrine
Quinethazone

Quinidine
Quinine
Rabies Immune Globulin and
  Vaccine
Radioactive Iodides
Rifampin
Rubella Virus Vaccine Live
Secobarbital
Smallpox Vaccine
Sodium Antimonylgluconate
Sodium Salicylate
Stibocaptate
Stibogluconate
Stibophen
Sulfacetamide
Sulfachlorpyridazine
Sulfacytine
Sulfadiazine
Sulfadimethoxine
Sulfamerazine
Sulfameter
Sulfamethazine
Sulfamethizole
Sulfamethoxazole
Sulfamethoxypyridazine
Sulfanilamide
Sulfaphenazole
Sulfapyridine
Sulfasalazine
Sulfathiazole
Sulfisoxazole
Suramin
Talbutal
Tetanus Toxoid
Tetracycline
Thiamylal
Thiopental
Thiotepa
Thiothixene
Timolol
Trichlormethiazide
Trimethaphan
Trimipramine
Tripelennamine

Triprolidine
Vancomycin
Vinbarbital
Warfarin

*Eyelids or Conjunctiva — Allergic
Reactions*
Acenocoumarol
Acetaminophen
Acetanilid
Acetazolamide
Acetohexamide
Acetophenazine
Acetyldigitoxin
Adiphenine
Allobarbital
Allopurinol
Aluminum Nicotinate
Ambutonium
Aminosalicylate (?)
Aminosalicylic Acid (?)
Amithiozone
Amobarbital
Amodiaquine
Amoxicillin
Amphotericin B
Ampicillin
Amyl Nitrite
Anisindione
Anisotropine
Antipyrine
Aprobarbital
Aspirin
Atropine
Aurothioglucose
Aurothioglycanide
Bacitracin
Barbital
BCNU
Belladonna
Bendroflumethiazide
Benoxinate
Benzathine Penicillin G
Benzthiazide

Eyelids or Conjunctiva — Allergic
Reactions (Cont'd)

Betamethasone
Bleomycin
Bromide
Bupivacaine
Busulfan
Butabarbital
Butacaine
Butalbital
Butallylonal
Butaperazine
Butethal
Cactinomycin
Carbachol
Carbamazepine
Carbenicillin
Carbimazole
Carisoprodol
Carmustine
Carphenazine
CCNU
Cefazolin
Cephalexin
Cephaloglycin
Cephaloridine
Cephalothin
Cephradine
Chloral Hydrate
Chlorambucil
Chloramphenicol
Chlordiazepoxide
Chloroprocaine
Chloroquine
Chlorothiazide
Chlorpromazine
Chlorpropamide
Chlorprothixene
Chlortetracycline
Chlorthalidone
Chrysarobin
Clidinium
Clindamycin
Clomiphene

Clonazepam
Clorazepate
Cloxacillin
Cocaine
Colistin
Colloidal Silver
Cortisone
Cyclobarbital
Cyclopentobarbital
Cyclopentolate
Cyclophosphamide
Cycloserine
Cyclothiazide
Cytarabine
Dacarbazine
Dactinomycin
Daunorubicin
Deferoxamine
Demecarium
Deslanoside
Dexamethasone
DFP
Diatrizoate Meglumine and
    Sodium
Diazepam
Diazoxide
Dibucaine
DIC
Dichlorphenamide
Dicloxacillin
Dicumarol
Dicyclomine
Diethazine
Diethylcarbamazine
Digitalis
Digitoxin
Digoxin
Dimercaprol
Diphemanil
Diphenadione
Diphtheria and Tetanus Toxoids
    and Pertussis (DPT) Vaccine
    Adsorbed
Disulfiram

Sulfachlorpyridazine
Sulfacytine
Sulfadiazine
Sulfadimethoxine
Sulfamerazine
Sulfameter
Sulfamethazine
Sulfamethizole
Sulfamethoxazole
Sulfamethoxypyridazine
Sulfanilamide
Sulfaphenazole
Sulfapyridine
Sulfasalazine
Sulfathiazole
Sulfisoxazole
Talbutal
Tetracaine
Tetracycline
Tetrahydrozoline
Thiabendazole
Thiamylal
Thiethylperazine
Thimerosal
Thiopental
Thiopropazate
Thioproperazine
Thioridazine
Thiotepa
Thiothixene
Timolol
Tolazamide
Tolbutamide
Trichlormethiazide
Tridihexethyl
Triethylenemelamine
Trifluoperazine
Trifluperidol
Triflupromazine
Trifluridine
Trimeprazine
Trimethadione
Tropicamide
Uracil Mustard

Vancomycin
Vidarabine
Vinbarbital
Warfarin

Eyelids or Conjunctiva — Angioneurotic Edema

Acetaminophen
Acetanilid
Acetophenazine
Acetyldigitoxin
Adrenal Cortex Injection
Aldosterone
Allobarbital
Aluminum Nicotinate
Amobarbital
Amoxicillin
Ampicillin
Aprobarbital
Aspirin
Bacitracin
Barbital
Benzathine Penicillin G
Betamethasone
Butabarbital
Butalbital
Butallylonal
Butaperazine
Butethal
Capreomycin
Carbenicillin
Carisoprodol
Carphenazine
Cefazolin
Cephalexin
Cephaloglycin
Cephaloridine
Cephalothin
Cephradine
Chloramphenicol
Chlordiazepoxide
Chlorpromazine
Chlorprothixene
Chlortetracycline

Eyelids or Conjunctiva — Angioneurotic Edema (Cont'd)

Clindamycin
Clonazepam
Clonidine
Clorazepate
Cloxacillin
Cortisone
Cyclobarbital
Cyclopentobarbital
Daunorubicin
Demeclocycline
Deslanoside
Desoxycorticosterone
Dexamethasone
Dextran
Diatrizoate Meglumine and
     Sodium
Diazepam
Dicloxacillin
Diethazine
Digitalis
Digitoxin
Digoxin
Doxycycline
Droperidol
Erythromycin
Ethopropazine
Ethosuximide
Ethotoin
Fludrocortisone
Fluorescein
Fluphenazine
Fluprednisolone
Flurazepam
Gitalin
Griseofulvin
Haloperidol
Heparin
Heptabarbital
Hetacillin
Hexethal
Hexobarbital
Hydrabamine Penicillin V

Hydrocortisone
Indomethacin
Insulin
Iodide and Iodine Solutions and
     Compounds
Iron Dextran
Isoniazid
Ketoprofen
Lanatoside C
Lincomycin
Lorazepam
Mephenytoin
Mephobarbital
Meprednisone
Meprobamate
Mesoridazine
Methacycline
Metharbital
Methdilazine
Methicillin
Methitural
Methohexital
Methotrimeprazine
Methsuximide
Methylprednisolone
Minocycline
Nafcillin
Nalidixic Acid
Naproxen
Niacin
Niacinamide
Nicotinyl Alcohol
Nitrazepam
Nitrofurantoin
Oral Contraceptives
Ouabain
Oxacillin
Oxazepam
Oxytetracycline
Paramethadione
Paramethasone
Pentobarbital
Perazine
Periciazine

Perphenazine
Phenacetin
Phenobarbital
Phensuximide
Piperacetazine
Potassium Penicillin G
Potassium Penicillin V
Potassium Phenethicillin
Prazepam
Prednisolone
Prednisone
Primidone
Probarbital
Procaine Penicillin G
Prochlorperazine
Promazine
Promethazine
Propiomazine
Quinidine
Quinine
Radioactive Iodides
Rifampin
Secobarbital
Sodium Salicylate
Streptomycin
Sulindac
Talbutal
Tetracycline
Thiabendazole
Thiamylal
Thiethylperazine
Thiopental
Thiopropazate
Thioproperazine
Thioridazine
Thiothixene
Triamcinolone
Trifluoperazine
Trifluperidol
Triflupromazine
Trimeprazine
Trimethadione
Vancomycin
Vinbarbital

Eyelids or Conjunctiva —
Depigmentation
Betamethasone
Carbimazole
Chloramphenicol
Cortisone
Dexamethasone
Fluorometholone
Gentamicin (?)
Hydrocortisone
Isoflurophate
Medrysone
Methimazole
Methotrexate
Methylthiouracil
Neostigmine
Physostigmine
Prednisolone
Propylthiouracil
Thiotepa

Eyelids or Conjunctiva — Deposits
Amiodarone
Aurothioglucose
Aurothioglycanide
Calcitriol
Cholecalciferol
Colloidal Silver
Epinephrine
Ergocalciferol
Ferrocholinate
Ferrous Fumarate
Ferrous Gluconate
Ferrous Succinate
Ferrous Sulfate
Gold Au^{198}
Gold Sodium Thiomalate
Gold Sodium Thiosulfate
Iron Dextran
Iron Sorbitex
Mercuric Oxide
Nitromersol
Phenylmercuric Acetate
Phenylmercuric Nitrate

Eyelids or Conjunctiva — Deposits (Cont'd)
Polysaccharide-Iron Complex
Quinacrine
Silver Nitrate
Silver Protein
Sulfacetamide
Sulfamethizole
Sulfisoxazole
Thimerosal
Vitamin D$_2$
Vitamin D$_3$

Eyelids or Conjunctiva — Discoloration
Acid Bismuth Sodium
  Tartrate (?)
Alcian Blue
Amphotericin B
Antimony Lithium Thiomalate
Antimony Potassium Tartrate
Antimony Sodium Tartrate
Antimony Sodium Thioglycollate
Antipyrine
Bismuth Oxychloride (?)
Bismuth Sodium Tartrate (?)
Bismuth Sodium Thioglycol-
  late (?)
Bismuth Sodium Triglycolla-
  mate (?)
Bismuth Subcarbonate (?)
Bismuth Subsalicylate (?)
Chlortetracycline
Chrysarobin
Clofazimine
Demeclocycline
Diethazine
Doxycycline
Ethopropazine
Ferrocholinate
Ferrous Fumarate
Ferrous Gluconate
Ferrous Succinate
Ferrous Sulfate

Fluorescein
Iron Dextran
Iron Sorbitex
Methacycline
Methylene Blue
Minocycline
Oxytetracycline
Penicillamine
Polysaccharide-Iron Complex
Quinacrine
Rifampin
Rose Bengal
Sodium Antimonylgluconate
Stibocaptate
Stibogluconate
Stibophen
Tetracycline
Trypan Blue
Vitamin A

Eyelids or Conjunctiva — Edema
Acetohexamide
Acetophenazine
Adrenal Cortex Injection
Aldosterone
Allobarbital
Aminosalicylate (?)
Aminosalicylic Acid (?)
Amitriptyline
Amobarbital
Amoxapine
Amoxicillin
Ampicillin
Antimony Lithium Thiomalate
Antimony Potassium Tartrate
Antimony Sodium Tartrate
Antimony Sodium Thioglycollate
Antipyrine
Aprobarbital
Aspirin
Aurothioglucose
Aurothioglycanide
Bacitracin
Barbital

Benzathine Penicillin G
Betamethasone
Bleomycin
Bupivacaine
Butabarbital
Butalbital
Butallylonal
Butaperazine
Butethal
Cactinomycin
Carbenicillin
Carphenazine
Chloral Hydrate
Chloroprocaine
Chlorpromazine
Chlorpropamide
Chlortetracycline
Chrysarobin
Clofibrate
Clomipramine
Cloxacillin
Colloidal Silver
Cortisone
Cyclobarbital
Cyclopentobarbital
Dactinomycin
Daunorubicin
Demecarium
Demeclocycline
Desipramine
Desoxycorticosterone
Dexamethasone
Dextrothyroxine
DFP
Diacetylmorphine
Diatrizoate Meglumine and
  Sodium
Dicloxacillin
Diethazine
Diethylcarbamazine
Doxepin
Doxorubicin
Doxycycline
Echothiophate

Emetine
Ergonovine
Ergotamine
Ethopropazine
Etidocaine
Floxuridine
Fludrocortisone
Fluorouracil
Fluphenazine
Fluprednisolone
F_3T
Gold Au^{198}
Gold Sodium Thiomalate
Gold Sodium Thiosulfate
Griseofulvin
Heptabarbital
Hetacillin
Hexamethonium
Hexethal
Hexobarbital
Hydrabamine Penicillin V
Hydralazine
Hydrocortisone
Ibuprofen
Idoxuridine
IDU
Imipramine
Iodide and Iodine Solutions and
  Compounds
Iron Dextran
Isoflurophate
Levodopa
Levothyroxine
Lidocaine
Liothyronine
Liotrix
Lithium Carbonate
Loxapine
Mecamylamine
Medrysone
Mephobarbital
Mepivacaine
Meprednisone
Mercuric Oxide

Eyelids or Conjunctiva — Edema
(Cont'd)

Mesoridazine
Methacycline
Metharbital
Methdilazine
Methicillin
Methitural
Methohexital
Methotrimeprazine
Methyldopa
Methylergonovine
Methylpentynol
Methylprednisolone
Methysergide
Metoclopramide
Minocycline
Mitomycin
Nafcillin
Naproxen
Nitromersol
Nortriptyline
Oral Contraceptives
Oxacillin
Oxprenolol
Oxyphenbutazone
Oxytetracycline
Paramethasone
Pentobarbital
Pentolinium
Perazine
Periciazine
Perphenazine
Phenobarbital
Phenylbutazone
Phenylmercuric Acetate
Phenylmercuric Nitrate
Piperacetazine
Piperazine
Poliovirus Vaccine
Potassium Penicillin G
Potassium Penicillin V
Potassium Phenethicillin
Practolol

Prednisolone
Prednisone
Prilocaine
Primidone
Probarbital
Procaine
Procaine Penicillin G
Prochlorperazine
Promazine
Promethazine
Propiomazine
Propoxycaine
Protriptyline
Quinacrine
Radioactive Iodides
Rifampin
Secobarbital
Silver Nitrate
Silver Protein
Smallpox Vaccine
Sodium Antimonylgluconate
Sodium Salicylate
Stibocaptate
Stibogluconate
Stibophen
Streptomycin
Succinylcholine
Suramin
Talbutal
Tetracycline
Tetraethylammonium
Thiamylal
Thiethylperazine
Thimerosal
Thiopental
Thiopropazate
Thioproperazine
Thioridazine
Thyroglobulin
Thyroid
Tolazamide
Tolbutamide
Triamcinolone
Trifluoperazine

Triflupromazine
Trifluridine
Trimeprazine
Trimethaphan
Trimethidinium
Trimipramine
Vidarabine
Vinbarbital

Eyelids or Conjunctiva — Erythema
Multiforme
  Acetaminophen
  Acetanilid
  Acetohexamide
  Allobarbital
  Amithiozone
  Amobarbital
  Amodiaquine
  Amoxicillin
  Ampicillin
  Aprobarbital
  Aurothioglucose
  Aurothioglycanide
  Barbital
  Bendroflumethiazide
  Benzthiazide
  Butabarbital
  Butalbital
  Butallylonal
  Butethal
  Carbamazepine
  Carbenicillin
  Carisoprodol
  Chlordiazepoxide
  Chloroquine
  Chlorothiazide
  Chlorpropamide
  Chlortetracycline
  Chlorthalidone
  Clonazepam
  Clorazepate
  Cloxacillin
  Cyclobarbital
  Cyclopentobarbital

Cyclopromazine
Cyclothiazide
Demeclocycline
Diazepam
Dicloxacillin
Doxycycline
Ethosuximide
Ethotoin
Flurazepam
Furosemide
Gold Au^{198}
Gold Sodium Thiomalate
Gold Sodium Thiosulfate
Heptabarbital
Hetacillin
Hexethal
Hexobarbital
Hydrochlorothiazide
Hydroflumethiazide
Hydroxychloroquine
Ibuprofen
Lorazepam
Mephenytoin
Mephobarbital
Meprobamate
Methacycline
Metharbital
Methicillin
Methitural
Methohexital
Methsuximide
Methyclothiazide
Methylphenidate
Metolazone
Minocycline
Nafcillin
Nitrazepam
Oral Contraceptives
Oxacillin
Oxazepam
Oxytetracycline
Paramethadione
Pentobarbital
Phenacetin

Eyelids or Conjunctiva — Erythema Multiforme (Cont'd)

Phenobarbital
Phensuximide
Phenytoin
Piperazine
Polythiazide
Prazepam
Primidone
Probarbital
Propranolol
Quinethazone
Quinine
Secobarbital
Smallpox Vaccine
Sulfacetamide
Sulfachlorpyridazine
Sulfacytine
Sulfadiazine
Sulfadimethoxine
Sulfamerazine
Sulfameter
Sulfamethazine
Sulfamethizole
Sulfamethoxazole
Sulfamethoxypyridazine
Sulfanilamide
Sulfaphenazole
Sulfapyridine
Sulfasalazine
Sulfathiazole
Sulfisoxazole
Talbutal
Tetracycline
Thiabendazole
Thiamylal
Thiopental
Timolol
Tolazamide
Tolbutamide
Trichlormethiazide
Trimethadione
Vinbarbital

Eyelids or Conjunctiva — Hyperpigmentation

Acetophenazine
Aluminum Nicotinate
Bleomycin
Busulfan
Butaperazine
Cactinomycin
Carphenazine
Chlorambucil
Chlorpromazine
Clofazimine
Cyclophosphamide
Cytarabine
Dactinomycin
Dapsone
Daunorubicin
Diethazine
Doxorubicin
Ethopropazine
Floxuridine
Fluorouracil
Fluphenazine
Hydroxyurea
Loxapine
Mercaptopurine
Mesoridazine
Methdilazine
Methotrexate
Methotrimeprazine
Methoxsalen
Mitomycin
Niacin
Niacinamide
Nicotinyl Alcohol
Oxprenolol
Perazine
Periciazine
Perphenazine
Piperacetazine
Practolol
Procarbazine
Prochlorperazine
Promazine

Promethazine
Propiomazine
Quinacrine
Thiethylperazine
Thioguanine
Thiopropazate
Thioproperazine
Thioridazine
Trifluoperazine
Triflupromazine
Trimeprazine
Trioxsalen
Uracil Mustard

Eyelids or Conjunctiva — Lupoid Syndrome
Acetophenazine
Allobarbital
Alseroxylon
Aminosalicylate
Aminosalicylic Acid
Amobarbital
Aprobarbital
Aurothioglucose
Aurothioglycanide
Barbital
Bendroflumethiazide
Benzathine Penicillin G
Benzthiazide
Butabarbital
Butalbital
Butallylonal
Butaperazine
Butethal
Carbamazepine
Carbimazole
Carphenazine
Chlorothiazide
Chlorpromazine
Chlorprothixene
Chlortetracycline
Chlorthalidone
Clofibrate
Cyclobarbital

Cyclopentobarbital
Cyclothiazide
Demeclocycline
Deserpidine
Diethazine
Digitalis
Doxycycline
Ergonovine
Ergotamine
Ethopropazine
Ethosuximide
Ethotoin
Fluphenazine
Gold Au^{198}
Gold Sodium Thiomalate
Gold Sodium Thiosulfate
Griseofulvin
Heptabarbital
Hexethal
Hexobarbital
Hydrabamine Penicillin V
Hydralazine
Hydrochlorothiazide
Hydroflumethiazide
Ibuprofen
Isoniazid
Levodopa
Mephenytoin
Mephobarbital
Mesoridazine
Methacycline
Metharbital
Methdilazine
Methimazole
Methitural
Methohexital
Methotrimeprazine
Methsuximide
Methyclothiazide
Methyldopa
Methylergonovine
Methylthiouracil
Methysergide
Metolazone

Eyelids or Conjunctiva — Lupoid
Syndrome (Cont'd)
  Minocycline
  Oral Contraceptives
  Oxyphenbutazone
  Oxytetracycline
  Paramethadione
  Penicillamine
  Pentobarbital
  Perazine
  Periciazine
  Perphenazine
  Phenobarbital
  Phensuximide
  Phenylbutazone
  Phenytoin
  Piperacetazine
  Polythiazide
  Potassium Penicillin G
  Potassium Penicillin V
  Potassium Phenethicillin
  Practolol
  Primidone
  Probarbital
  Procaine Penicillin G
  Prochlorperazine
  Promazine
  Promethazine
  Propiomazine
  Propranolol
  Propylthiouracil
  Quinethazone
  Quinidine
  Rauwolfia Serpentina
  Rescinnamine
  Reserpine
  Secobarbital
  Streptomycin
  Sulfacetamide
  Sulfachlorpyridazine
  Sulfacytine
  Sulfadiazine
  Sulfadimethoxine
  Sulfamerazine

  Sulfameter
  Sulfamethazine
  Sulfamethizole
  Sulfamethoxazole
  Sulfamethoxypyridazine
  Sulfanilamide
  Sulfaphenazole
  Sulfapyridine
  Sulfasalazine
  Sulfathiazole
  Sulfisoxazole
  Syrosingopine
  Talbutal
  Tetracycline
  Thiamylal
  Thiethylperazine
  Thiopental
  Thiopropazate
  Thioproperazine
  Thioridazine
  Thiothixene
  Tolazamide
  Trichlormethiazide
  Trifluoperazine
  Triflupromazine
  Trimeprazine
  Trimethadione
  Vinbarbital

Eyelids or Conjunctiva — Lyell's
Syndrome
  Acetazolamide
  Acid Bismuth Sodium Tartrate
  Adrenal Cortex Injection
  Aldosterone
  Allobarbital
  Allopurinol
  Amobarbital
  Amoxicillin
  Ampicillin
  Antipyrine
  Aprobarbital
  Aurothioglucose
  Aurothioglycanide

Barbital
Benzathine Penicillin G
Betamethasone
Bismuth Oxychloride
Bismuth Sodium Tartrate
Bismuth Sodium Thioglycollate
Bismuth Sodium Triglycollamate
Bismuth Subcarbonate
Bismuth Subsalicylate
Butabarbital
Butalbital
Butallylonal
Butethal
Carbamazepine
Carbenicillin
Chlortetracycline
Cloxacillin
Cortisone
Cyclobarbital
Cyclopentobarbital
Demeclocycline
Desoxycorticosterone
Dexamethasone
Dichlorphenamide
Dicloxacillin
Doxycycline
Ethoxzolamide
Fludrocortisone
Fluprednisolone
Gold Au^{198}
Gold Sodium Thiomalate
Gold Sodium Thiosulfate
Heptabarbital
Hetacillin
Hexethal
Hexobarbital
Hydrabamine Penicillin V
Hydrocortisone
Kanamycin
Mephobarbital
Meprednisone
Methacycline
Metharbital
Methazolamide

Methicillin
Methitural
Methohexital
Methotrexate
Methylprednisolone
Minocycline
Nafcillin
Nitrofurantoin
Oxacillin
Oxyphenbutazone
Oxytetracycline
Paramethadione
Paramethasone
Penicillamine
Pentobarbital
Phenobarbital
Phenylbutazone
Phenytoin
Potassium Penicillin G
Potassium Penicillin V
Potassium Phenethicillin
Prednisolone
Prednisone
Primidone
Probarbital
Procaine Penicillin G
Procarbazine
Secobarbital
Sulfacetamide
Sulfachlorpyridazine
Sulfacytine
Sulfadiazine
Sulfadimethoxine
Sulfamerazine
Sulfameter
Sulfamethazine
Sulfamethizole
Sulfamethoxazole
Sulfamethoxypyridazine
Sulfanilamide
Sulfaphenazole
Sulfapyridine
Sulfasalazine
Sulfathiazole

Eyelids or Conjunctiva — Lyell's Syndrome (Cont'd)

Sulfisoxazole
Sulindac
Talbutal
Tetracycline
Thiabendazole
Thiamylal
Thiopental
Triamcinolone
Trimethadione
Vinbarbital

Eyelids or Conjunctiva — Necrosis

Acenocoumarol
Amphotericin B
Anisindione
Dicumarol
Diphenadione
Ethyl Biscoumacetate
Nafcillin
Phenindione
Phenprocoumon
Warfarin

Eyelids or Conjunctiva — Purpura

Acetazolamide
Acetohexamide
Allopurinol
Amantadine
Amitriptyline
Aurothioglucose
Aurothioglycanide
Bendroflumethiazide
Benzthiazide
Carbamazepine
Chlordiazepoxide
Chlorothiazide
Chlorpropamide
Chlorthalidone
Clofibrate
Clonazepam
Clorazepate
Cyclothiazide

Cytarabine
Dapsone
Desipramine
Diazepam
Dichlorphenamide
Emetine
Ethoxzolamide
Flurazepam
Glutethimide
Gold Au[198]
Gold Sodium Thiomalate
Gold Sodium Thiosulfate
Hydrochlorothiazide
Hydroflumethiazide
Ibuprofen
Imipramine
Lorazepam
Methazolamide
Methyclothiazide
Methyprylon
Metolazone
Metoprolol
Naproxen
Nitrazepam
Nortriptyline
Oxazepam
Oxprenolol
Phenytoin
Piperazine
Polythiazide
Prazepam
Procarbazine
Propranolol
Protriptyline
Quinethazone
Quinine
Rifampin
Rubella Virus Vaccine Live
Smallpox Vaccine
Sulfacetamide
Sulfachlorpyridazine
Sulfacytine
Sulfadiazine
Sulfadimethoxine

Sulfamerazine
Sulfameter
Sulfamethazine
Sulfamethizole
Sulfamethoxazole
Sulfamethoxypyridazine
Sulfanilamide
Sulfaphenazole
Sulfapyridine
Sulfasalazine
Sulfathiazole
Sulfisoxazole
Timolol
Tolazamide
Tolbutamide
Trichlormethiazide

Eyelids or Conjunctiva — Stevens-Johnson Syndrome
Acetaminophen
Acetanilid
Acetohexamide
Acetophenazine
Allobarbital
Allopurinol
Aminosalicylate (?)
Aminosalicylic Acid (?)
Amiodarone
Amithiozone
Amobarbital
Amodiaquine
Amoxicillin
Ampicillin
Antipyrine
Aprobarbital
Aspirin
Aurothioglucose
Aurothioglycanide
Barbital
Belladonna
Bendroflumethiazide
Benzathine Penicillin G
Benzthiazide
Bromide

Bromisovalum
Butabarbital
Butalbital
Butallylonal
Butaperazine
Butethal
Carbamazepine
Carbenicillin
Carbromal
Carisoprodol
Carphenazine
Chloroquine
Chlorothiazide
Chlorpromazine
Chlorpropamide
Chlortetracycline
Chlorthalidone
Cimetidine
Clindamycin
Cloxacillin
Cyclobarbital
Cyclopentobarbital
Cyclothiazide
Demeclocycline
Dicloxacillin
Diethazine
Doxycycline
Erythromycin
Ethopropazine
Ethosuximide
Ethotoin
Fluphenazine
Gold Au[198]
Gold Sodium Thiomalate
Gold Sodium Thiosulfate
Heptabarbital
Hetacillin
Hexethal
Hexobarbital
Hydrabamine Penicillin V
Hydrochlorothiazide
Hydroflumethiazide
Hydroxychloroquine
Ibuprofen

Eyelids or Conjunctiva — Stevens-Johnson Syndrome (Cont'd)

Isoniazid
Lincomycin
Mephenytoin
Mephobarbital
Meprobamate
Mesoridazine
Methacycline
Metharbital
Methdilazine
Methicillin
Methitural
Methohexital
Methotrimeprazine
Methsuximide
Methyclothiazide
Methylphenidate
Metolazone
Minocycline
Nafcillin
Oxacillin
Oxyphenbutazone
Oxytetracycline
Paramethadione
Pentobarbital
Perazine
Periciazine
Perphenazine
Phenacetin
Phenobarbital
Phensuximide
Phenylbutazone
Phenytoin
Piperacetazine
Polythiazide
Potassium Penicillin G
Potassium Penicillin V
Potassium Phenethicillin
Primidone
Probarbital
Procaine Penicillin G
Prochlorperazine
Promazine

Promethazine
Propiomazine
Propranolol
Quinethazone
Quinine
Rifampin
Secobarbital
Smallpox Vaccine
Sodium Salicylate
Sulfacetamide
Sulfachlorpyridazine
Sulfacytine
Sulfadiazine
Sulfadimethoxine
Sulfamerazine
Sulfameter
Sulfamethazine
Sulfamethizole
Sulfamethoxazole
Sulfamethoxypyridazine
Sulfanilamide
Sulfaphenazole
Sulfapyridine
Sulfasalazine
Sulfathiazole
Sulfisoxazole
Sulindac
Sulthiame
Talbutal
Tetracycline
Thiabendazole
Thiamylal
Thiethylperazine
Thiopental
Thiopropazate
Thioproperazine
Thioridazine
Tolazamide
Tolbutamide
Trichlormethiazide
Trifluoperazine
Triflupromazine
Trimeprazine
Trimethadione

Vancomycin
Vinbarbital

Eyelids or Conjunctiva — Ulceration
Amphotericin B
Ferrocholinate
Ferrous Fumarate
Ferrous Gluconate
Ferrous Succinate
Ferrous Sulfate
Floxuridine
Fluorouracil
Iron Dextran
Iron Sorbitex
Phenytoin
Polysaccharide-Iron Complex

Heightened Color Perception
Ethionamide
Hashish
LSD
Lysergide
Marihuana
Mescaline
Oxygen
Psilocybin
Tetrahydrocannabinol
THC

Hippus
Allobarbital
Amobarbital
Aprobarbital
Barbital
Butabarbital
Butalbital
Butallylonal
Butethal
Cyclobarbital
Cyclopentobarbital
Heptabarbital
Hexethal
Hexobarbital

Mephobarbital
Metharbital
Methitural
Methohexital
Pentobarbital
Pentylenetetrazol
Phenobarbital
Primidone
Probarbital
Secobarbital
Talbutal
Thiamylal
Thiopental
Vinbarbital

Horner's Syndrome
Acetophenazine
Alseroxylon
Bupivacaine
Butaperazine
Carphenazine
Chloroprocaine
Chlorpromazine
Deserpidine
Diacetylmorphine
Diethazine
Ethopropazine
Etidocaine
Fluphenazine
Guanethidine
Levodopa
Lidocaine
Mepivacaine
Mesoridazine
Methdilazine
Methotrimeprazine
Perazine
Periciazine
Perphenazine
Piperacetazine
Prilocaine
Procaine
Prochlorperazine
Promazine

Horner's Syndrome (Cont'd)
Promethazine
Propiomazine
Propoxycaine
Rauwolfia Serpentina
Rescinnamine
Reserpine
Syrosingopine
Thiethylperazine
Thiopropazate
Thioproperazine
Thioridazine
Trifluoperazine
Triflupromazine
Trimeprazine

Hypermetropia
Ergot
Penicillamine
Sulfacetamide (?)
Sulfachlorpyridazine (?)
Sulfacytine (?)
Sulfadiazine (?)
Sulfadimethoxine (?)
Sulfamerazine (?)
Sulfameter (?)
Sulfamethazine (?)
Sulfamethizole (?)
Sulfamethoxazole (?)
Sulfamethoxypyridazine (?)
Sulfanilamide (?)
Sulfaphenazole (?)
Sulfapyridine (?)
Sulfasalazine (?)
Sulfathiazole (?)
Sulfisoxazole (?)
Tolbutamide (?)

Hypopyon
Benoxinate
Butacaine
Cocaine
Colchicine (?)
Dibucaine

Dyclonine
Ferrocholinate
Ferrous Fumarate
Ferrous Gluconate
Ferrous Succinate
Ferrous Sulfate
Iodide and Iodine Solutions and
    Compounds
Iron Dextran
Iron Sorbitex
Phenacaine
Piperocaine
Polysaccharide-Iron Complex
Proparacaine
Radioactive Iodides
Tetracaine
Urokinase

Impaired Oculomotor Coordination
Alcohol
Hashish
Marihuana
Tetrahydrocannabinol
THC

Increased Intraocular Pressure
Adrenal Cortex Injection
Aldosterone
Aluminum Nicotinate (?)
Atropine
Betamethasone
Carbon Dioxide
Chymotrypsin
Cortisone
Cyclopentolate
Demecarium
Desoxycorticosterone
Dexamethasone
DFP
Echothiophate
Erythrityl Tetranitrate (?)
Fludrocortisone
Fluorometholone

Fluprednisolone
Homatropine
Hydrocortisone
Insulin
Isoflurophate
Isosorbide Dinitrate (?)
Ketamine
Mannitol Hexanitrate (?)
Medrysone
Meprednisone
Methylphenidate (?)
Methylprednisolone
Mitomycin
Morphine (?)
Niacin (?)
Niacinamide (?)
Nicotinyl Alcohol (?)
Nitroglycerin (?)
Nitrous Oxide
Oxyphenonium
Paramethasone
Pentaerythritol Tetranitrate (?)
Phencyclidine
Pilocarpine
Prednisolone
Prednisone
Scopolamine
Sodium Chloride
Succinylcholine
Tolazoline
Triamcinolone
Trolnitrate (?)
Tropicamide
Urokinase

Iris or Ciliary Body Cysts
Adrenal Cortex Injection
Aldosterone
Betamethasone
Cortisone
Demecarium
Desoxycorticosterone
Dexamethasone
DFP

Echothiophate
Edrophonium
Epinephrine
Fludrocortisone
Fluprednisolone
Hydrocortisone
Isoflurophate
Meprednisone
Methylprednisolone
Neostigmine
Paramethasone
Physostigmine
Pilocarpine
Prednisolone
Prednisone
Triamcinolone

Iritis
Acetazolamide
Aurothioglucose
Aurothioglycanide
Benoxinate
Butacaine
Cocaine
Cytarabine
Demecarium
DFP
Dibucaine
Dichlorphenamide
Dyclonine
Echothiophate
Edrophonium
Emetine
Epinephrine
Ethoxzolamide
Gold Au[198]
Gold Sodium Thiomalate
Gold Sodium Thiosulfate
Iodide and Iodine Solutions and
    Compounds
Isoflurophate
Methazolamide
Neostigmine
Phenacaine

Iritis (Cont'd)
Physostigmine
Piperocaine
Pralidoxime
Proparacaine
Radioactive Iodides
Suramin
Tetracaine

Jerky Pursuit Movements
Acetophenazine
Alcohol
Allobarbital
Alseroxylon
Amitriptyline
Amobarbital
Aprobarbital
Barbital
Bromide
Bupivacaine
Butabarbital
Butalbital
Butallylonal
Butaperazine
Butethal
Carphenazine
Chlordiazepoxide
Chloroprocaine
Chlorpromazine
Clonazepam
Clorazepate
Cyclobarbital
Cyclopentobarbital
Deserpidine
Desipramine
Diazepam
Diethazine
Ethopropazine
Etidocaine
Fluphenazine
Flurazepam
Heptabarbital
Hexethal
Hexobarbital

Imipramine
Lidocaine
Lithium Carbonate
Lorazepam
Mephobarbital
Mepivacaine
Mesoridazine
Metharbital
Methdilazine
Methitural
Methohexital
Methotrimeprazine
Nitrazepam
Nortriptyline
Oxazepam
Pentobarbital
Perazine
Periciazine
Perphenazine
Phencyclidine
Phenobarbital
Piperacetazine
Prazepam
Prilocaine
Primidone
Probarbital
Procaine
Prochlorperazine
Promazine
Promethazine
Propiomazine
Propoxycaine
Protriptyline
Rauwolfia Serpentina
Rescinnamine
Reserpine
Secobarbital
Syrosingopine
Talbutal
Thiamylal
Thiethylperazine
Thiopental
Thiopropazate
Thioproperazine

Keratitis (Cont'd)
Sodium Salicylate
Sulfacetamide
Sulfachlorpyridazine
Sulfacytine
Sulfadiazine
Sulfadimethoxine
Sulfamerazine
Sulfameter
Sulfamethazine
Sulfamethizole
Sulfamethoxazole
Sulfamethoxypyridazine
Sulfanilamide
Sulfaphenazole
Sulfapyridine
Sulfasalazine
Sulfathiazole
Sulfisoxazole
Suramin
Tetracaine
Tetrahydrozoline
Thiethylperazine
Thiopropazate
Thioproperazine
Thioridazine
Thiotepa
Thiothixene
Timolol
Trichloroethylene
Trifluoperazine
Triflupromazine
Trifluridine
Trimeprazine
Tropicamide
Vinblastine
Vidarabine

Keratoconjunctivitis
Aurothioglucose (?)
Aurothioglycanide (?)
Chrysarobin
Gold Au[198] (?)
Gold Sodium Thiomalate (?)

Gold Sodium Thiosulfate (?)
Morphine
Opium
Vinblastine

Keratoconjunctivitis Sicca
Busulfan
Chlorambucil
Clonidine (?)
Doxepin
Methyldopa
Metoprolol (?)
Oxprenolol (?)
Practolol
Thiabendazole
Timolol
Vinblastine (?)

Lacrimation
Acetophenazine
Acetylcholine
Alcohol
Ambenonium
Amoxapine
Butaperazine
Carphenazine
Chloral Hydrate
Chlorpromazine
Dantrolene
Diazoxide
Dicumarol
Diethazine
Doxorubicin
Edrophonium
Epinephrine
Ether
Ethopropazine
Fluphenazine
Heparin
Indomethacin (?)
Ketamine
Levallorphan
Mesoridazine
Methacholine

Methaqualone
Methdilazine
Methotrimeprazine
Morphine
Nalorphine
Naloxone
Opium
Pentazocine
Perazine
Periciazine
Perphenazine
Piperacetazine
Piperazine
Prochlorperazine
Promazine
Promethazine
Propiomazine
Pyridostigmine
Rifampin
Thiethylperazine
Thiopropazate
Thioproperazine
Thioridazine
Trifluoperazine
Triflupromazine
Trimeprazine
Warfarin

Lens Deposits
Amiodarone
Aurothioglucose
Aurothioglycanide
Chlorprothixene
Colloidal Silver
Diazepam (?)
Gold Au^{198}
Gold Sodium Thiomalate
Gold Sodium Thiosulfate
Mercuric Oxide
Phenylmercuric Acetate
Phenylmercuric Nitrate
Silver Nitrate
Silver Protein
Thiothixene

Loss of Eyelashes or Eyebrows
Acenocoumarol (?)
Acetohexamide (?)
Alcohol (?)
Allopurinol (?)
Aluminum Nicotinate (?)
Amantadine (?)
Amithiozone (?)
Amitriptyline (?)
Amodiaquine (?)
Amphetamine (?)
Anisindione (?)
Aspirin (?)
Aurothioglucose (?)
Aurothioglycanide (?)
Azathioprine (?)
BCNU
Benzphetamine (?)
Bleomycin
Broxyquinoline (?)
Busulfan
Cactinomycin
Carbamazepine (?)
Carbimazole (?)
Carmustine
CCNU
Chlorambucil
Chloroquine (?)
Chlorphentermine (?)
Chlorpropamide (?)
Clofibrate (?)
Clomiphene (?)
Clonazepam (?)
Colchicine (?)
Cyclophosphamide
Cytarabine (?)
Dacarbazine
Dactinomycin
Daunorubicin
Desipramine (?)
Dextroamphetamine (?)
Dextrothyroxine (?)
DIC
Dicumarol (?)

Loss of Eyelashes or Eyebrows
(Cont'd)
Diethylcarbamazine
Diethylpropion (?)
Diphenadione (?)
Doxepin (?)
Doxorubicin
Droperidol (?)
Epinephrine
Ergonovine (?)
Ergotamine (?)
Ethionamide (?)
Ethotoin (?)
Ethyl Biscoumacetate (?)
Fenfluramine (?)
Floxuridine
Fluorouracil
Gentamicin
Glycopyrrolate (?)
Gold Au^{198} (?)
Gold Sodium Thiomalate (?)
Gold Sodium Thiosulfate (?)
Guanethidine (?)
Haloperidol (?)
Heparin (?)
Hydroxychloroquine (?)
Hydroxyurea (?)
Ibuprofen (?)
Imipramine (?)
Indomethacin (?)
Iodochlorhydroxyquin (?)
Iodoquinol (?)
Levodopa (?)
Lithium Carbonate (?)
Lomustine
Mechlorethamine
Melphalan
Mephenytoin (?)
Methamphetamine (?)
Methimazole (?)
Methotrexate
Methylergonovine (?)
Methylthiouracil (?)
Methysergide (?)

Metoprolol (?)
Minocycline (?)
Mitomycin
Niacin (?)
Niacinamide (?)
Nicotinyl Alcohol (?)
Nitrofurantoin (?)
Nortriptyline (?)
Oxprenolol (?)
Paramethadione (?)
Penicillamine (?)
Phendimetrazine (?)
Phenindione (?)
Phenmetrazine (?)
Phenprocoumon (?)
Phentermine (?)
Procarbazine (?)
Propranolol (?)
Propylthiouracil (?)
Protriptyline (?)
Semustine
Sodium Salicylate (?)
Streptomycin (?)
Tetracycline (?)
Thiotepa
Timolol (?)
Tolazamide (?)
Tolbutamide (?)
Triethylenemelamine
Trifluperidol (?)
Trimethadione (?)
Uracil Mustard
Valproate Sodium (?)
Valproic Acid (?)
Vinblastine
Vincristine
Vitamin A
Warfarin (?)

Macular Edema
Acetazolamide
Aluminum Nicotinate
Broxyquinoline
Dichlorphenamide

Dipivefrin (?)
DPE (?)
Epinephrine
Ethoxzolamide
Griseofulvin
Hexamethonium
Indomethacin (?)
Iodide and Iodine Solutions and
   Compounds
Iodochlorhydroxyquin
Iodoquinol
Methazolamide
Niacin
Niacinamide
Nicotinyl Alcohol
Phenylephrine (?)
Quinine
Radioactive Iodides
Tamoxifen

Macular or Paramacular Degeneration
Allopurinol (?)
Broxyquinoline
Clonidine (?)
Griseofulvin (?)
Ibuprofen (?)
Indomethacin (?)
Iodochlorhydroxyquin
Iodoquinol
Quinine

Miosis
Aceclidine
Acetophenazine
Acetylcholine
Alcohol
Allobarbital
Ambenonium
Amobarbital
Aprobarbital
Baclofen
Barbital
Bromide

Bromisovalum
Butabarbital
Butalbital
Butallylonal
Butaperazine
Butethal
Carbachol
Carbromal
Carisoprodol
Carphenazine
Chloral Hydrate
Chloroform
Chlorpromazine
Chlorprothixene
Clonidine
Codeine
Cyclobarbital
Cyclopentobarbital
Demecarium
DFP
Diacetylmorphine
Dibucaine
Diethazine
Droperidol
Echothiophate
Edrophonium
Ephedrine (?)
Ergot
Ergotamine
Ether
Ethopropazine
Fluphenazine
Haloperidol
Hashish
Heptabarbital
Hexachlorophene
Hexethal
Hexobarbital
Hydromorphone
Isocarboxazid
Isoflurophate
Levallorphan
Levodopa
Marihuana

Miosis (Cont'd)
Meperidine
Mephobarbital
Meprobamate
Mesoridazine
Methacholine
Methadone
Metharbital
Methdilazine
Methitural
Methohexital
Methotrimeprazine
Methyprylon
Morphine
Nalorphine
Naloxone
Neostigmine
Nialamide
Nitrous Oxide
Opium
Oxprenolol
Oxymorphone
Paraldehyde
Pentazocine
Pentobarbital
Perazine
Periciazine
Perphenazine
Phencyclidine
Phenelzine
Phenobarbital
Phenoxybenzamine
Phenylephrine
Physostigmine
Pilocarpine
Piperacetazine
Piperazine
Piperocaine
Primidone
Probarbital
Prochlorperazine
Promazine
Promethazine
Propiomazine

Propoxyphene
Propranolol
Pyridostigmine
Secobarbital
Sulindac
Talbutal
Tetracaine
Tetrahydrocannabinol
THC
Thiamylal
Thiethylperazine
Thiopental
Thiopropazate
Thioproperazine
Thioridazine
Thiothixene
Tolazoline
Tranylcypromine
Trifluoperazine
Trifluperidol
Triflupromazine
Trimeprazine
Vinbarbital
Vitamin A

Myasthenic Neuromuscular Blocking Effect
Acetophenazine
Adrenal Cortex Injection
Aldosterone
Bacitracin
Betamethasone
Butaperazine
Carphenazine
Chlorpromazine
Chlortetracycline
Colistimethate
Colistin
Cortisone
Demeclocycline
Desoxycorticosterone
Dexamethasone
Dextrothyroxine
Diethazine

Doxycycline
Ethopropazine
Ethotoin (?)
Fludrocortisone
Fluphenazine
Fluprednisolone
Gentamicin
Hydrocortisone
Kanamycin
Levothyroxine
Liothyronine
Liotrix
Lithium Carbonate
Mephenytoin (?)
Meprednisone
Mesoridazine
Methacycline
Methdilazine
Methotrimeprazine
Methoxyflurane
Methylprednisolone
Minocycline
Neomycin
Oxprenolol (?)
Oxytetracycline
Paramethadione
Paramethasone
Penicillamine
Perazine
Periciazine
Perphenazine
Phenytoin
Piperacetazine
Polymyxin B
Practolol (?)
Prednisolone
Prednisone
Prochlorperazine
Promazine
Promethazine
Propiomazine
Propranolol
Quinidine
Streptomycin

Sulfacetamide
Sulfachlorpyridazine
Sulfacytine
Sulfadiazine
Sulfadimethoxine
Sulfamerazine
Sulfameter
Sulfamethazine
Sulfamethizole
Sulfamethoxazole
Sulfamethoxypyridazine
Sulfanilamide
Sulfaphenazole
Sulfapyridine
Sulfasalazine
Sulfathiazole
Sulfisoxazole
Tetracycline
Tetraethylammonium
Thiethylperazine
Thiopropazate
Thioproperazine
Thioridazine
Thyroglobulin
Thyroid
Timolol
Triamcinolone
Trifluoperazine
Triflupromazine
Trimeprazine
Trimethadione
Trimethaphan

Mydriasis
Acetaminophen
Acetanilid
Acetophenazine
Acetylcholine
Adiphenine
Adrenal Cortex Injection
Alcohol
Aldosterone
Alkavervir
Allobarbital

Mydriasis (Cont'd)

Alseroxylon
Amantadine
Ambutonium
Amitriptyline
Amobarbital
Amoxapine
Amphetamine
Amyl Nitrite
Anisotropine
Antazoline
Antimony Lithium Thiomalate
Antimony Potassium Tartrate
Antimony Sodium Tartrate
Antimony Sodium Thioglycollate
Aprobarbital
Aspirin
Atropine
Azatadine
Baclofen
Barbital
Belladonna
Benzathine Penicillin G
Benzphetamine
Benztropine
Betamethasone
Biperiden
Bromide
Bromisovalum
Brompheniramine
Butabarbital
Butalbital
Butallylonal
Butaperazine
Butethal
Caramiphen
Carbamazepine
Carbinoxamine
Carbon Dioxide
Carbromal
Carisoprodol
Carphenazine
Chloral Hydrate
Chloramphenicol

Chlorcyclizine
Chlordiazepoxide
Chloroform
Chlorpheniramine
Chlorphenoxamine
Chlorphentermine
Chlorpromazine
Chlorprothixene
Clemastine
Clidinium
Clomiphene
Clomipramine
Clonazepam
Clonidine
Clorazepate
Cocaine
Colistimethate
Colistin
Cortisone
Cryptenamine
Cyclizine
Cyclobarbital
Cyclopentobarbital
Cyclopentolate
Cycrimine
Cyproheptadine
Deserpidine
Desipramine
Desoxycorticosterone
Dexamethasone
Dexbrompheniramine
Dexchlorpheniramine
Dextroamphetamine
Diacetylmorphine
Diazepam
Dicyclomine
Diethazine
Diethylpropion
Digitalis
Digoxin
Dimethindene
Diphemanil
Diphenhydramine
Diphenylpyraline

Myopia (Cont'd)
Sulfadiazine
Sulfadimethoxine
Sulfamerazine
Sulfameter
Sulfamethazine
Sulfamethizole
Sulfamethoxazole
Sulfamethoxypyridazine
Sulfanilamide
Sulfaphenazole
Sulfapyridine
Sulfasalazine
Sulfathiazole
Sulfisoxazole
Tetracycline
Thiethylperazine
Thiopropazate
Thioproperazine
Thioridazine
Timolol
Triamcinolone
Trichlormethiazide
Trifluoperazine
Trifluperidol (?)
Triflupromazine
Trimeprazine

Narrowing or Occlusion of
Lacrimal Canaliculi or Puncta
Colloidal Silver
Demecarium
DFP
Echothiophate
Epinephrine
Floxuridine
Fluorouracil
F_3T
Idoxuridine
IDU
Isoflurophate
Neostigmine
Physostigmine
Quinacrine

Silver Nitrate
Silver Protein
Thiotepa
Trifluridine
Vidarabine

Night Blindness
Acetophenazine
Amodiaquine
Butaperazine
Carphenazine
Chloroquine
Chlorpromazine
Diethazine
Ethopropazine
Fluphenazine
Hydroxychloroquine
Mesoridazine
Methdilazine
Methotrimeprazine
Paramethadione
Perazine
Periciazine
Perphenazine
Piperacetazine
Prochlorperazine
Promazine
Promethazine
Propiomazine
Quinidine
Quinine
Thiethylperazine
Thiopropazate
Thioproperazine
Thioridazine
Trifluoperazine
Triflupromazine
Trimeprazine
Trimethadione

Nystagmus
Acetophenazine
Alcohol
Allobarbital

Amitriptyline
Amobarbital
Amodiaquine
Amoxapine
Aprobarbital
Aspirin
Aurothioglucose
Aurothioglycanide
Baclofen
Barbital
Bromide
Bromisovalum
Broxyquinoline
Bupivacaine
Butabarbital
Butalbital
Butallylonal
Butaperazine
Butethal
Calcitriol
Carbamazepine
Carbinoxamine
Carbromal
Carisoprodol
Carphenazine
Cefazolin
Cephalexin
Cephaloglycin
Cephaloridine
Cephalothin
Cephradine
Chloral Hydrate
Chloramphenicol (?)
Chlordiazepoxide
Chloroform
Chloroprocaine
Chloroquine
Chlorpromazine
Cholecalciferol
Clemastine
Clomipramine
Clonazepam
Clorazepate
Colistimethate

Colistin
Cyclobarbital
Cyclopentobarbital
Desipramine
Diazepam
Diethazine
Diphenhydramine
Diphenylpyraline
Disulfiram
Doxepin
Doxylamine
Ergocalciferol
Ergot (?)
Ethacrynic Acid
Ethchlorvynol
Ethopropazine
Ethotoin
Etidocaine
Fenfluramine
Floxuridine
Fluorouracil
Fluphenazine
Flurazepam
Glutethimide
Gold Au[198]
Gold Sodium Thiomalate
Gold Sodium Thiosulfate
Hashish
Heptabarbital
Hexethal
Hexobarbital
Hydroxychloroquine
Imipramine
Influenza Virus Vaccine
Insulin
Iodochlorhydroxyquin
Iodoquinol
Isoniazid
Ketamine
Lidocaine
Lithium Carbonate
Lorazepam
Marihuana
Measles Virus Vaccine Live

Nystagmus (Cont'd)

Mephenesin
Mephentermine
Mephenytoin
Mephobarbital
Mepivacaine
Meprobamate
Mesoridazine
Metaraminol
Methaqualone
Metharbital
Methdilazine
Methitural
Methocarbamol
Methohexital
Methotrimeprazine
Methoxamine
Methyl Alcohol
Methylpentynol
Methylthiouracil
Methyprylon
Metoclopramide
Metocurine Iodide
Nalidixic Acid
Nitrazepam
Nitrofurantoin
Norepinephrine
Nortriptyline
Oxazepam
Paramethadione
Pentazocine
Pentobarbital
Perazine
Perhexilene
Periciazine
Perphenazine
Phencyclidine
Phenelzine
Phenobarbital
Phenytoin
Piperacetazine
Piperazine
Poliovirus Vaccine
Polymyxin B

Prazepam
Prilocaine
Primidone
Probarbital
Procaine
Procarbazine
Prochlorperazine
Promazine
Promethazine
Propiomazine
Propoxycaine
Protriptyline
Quinine
Rabies Immune Globulin and
   Vaccine
Rubella Virus Vaccine Live
Secobarbital
Sodium Salicylate
Streptomycin
Talbutal
Tetanus Toxoid
Tetrahydrocannabinol
THC
Thiamylal
Thiethylperazine
Thiopental
Thiopcrazine
Thiopropazate
Thioproperazine
Thioridazine
Tranylcypromine
Trichloroethylene
Trifluoperazine
Triflupromazine
Trimeprazine
Trimethadione
Trimipramine
Tripelennamine
Tubocurarine
Urea (?)
Urethan
Valproate Sodium
Valproic Acid
Vinbarbital

Vitamin A
Vitamin D$_2$
Vitamin D$_3$

Objects Have Blue Tinge
Acetyldigitoxin
Alcohol
Amodiaquine
Amphetamine
Chloroquine
Deslanoside
Digitalis
Digitoxin
Digoxin
Gitalin
Hydroxyamphetamine
Hydroxychloroquine
Lanatoside C
Methylene Blue
Nalidixic Acid
Oral Contraceptives
Ouabain
Quinacrine

Objects Have Brown Tinge
Acetophenazine
Butaperazine
Carphenazine
Chlorpromazine
Diethazine
Ethopropazine
Fluphenazine
Mesoridazine
Methdilazine
Methotrimeprazine
Perazine
Periciazine
Perphenazine
Piperacetazine
Prochlorperazine
Promazine
Promethazine
Propiomazine
Thiethylperazine

Thiopropazate
Thioproperazine
Thioridazine
Trifluoperazine
Triflupromazine
Trimeprazine

Objects Have Green Tinge
Acetyldigitoxin
Allobarbital
Amobarbital
Amodiaquine
Aprobarbital
Barbital
Butabarbital
Butalbital
Butallylonal
Butethal
Chloroquine
Cyclobarbital
Cyclopentobarbital
Deslanoside
Digitalis
Digitoxin
Digoxin
Epinephrine
Gitalin
Griseofulvin
Heptabarbital
Hexethal
Hexobarbital
Hydroxychloroquine
Iodide and Iodine Solutions and
    Compounds
Lanatoside C
Mephobarbital
Metharbital
Methitural
Methohexital
Nalidixic Acid
Ouabain
Pentobarbital
Phenobarbital
Primidone

Objects Have Green Tinge
(*Cont'd*)
   Probarbital
   Quinacrine
   Quinine
   Radioactive Iodides
   Secobarbital
   Talbutal
   Thiamylal
   Thiopental
   Vinbarbital

Objects Have Red Tinge
   Acetyldigitoxin
   Atropine
   Belladonna
   Deslanoside
   Digitalis
   Digitoxin
   Digoxin
   Ergonovine
   Ergotamine
   Gitalin
   Homatropine
   Lanatoside C
   Methylergonovine
   Methysergide
   Ouabain
   Quinine
   Sulfacetamide
   Sulfachlorpyridazine
   Sulfacytine
   Sulfadiazine
   Sulfadimethoxine
   Sulfamerazine
   Sulfameter
   Sulfamethazine
   Sulfamethizole
   Sulfamethoxazole
   Sulfamethoxypyridazine
   Sulfanilamide
   Sulfaphenazole
   Sulfapyridine
   Sulfasalazine

   Sulfathiazole
   Sulfisoxazole
   Sulthiame

Objects Have Violet Tinge
   Hashish
   Marihuana
   Nalidixic Acid
   Quinacrine
   Tetrahydrocannabinol
   THC

Objects Have White Tinge
   Capreomycin
   Paramethadione
   Phenytoin
   Trimethadione

Objects Have Yellow Tinge
   Acetophenazine
   Acetyldigitoxin
   Allobarbital
   Alseroxylon
   Amobarbital
   Amodiaquine
   Amyl Nitrite
   Aprobarbital
   Aspirin
   Barbital
   Bendroflumethiazide
   Benzthiazide
   Butabarbital
   Butalbital
   Butallylonal
   Butaperazine
   Butethal
   Carbon Dioxide
   Carphenazine
   Chloramphenicol
   Chloroquine
   Chlorothiazide
   Chlorpromazine
   Chlortetracycline
   Chlorthalidone

Objects Have Yellow Tinge
(Cont'd)
   Thioproperazine
   Thioridazine
   Trichlormethiazide
   Trifluoperazine
   Triflupromazine
   Trimeprazine
   Vinbarbital
   Vitamin A

Ocular Exposure — Irritation
   Aceclidine
   Alcian Blue
   Alcohol
   Amoxicillin
   Amphotericin B
   Ampicillin
   Atropine
   Aurothioglucose
   Aurothioglycanide
   Bacitracin
   Benoxinate
   Benzalkonium
   Benzathine Penicillin G
   Betamethasone
   Butacaine
   Carbachol
   Carbenicillin
   Cefazolin
   Cephalexin
   Cephaloglycin
   Cephaloridine
   Cephalothin
   Cephradine
   Chloramphenicol
   Chloroform
   Chlortetracycline
   Chrysarobin
   Clindamycin
   Cloxacillin
   Cocaine
   Colistin
   Colloidal Silver

Cortisone
Cyclopentolate
Cytarabine
Demecarium
Dexamethasone
DFP
Dibucaine
Dicloxacillin
Dimercaprol
Dimethyl Sulfoxide
Dipivefrin
DMSO
DPE
Dyclonine
Echothiophate
Emetine
Ephedrine
Epinephrine
Erythromycin
Ether
Ferrocholinate
Ferrous Fumarate
Ferrous Gluconate
Ferrous Succinate
Ferrous Sulfate
Fluorescein
Fluorometholone
Framycetin
F_3T
Gentamicin
Glycerin
Gold Au[198]
Gold Sodium Thiomalate
Gold Sodium Thiosulfate
Guanethidine
Hetacillin
Hexachlorophene
Homatropine
Hyaluronidase
Hydrabamine Penicillin V
Hydrocortisone
Hydroxyamphetamine
Idoxuridine
IDU

Ocular Teratogenic Effects

Ocular Teratogenic Effects (Cont'd)

Diethazine
Doxorubicin (?)
Doxycycline (?)
Ethopropazine
Floxuridine (?)
Fludrocortisone (?)
Fluorouracil (?)
Fluphenazine
Fluprednisolone (?)
Furosemide (?)
Hashish (?)
Hexachlorophene (?)
Hydrocortisone (?)
Hydroxychloroquine (?)
Hydroxyurea (?)
Lomustine (?)
LSD (?)
Lysergide (?)
Marihuana (?)
Mechlorethamine (?)
Meclizine (?)
Melphalan (?)
Meprednisone (?)
Mercaptopurine (?)
Mescaline (?)
Mesoridazine
Methacycline (?)
Methdilazine
Methotrexate (?)
Methotrimeprazine
Methylprednisolone (?)
Minocycline (?)
Mithramycin (?)
Mitomycin (?)
Mitotane (?)
Nalidixic Acid (?)
Oxytetracycline (?)
Paramethasone (?)
Perazine
Periciazine
Perphenazine
Phenytoin

Piperacetazine
Prednisolone (?)
Prednisone (?)
Primidone (?)
Procarbazine (?)
Prochlorperazine
Promazine
Promethazine
Propiomazine
Psilocybin (?)
Quinacrine (?)
Quinine
Radioactive Iodides
Semustine (?)
Sodium Salicylate (?)
Tamoxifen (?)
Tetracycline (?)
Tetrahydrocannabinol (?)
THC (?)
Thiethylperazine
Thioguanine (?)
Thiopropazate
Thioproperazine
Thioridazine
Thiotepa (?)
Triamcinolone (?)
Triethylenemelamine (?)
Trifluoperazine
Triflupromazine
Trimeprazine
Trimethadione
Uracil Mustard (?)
Urethan (?)
Vinblastine (?)
Vincristine (?)
Vitamin A (?)
Warfarin

Oculogyric Crises

Acetophenazine
Alseroxylon
Amantadine
Amitriptyline
Amodiaquine

Butaperazine
Carphenazine
Chlordiazepoxide
Chloroquine
Chlorpromazine
Chlorprothixene
Clonazepam
Clorazepate
Deserpidine
Desipramine
Diazepam
Diethazine
Doxepin
Droperidol
Ethopropazine
Fluphenazine
Flurazepam
Haloperidol
Hydroxychloroquine
Imipramine
Levodopa
Lithium Carbonate
Lorazepam
Loxapine
Mesoridazine
Methdilazine
Methotrimeprazine
Metoclopramide
Nitrazepam
Nortriptyline
Oxazepam
Perazine
Periciazine
Perphenazine
Piperacetazine
Prazepam
Prochlorperazine
Promazine
Promethazine
Propiomazine
Protriptyline
Rauwolfia Serpentina
Rescinnamine
Reserpine

Syrosingopine
Thiethylperazine
Thiopropazate
Thioproperazine
Thioridazine
Thiothixene
Trifluoperazine
Trifluperidol
Triflupromazine
Trimeprazine

Optic Atrophy
Acetophenazine
Allobarbital
Alseroxylon (?)
Aminosalicylate (?)
Aminosalicylic Acid (?)
Amobarbital
Amodiaquine
Antimony Lithium Thiomalate
Antimony Potassium Tartrate
Antimony Sodium Tartrate
Antimony Sodium Thioglycollate
Antipyrine
Aprobarbital
Aspirin
Barbital
Betamethasone
Bromide (?)
Broxyquinoline
Bupivacaine (?)
Butabarbital
Butalbital
Butallylonal
Butaperazine
Butethal
Calcitriol
Carphenazine
Chloramphenicol
Chloroprocaine (?)
Chloroquine
Chlorpromazine
Cholecalciferol
Clindamycin

Optic Atrophy (Cont'd)
Cobalt (?)
Cortisone
Cyclobarbital
Cyclopentobarbital
Cycloserine (?)
Dapsone
Deserpidine (?)
Dexamethasone
Dextrothyroxine (?)
Diethazine
Ergocalciferol
Ergot (?)
Ethambutol
Ethopropazine
Etidocaine (?)
Ferrocholinate (?)
Ferrous Fumarate (?)
Ferrous Gluconate (?)
Ferrous Succinate (?)
Ferrous Sulfate (?)
Fluorometholone
Fluphenazine
Heptabarbital
Hexachlorophene
Hexamethonium
Hexethal
Hexobarbital
Hydrocortisone
Hydroxychloroquine
Iodide and Iodine Solutions and
   Compounds
Iodochlorhydroxyquin
Iodoquinol
Iron Dextran (?)
Iron Sorbitex (?)
Isoniazid
Levothyroxine (?)
Lidocaine (?)
Liothyronine (?)
Liotrix (?)
Medrysone
Mephobarbital
Mepivacaine (?)

Mesoridazine
Metharbital
Methdilazine
Methitural
Methohexital
Methotrimeprazine
Methyl Alcohol
Methylene Blue
Nitroglycerin (?)
Oxyphenbutazone
Pentobarbital
Perazine
Periciazine
Perphenazine
Phenobarbital
Phenylbutazone
Piperacetazine
Polysaccharide-Iron Complex (?)
Prednisolone
Prilocaine (?)
Primidone
Probarbital
Procaine (?)
Prochlorperazine
Promazine
Promethazine
Propiomazine
Propoxycaine (?)
Quinine
Radioactive Iodides
Rauwolfia Serpentina (?)
Rescinnamine (?)
Reserpine (?)
Secobarbital
Sodium Antimonylgluconate
Sodium Salicylate
Stibocaptate
Stibogluconate
Stibophen
Streptomycin
Sulfacetamide (?)
Sulfachlorpyridazine (?)
Sulfacytine (?)
Sulfadiazine (?)

Sulfadimethoxine (?)
Sulfamerazine (?)
Sulfameter (?)
Sulfamethazine
Sulfamethizole (?)
Sulfamethoxazole (?)
Sulfamethoxypyridazine (?)
Sulfanilamide (?)
Sulfaphenazole (?)
Sulfapyridine (?)
Sulfasalazine (?)
Sulfathiazole (?)
Sulfisoxazole (?)
Suramin
Syrosingopine (?)
Talbutal
Thiamylal
Thiethylperazine
Thiopental
Thiopropazate
Thioproperazine
Thioridazine
Thyroglobulin (?)
Thyroid (?)
Trichloroethylene
Trifluoperazine
Triflupromazine
Trimeprazine
Tryparsamide
Vinbarbital
Vinblastine
Vincristine
Vitamin D_2
Vitamin D_3

Oscillopsia
Allobarbital
Amobarbital
Aprobarbital
Barbital
Butabarbital
Butalbital
Butallylonal
Butethal

Cyclobarbital
Cyclopentobarbital
Heptabarbital
Hexethal
Hexobarbital
Mephobarbital
Metharbital
Methitural
Methohexital
Pentobarbital
Phenobarbital
Primidone
Probarbital
Secobarbital
Talbutal
Thiamylal
Thiopental
Vinbarbital

Papilledema
Acetophenazine
Allobarbital
Amobarbital
Antimony Lithium Thiomalate
Antimony Potassium Tartrate
Antimony Sodium Tartrate
Antimony Sodium Thioglycollate
Aprobarbital
Aspirin
Aurothioglucose (?)
Aurothioglycanide (?)
Barbital
Benzathine Penicillin G
Bromide (?)
Bupivacaine (?)
Butabarbital
Butalbital
Butallylonal
Butaperazine
Butethal
Calcitriol
Carbamazepine
Carbon Dioxide
Carphenazine

Papilledema (Cont'd)
Cephaloridine (?)
Chloramphenicol (?)
Chloroprocaine (?)
Chlorpromazine
Cholecalciferol
Colchicine
Cortisone
Cyclobarbital
Cyclopentobarbital
Diethazine
Ergocalciferol
Ethambutol
Ethopropazine
Etidocaine (?)
Fluorometholone
Fluphenazine
Glutethimide
Gold Au^{198} (?)
Gold Sodium Thiomalate (?)
Gold Sodium Thiosulfate (?)
Heptabarbital
Hexethal
Hexobarbital
Hydrabamine Penicillin V
Ibuprofen (?)
Indomethacin (?)
Isocarboxazid (?)
Isoniazid
Ketoprofen (?)
Lidocaine (?)
Lithium Carbonate (?)
Mephobarbital
Mepivacaine (?)
Mesoridazine
Metharbital
Methdilazine
Methitural
Methohexital
Methotrimeprazine
Methylene Blue
Methyprylon
Mitotane
Penicillamine

Pentobarbital
Perazine
Periciazine
Perhexilene
Perphenazine
Phenobarbital
Piperacetazine
Potassium Penicillin G
Potassium Penicillin V
Potassium Phenethicillin
Prilocaine (?)
Primidone
Probarbital
Procaine (?)
Procaine Penicillin G
Procarbazine
Prochlorperazine
Promazine
Promethazine
Propiomazine
Propoxycaine (?)
Quinine
Secobarbital
Sodium Antimonylgluconate
Sodium Salicylate
Stibocaptate
Stibogluconate
Stibophen
Sulfacetamide
Sulfachlorpyridazine
Sulfacytine
Sulfadiazine
Sulfadimethoxine
Sulfamerazine
Sulfameter
Sulfamethazine
Sulfamethizole
Sulfamethoxazole
Sulfamethoxypyridazine
Sulfanilamide
Sulfaphenazole
Sulfapyridine
Sulfasalazine
Sulfathiazole

Sulfisoxazole
Sulthiame
Talbutal
Thiamylal
Thiethylperazine
Thiopental
Thiopropazate
Thioproperazine
Thioridazine
Tranylcypromine (?)
Trifluoperazine
Triflupromazine
Trimeprazine
Vinbarbital
Vitamin D$_2$
Vitamin D$_3$

Papilledema Secondary to Pseudo-tumor Cerebri
Adrenal Cortex Injection
Aldosterone
Betamethasone
Chlortetracycline
Cortisone
Demeclocycline
Desoxycorticosterone
Dexamethasone
Diphtheria and Tetanus Toxoids
   and Pertussis (DPT) Vaccine
   Adsorbed
Doxycycline
Fludrocortisone
Fluprednisolone
Gentamicin
Griseofulvin
Hydrocortisone
Levodopa (?)
Meprednisone
Methacycline
Methylprednisolone
Minocycline
Nalidixic Acid
Nitrofurantoin
Oral Contraceptives

Oxytetracycline
Paramethasone
Prednisolone
Prednisone
Tetracycline
Triamcinolone
Vitamin A

Paresis or Paralysis of Extraocular Muscles
Acetohexamide
Alcohol
Allobarbital
Amitriptyline
Amobarbital
Amodiaquine
Amphotericin B
Aprobarbital
Aspirin
Aurothioglucose
Aurothioglycanide
Barbital
Bupivacaine
Butabarbital
Butalbital
Butallylonal
Butethal
Calcitriol (?)
Carisoprodol
Chloral Hydrate
Chlordiazepoxide
Chloroprocaine
Chloroquine
Chlorpropamide
Cholecalciferol (?)
Clonazepam
Clorazepate
Colchicine
Cyclobarbital
Cyclopentobarbital
Desipramine
Diazepam
Digitalis
Digitoxin

Epinephrine
Isoflurophate
Penicillamine
Rifampin
Sulfacetamide
Sulfachlorpyridazine
Sulfacytine
Sulfadiazine
Sulfadimethoxine
Sulfamerazine
Sulfameter
Sulfamethazine
Sulfamethizole
Sulfamethoxazole
Sulfamethoxypyridazine
Sulfanilamide
Sulfaphenazole
Sulfapyridine
Sulfasalazine
Sulfathiazole
Sulfisoxazole

Periorbital Edema
Carisoprodol
Epinephrine
Ethosuximide
Fluorouracil
Hexamethonium (?)
Hydralazine
Meprobamate
Methotrexate
Methsuximide
Phensuximide
Sulfacetamide
Sulfachlorpyridazine
Sulfacytine
Sulfadiazine
Sulfadimethoxine
Sulfamerazine
Sulfameter
Sulfamethazine
Sulfamethizole
Sulfamethoxazole
Sulfamethoxypyridazine

Sulfanilamide
Sulfaphenazole
Sulfapyridine
Sulfasalazine
Sulfathiazole
Sulfisoxazole

Photophobia
Acetohexamide
Acetophenazine
Adiphenine
Ambutonium
Amitriptyline
Amodiaquine
Anisotropine
Atropine
Aurothioglucose
Aurothioglycanide
Belladonna
Bromide
Butaperazine
Carbon Dioxide
Carphenazine
Chloroquine
Chlorpromazine
Chlorpropamide
Chlortetracycline
Cimetidine
Clidinium
Clomiphene
Demeclocycline
Desipramine
Dicyclomine
Diethazine
Digitalis
Digitoxin
Diphemanil
Doxepin
Doxycycline
Edrophonium
Ethambutol
Ethionamide
Ethopropazine
Ethosuximide

Photophobia (Cont'd)
Ethotoin
Fluphenazine
Furosemide (?)
Glycopyrrolate
Gold Au^{198}
Gold Sodium Thiomalate
Gold Sodium Thiosulfate
Hexocyclium
Homatropine
Hydroxychloroquine
Imipramine
Isocarboxazid
Isoniazid
Isopropamide
Lithium Carbonate
Mepenzolate
Mephenytoin
Mesoridazine
Methacycline
Methantheline
Methdilazine
Methixene
Methotrimeprazine
Methsuximide
Methylatropine Nitrate
Minocycline
Nalidixic Acid
Nialamide
Norepinephrine
Nortriptyline
Oxyphencyclimine
Oxyphenonium
Oxytetracycline
Paramethadione
Perazine
Periciazine
Perphenazine
Phenelzine
Phensuximide
Pipenzolate
Piperacetazine
Piperidolate
Poldine

Practolol
Procarbazine
Prochlorperazine
Promazine
Promethazine
Propantheline
Propiomazine
Protriptyline
Quinacrine
Quinidine
Rabies Vaccine
Streptomycin
Tetracycline
Thiethylperazine
Thiopropazate
Thioproperazine
Thioridazine
Tolazamide
Tolbutamide
Tranylcypromine
Trichloroethylene
Tridihexethyl
Trifluoperazine
Triflupromazine
Trimeprazine
Trimethadione

Photosensitivity
Acetohexamide
Acetophenazine
Allobarbital
Amantadine
Amiodarone
Amitriptyline
Amobarbital
Amodiaquine
Amoxapine
Amoxicillin
Ampicillin
Antazoline
Aprobarbital
Aurothioglucose
Aurothioglycanide
Azatadine

Barbital
Bendroflumethiazide
Benzthiazide
Brompheniramine
Butabarbital
Butalbital
Butallylonal
Butaperazine
Butethal
Carbamazepine
Carbenicillin
Carbinoxamine
Carphenazine
Chlordiazepoxide
Chloroquine
Chlorothiazide
Chlorpheniramine
Chlorpromazine
Chlorpropamide
Chlorprothixene
Chlortetracycline
Chlorthalidone
Clemastine
Clindamycin
Clomipramine
Clonazepam
Clorazepate
Cloxacillin
Cocaine
Cyclobarbital
Cyclopentobarbital
Cyclophosphamide
Cycloserine
Cyclothiazide
Cyproheptadine
Dacarbazine
Dantrolene
Demeclocycline
Desipramine
Dexbrompheniramine
Dexchlorpheniramine
Diazepam
Dibucaine
DIC

Dicloxacillin
Diethazine
Dimethindene
Dimethyl Sulfoxide
Diphenhydramine
Diphenylpyraline
Disopyramide
DMSO
Doxepin
Doxycycline
Doxylamine
Droperidol
Erythromycin
Ethopropazine
Floxuridine
Fluorouracil
Fluphenazine
Flurazepam
Furosemide
Gentamicin
Gold Au[198]
Gold Sodium Thiomalate
Gold Sodium Thiosulfate
Griseofulvin
Haloperidol
Heptabarbital
Hetacillin
Hexachlorophene
Hexethal
Hexobarbital
Hydrochlorothiazide
Hydroflumethiazide
Hydroxychloroquine
Imipramine
Isocarboxazid
Lincomycin
Lorazepam
Loxapine
Mephobarbital
Mesoridazine
Methacycline
Metharbital
Methdilazine
Methicillin

Photosensitivity (Cont'd)
  Methitural
  Methohexital
  Methotrexate
  Methotrimeprazine
  Methoxsalen
  Methyclothiazide
  Metolazone
  Minocycline
  Nafcillin
  Nalidixic Acid
  Nialamide
  Nitrazepam
  Nitrofurantoin
  Nortriptyline
  Oral Contraceptives
  Oxacillin
  Oxazepam
  Oxytetracycline
  Paramethadione
  Pentobarbital
  Perazine
  Periciazine
  Perphenazine
  Phenelzine
  Pheniramine
  Phenobarbital
  Piperacetazine
  Piperazine
  Polythiazide
  Prazepam
  Primidone
  Probarbital
  Procarbazine
  Prochlorperazine
  Promazine
  Promethazine
  Propiomazine
  Protriptyline
  Pyrilamine
  Quinethazone
  Quinidine
  Quinine
  Secobarbital

  Smallpox Vaccine
  Sulfacetamide
  Sulfachlorpyridazine
  Sulfacytine
  Sulfadiazine
  Sulfadimethoxine
  Sulfamerazine
  Sulfameter
  Sulfamethazine
  Sulfamethizole
  Sulfamethoxazole
  Sulfamethoxypyridazine
  Sulfanilamide
  Sulfaphenazole
  Sulfapyridine
  Sulfasalazine
  Sulfathiazole
  Sulfisoxazole
  Talbutal
  Tetracycline
  Thiamylal
  Thiethylperazine
  Thiopental
  Thiopropazate
  Thioproperazine
  Thioridazine
  Thiothixene
  Tolazamide
  Tolbutamide
  Tranylcypromine
  Trichlormethiazide
  Trifluoperazine
  Trifluperidol
  Triflupromazine
  Trimeprazine
  Trimethadione
  Trimipramine
  Trioxsalen
  Tripelennamine
  Triprolidine
  Vancomycin
  Vinbarbital
  Vinblastine
  Vincristine

Random Ocular Movements
Allobarbital
Amobarbital
Aprobarbital
Barbital
Butabarbital
Butalbital
Butallylonal
Butethal
Carisoprodol
Cyclobarbital
Cyclopentobarbital
Heptabarbital
Hexethal
Hexobarbital
Ketamine
Mephobarbital
Meprobamate
Metharbital
Methitural
Methohexital
Pentobarbital
Phenobarbital
Primidone
Probarbital
Secobarbital
Talbutal
Thiamylal
Thiopental
Vinbarbital

Retinal Degeneration
Betamethasone
Clonidine (?)
Cortisone
Dexamethasone
Ferrocholinate
Ferrous Fumarate
Ferrous Gluconate
Ferrous Succinate
Ferrous Sulfate
Hydrocortisone
Indomethacin (?)

Iodide and Iodine Solutions and
   Compounds
Iron Dextran
Iron Sorbitex
Nalidixic Acid (?)
Polysaccharide-Iron Complex
Prednisolone
Quinine
Radioactive Iodides

Retinal Detachment
Aceclidine (?)
Acetylcholine (?)
Betamethasone
Carbachol
Chymotrypsin (?)
Cortisone
Demecarium (?)
Dexamethasone
DFP (?)
Echothiophate (?)
Hydrocortisone
Isoflurophate (?)
Methylphenidate
Neostigmine (?)
Oxygen
Physostigmine (?)
Pilocarpine
Prednisolone

Retinal Edema
Acetazolamide
Acetophenazine
Adrenal Cortex Injection
Aldosterone
Amithiozone
Amodiaquine
Aspirin
Bendroflumethiazide
Benzthiazide
Betamethasone
Butaperazine
Carphenazine
Chloramphenicol

Chloroquine
Chlorothiazide
Chlorpromazine
Chlorthalidone
Cobalt (?)
Cortisone
Cyclothiazide
Desoxycorticosterone
Dexamethasone
Dichlorphenamide
Diethazine
Ergot
Ethambutol
Ethopropazine
Ethoxzolamide
Fludrocortisone
Fluphenazine
Fluprednisolone
Hydrochlorothiazide
Hydrocortisone
Hydroflumethiazide
Hydroxychloroquine
Indomethacin (?)
Iodide and Iodine Solutions and
  Compounds
Meprednisone
Mesoridazine
Methazolamide
Methdilazine
Methotrimeprazine
Methyclothiazide
Methylprednisolone
Metolazone
Paramethasone
Perazine
Periciazine
Perphenazine
Piperacetazine
Polythiazide
Prednisolone
Prednisone
Prochlorperazine
Promazine
Promethazine

Propiomazine
Quinethazone
Quinine
Radioactive Iodides
Sodium Salicylate
Thiethylperazine
Thiopropazate
Thioproperazine
Thioridazine
Triamcinolone
Trichlormethiazide
Trichloroethylene
Trifluoperazine
Triflupromazine
Trimeprazine

Retinal or Macular Pigmentary
Changes or Deposits
  Acetophenazine
  Amiodarone (?)
  Amodiaquine
  Azathioprine
  Benztropine (?)
  Biperiden (?)
  Butaperazine
  Carphenazine
  Cephaloridine (?)
  Chloramphenicol
  Chloroquine
  Chlorphenoxamine (?)
  Chlorpromazine
  Chlorprothixene
  Clofazimine
  Clonidine (?)
  Cobalt (?)
  Cycrimine (?)
  Diethazine
  Diethylcarbamazine
  Ethambutol
  Ethopropazine
  Fluphenazine
  Hydroxychloroquine
  Indomethacin (?)
  Mesoridazine

Phendimetrazine (?)
Phenmetrazine (?)
Phenobarbital
Phentermine (?)
Prednisolone
Primidone
Probarbital
Procaine (?)
Quinine
Radioactive Iodides
Secobarbital
Streptomycin
Sulfacetamide
Sulfachlorpyridazine
Sulfacytine
Sulfadiazine
Sulfadimethoxine
Sulfamerazine
Sulfameter
Sulfamethazine
Sulfamethizole
Sulfamethoxazole
Sulfamethoxypyridazine
Sulfanilamide
Sulfaphenazole
Sulfapyridine
Sulfasalazine
Sulfathiazole
Sulfisoxazole
Talbutal
Thiamylal
Thiopental
Trichloroethylene
Vinbarbital

Retrobulbar or Optic Neuritis
Acetohexamide
Acetyldigitoxin
Alcohol
Allobarbital
Aminosalicylate (?)
Aminosalicylic Acid (?)
Amitriptyline
Amobarbital

Aprobarbital
Barbital
Benzphetamine (?)
Bromisovalum
Broxyquinoline
Bupivacaine (?)
Butabarbital
Butalbital
Butallylonal
Butethal
Calcitriol (?)
Caramiphen
Carbromal
Chloral Hydrate (?)
Chloramphenicol
Chloroprocaine (?)
Chlorphentermine (?)
Chlorpropamide
Cholecalciferol (?)
Clindamycin
Cyclobarbital
Cyclopentobarbital
Cycloserine (?)
Desipramine
Deslanoside
Dextrothyroxine (?)
Diethylpropion (?)
Digitalis
Digitoxin
Digoxin
Diphtheria and Tetanus Toxoids
  and Pertussis (DPT) Vaccine
  Adsorbed
Disulfiram
Ergocalciferol (?)
Ergonovine (?)
Ergotamine (?)
Ethambutol
Ethchlorvynol
Ethionamide
Etidocaine (?)
Fenfluramine (?)
Ferrocholinate (?)
Ferrous Fumarate (?)

Retrobulbar or Optic Neuritis
(Cont'd)
  Ferrous Gluconate (?)
  Ferrous Succinate (?)
  Ferrous Sulfate (?)
  Gitalin
  Heptabarbital
  Hexethal
  Hexobarbital
  Ibuprofen
  Imipramine
  Influenza Virus Vaccine
  Iodide and Iodine Solutions and
    Compounds
  Iodochlorhydroxyquin
  Iodoquinol
  Iron Dextran (?)
  Iron Sorbitex (?)
  Isocarboxazid (?)
  Isoniazid
  Kanamycin (?)
  Lanatoside C
  Levothyroxine (?)
  Lidocaine (?)
  Liothyronine (?)
  Liotrix (?)
  Measles Virus Vaccine Live
  Mephobarbital
  Mepivacaine (?)
  Metharbital
  Methitural
  Methohexital
  Methylergonovine (?)
  Methysergide (?)
  Naproxen (?)
  Nialamide (?)
  Nortriptyline
  Nystatin
  Oral Contraceptives
  Ouabain
  Oxyphenbutazone
  Penicillamine
  Pentobarbital
  Phendimetrazine (?)

  Phenelzine (?)
  Phenobarbital
  Phentermine (?)
  Phenylbutazone
  Poliovirus Vaccine
  Polysaccharide-Iron Complex (?)
  Prilocaine (?)
  Primidone
  Probarbital
  Procaine (?)
  Propoxycaine (?)
  Protriptyline
  Quinacrine
  Quinidine
  Rabies Immune Globulin And
    Vaccine
  Radioactive Iodides
  Rifampin (?)
  Rubella Virus Vaccine Live
  Secobarbital
  Smallpox Vaccine
  Streptomycin
  Sulfacetamide
  Sulfachlorpyridazine
  Sulfacytine
  Sulfadiazine
  Sulfadimethoxine
  Sulfamerazine
  Sulfameter
  Sulfamethazine
  Sulfamethizole
  Sulfamethoxazole
  Sulfamethoxypyridazine
  Sulfanilamide
  Sulfaphenazole
  Sulfapyridine
  Sulfasalazine
  Sulfathiazole
  Sulfisoxazole
  Talbutal
  Tetanus Toxoid (?)
  Thiamylal
  Thiopental
  Thyroglobulin (?)

Thyroid (?)
Tolazamide
Tolbutamide
Trichloroethylene
Tryparsamide
Vinbarbital
Vitamin D_2 (?)
Vitamin D_3 (?)

Strabismus
Alcohol
Baclofen
Calcitriol
Chloramphenicol (?)
Chloroform
Cholecalciferol
Ergocalciferol
Insulin
Isocarboxazid
Measles Virus Vaccine Live
Metoclopramide
Nialamide
Pentylenetetrazol
Phenelzine
Tranylcypromine
Tripelennamine
Vitamin A
Vitamin D_2
Vitamin D_3

Subconjunctival or Retinal
Hemorrhages
Acetylcholine
Acid Bismuth Sodium Tartrate
Adrenal Cortex Injection
Aldosterone
Allopurinol (?)
Alseroxylon
Aspirin
Benoxinate
Betamethasone
Bismuth Oxychloride
Bismuth Sodium Tartrate
Bismuth Sodium Thioglycollate

Bismuth Sodium Triglycollamate
Bismuth Subcarbonate
Bismuth Subsalicylate
Butacaine
Cobalt (?)
Cocaine
Cortisone
Deserpidine
Desoxycorticosterone
Dexamethasone
Dibucaine
Dyclonine
Epinephrine
Fludrocortisone
Fluorouracil
Fluprednisolone
Glycerin
Hydrocortisone
Isosorbide
Lincomycin
Mannitol
Meprednisone
Methylphenidate
Methylprednisolone
Mithramycin
Mitotane
Oxyphenbutazone
Paramethasone
Penicillamine
Phenacaine
Phenylbutazone
Piperocaine
Pralidoxime
Prednisolone
Prednisone
Proparacaine
Rauwolfia Serpentina
Rescinnamine
Reserpine
Sodium Chloride
Sodium Salicylate
Sulfacetamide
Sulfachlorpyridazine
Sulfacytine

Subconjunctival or Retinal Hemorrhages (Cont'd)
Sulfadiazine
Sulfadimethoxine
Sulfamerazine
Sulfameter
Sulfamethazine
Sulfamethizole
Sulfamethoxazole
Sulfamethoxypyridazine
Sulfanilamide
Sulfaphenazole
Sulfapyridine
Sulfasalazine
Sulfathiazole
Sulfisoxazole
Sulindac
Syrosingopine
Tetracaine
Triamcinolone
Trichloroethylene
Urea

Subconjunctival or Retinal Hemorrhages Secondary to Drug-Induced Anemia
Acenocoumarol
Acetaminophen
Acetanilid
Acetazolamide
Acetohexamide
Acetophenazine
Allobarbital
Allopurinol
Aminosalicylate (?)
Aminosalicylic Acid (?)
Amithiozone
Amitriptyline
Amobarbital
Amodiaquine
Amoxicillin
Amphotericin B
Ampicillin
Anisindione

Antazoline
Antimony Lithium Thiomalate
Antimony Potassium Tartrate
Antimony Sodium Tartrate
Antimony Sodium Thioglycollate
Antipyrine
Aprobarbital
Aurothioglucose
Aurothioglycanide
Azatadine
Azathioprine
Barbital
BCNU
Bendroflumethiazide
Benzathine Penicillin G
Benzthiazide
Bleomycin
Brompheniramine
Busulfan
Butabarbital
Butalbital
Butallylonal
Butaperazine
Butethal
Cactinomycin
Calcitriol
Carbamazepine
Carbenicillin
Carbimazole
Carbinoxamine
Carisoprodol
Carmustine
Carphenazine
CCNU
Cefazolin
Cephalexin
Cephaloglycin
Cephaloridine
Cephalothin
Cephradine
Chlorambucil
Chloramphenicol
Chlordiazepoxide
Chloroquine

Subconjunctical or Retinal
Hemorrhages Secondary to Drug-
Induced Anemia (Cont'd)
  Mefenamic Acid
  Melphalan
  Mephenytoin
  Mephobarbital
  Meprobamate
  Mercaptopurine
  Mesoridazine
  Methacycline
  Methaqualone
  Metharbital
  Methazolamide
  Methdilazine
  Methicillin
  Methimazole
  Methitural
  Methohexital
  Methotrexate
  Methotrimeprazine
  Methsuximide
  Methyclothiazide
  Methyldopa
  Methylene Blue
  Methylphenidate
  Methylthiouracil
  Methyprylon
  Metolazone
  Minocycline
  Mitomycin
  Nafcillin
  Nalidixic Acid
  Naproxen
  Nitrazepam
  Nitrofurantoin
  Nitroglycerin
  Nortriptyline
  Orphenadrine
  Oxacillin
  Oxazepam
  Oxyphenbutazone
  Oxytetracycline
  Paramethadione
  Penicillamine

Pentobarbital
Perazine
Periciazine
Perphenazine
Phenacetin
Phenindione
Pheniramine
Phenobarbital
Phenprocoumon
Phensuximide
Phenylbutazone
Phenytoin
Piperacetazine
Piperazine
Polythiazide
Potassium Penicillin G
Potassium Penicillin V
Potassium Phenethicillin
Prazepam
Primidone
Probarbital
Procaine Penicillin C
Procarbazine
Prochlorperazine
Promazine
Promethazine
Propiomazine
Propylthiouracil
Protriptyline
Pyrilamine
Quinacrine
Quinethazone
Quinidine
Quinine
Rifampin
Secobarbital
Semustine
Sodium Antimonylgluconate
Stibocaptate
Stibogluconate
Stibophen
Streptomycin
Suramin
Talbutal

Tetracycline
Thiabendazole
Thiamylal
Thiethylperazine
Thioguanine
Thiopental
Thiopropazate
Thioproperazine
Thioridazine
Thiotepa
Thiothixene
Tolazamide
Tolazoline
Tolbutamide
Trichlormethiazide
Triethylenemelamine
Trifluoperazine
Trifluperidol
Triflupromazine
Trimeprazine
Trimethadione
Tripelennamine
Triprolidine
Uracil Mustard
Urethan
Vancomycin
Vinbarbital
Vinblastine
Vincristine
Vitamin A
Vitamin D_2
Vitamin D_3
Warfarin

Symblepharon
Aurothioglucose
Aurothioglycanide
Clonidine (?)
Colloidal Silver
Gold Au[198]
Gold Sodium Thiomalate
Gold Sodium Thiosulfate
Oxyphenbutazone
Phenylbutazone
Silver Nitrate

Silver Protein
Sulfacetamide
Sulfachlorpyridazine
Sulfacytine
Sulfadiazine
Sulfadimethoxine
Sulfamerazine
Sulfameter
Sulfamethazine
Sulfamethizole
Sulfamethoxazole
Sulfamethoxypyridazine
Sulfanilamide
Sulfaphenazole
Sulfapyridine
Sulfasalazine
Sulfathiazole
Sulfisoxazole

Systemic Administration — Non-specific Ocular Irritation
Alseroxylon
Amithiozone
Bethanechol
Carisoprodol
Chloral Hydrate
Clonidine
Clorazepate
Cyclophosphamide
Deserpidine
Dextran
Diacetylmorphine
Diatrizoate Meglumine and
    Sodium
Dimercaprol
Emetine
Ether
Floxuridine
Fluorouracil
Flurazepam
Guanethidine
Hashish
Hydralazine
Iodide and Iodine Solutions and
    Compounds

Hydroxychloroquine
Ibuprofen
Imipramine
Indomethacin (?)
Influenza Virus Vaccine
Iodide and Iodine Solutions and
  Compounds
Iodochlorhydroxyquin
Iodoquinol
Isoniazid
Medrysone
Mephobarbital
Meprednisone
Mesoridazine
Metharbital
Methdilazine
Methitural
Methohexital
Methotrimeprazine
Methyl Alcohol
Methylprednisolone
Niacin
Niacinamide
Nicotinyl Alcohol
Nortriptyline
Oxyphenbutazone
Paramethasone
Pentobarbital
Perazine
Periciazine
Perphenazine
Phenobarbital
Phenylbutazone
Piperacetazine
Prednisolone
Prednisone
Primidone
Probarbital
Prochlorperazine
Promazine
Promethazine
Propiomazine
Protriptyline
Quinidine

Quinine
Radioactive Iodides
Secobarbital
Sodium Antimonylgluconate
Sodium Salicylate
Stibocaptate
Stibogluconate
Stibophen
Streptomycin
Sulfacetamide (?)
Sulfachlorpyridazine (?)
Sulfacytine (?)
Sulfadiazine (?)
Sulfadimethoxine (?)
Sulfamerazine (?)
Sulfameter (?)
Sulfamethazine (?)
Sulfamethizole (?)
Sulfamethoxazole (?)
Sulfamethoxypyridazine (?)
Sulfanilamide (?)
Sulfaphenazole (?)
Sulfapyridine (?)
Sulfasalazine (?)
Sulfathiazole (?)
Sulfisoxazole (?)
Talbutal
Thiamylal
Thiethylperazine
Thiopental
Thiopropazate
Thioproperazine
Thioridazine
Triamcinolone
Trichloroethylene
Trifluoperazine
Triflupromazine
Trimeprazine
Tryparsamide
Vinbarbital

Uveitis
  Alseroxylon (?)
  Amodiaquine (?)

17

Uveitis (Cont'd)
  Amphotericin B
  Bacitracin
  Benzathine Penicillin G
  Chloramphenicol
  Chloroquine (?)
  Chlortetracycline
  Chymotrypsin
  Colistin
  Demecarium
  Deserpidine (?)
  DFP
  Diethylcarbamazine
  Diphtheria and Tetanus Toxoids
    and Pertussis (DPT) Vaccine
    Adsorbed
  Echothiophate
  Erythromycin
  Hydrabamine Penicillin V
  Hydroxychloroquine (?)
  Influenza Virus Vaccine
  Isoflurophate
  Measles Virus Vaccine Live
  Methicillin
  Mitomycin
  Neomycin
  Poliovirus Vaccine
  Polymyxin B
  Potassium Penicillin G
  Potassium Penicillin V
  Potassium Phenethicillin
  Procaine Penicillin G
  Quinidine
  Rabies Immune Globulin and
    Vaccine
  Rauwolfia Serpentina (?)
  Rescinnamine (?)
  Reserpine (?)
  Rifampin
  Rubella Virus Vaccine Live
  Smallpox Vaccine
  Streptomycin
  Sulfacetamide
  Sulfachlorpyridazine

  Sulfacytine
  Sulfadiazine
  Sulfadimethoxine
  Sulfamerazine
  Sulfameter
  Sulfamethazine
  Sulfamethizole
  Sulfamethoxazole
  Sulfamethoxypyridazine
  Sulfanilamide
  Sulfaphenazole
  Sulfapyridine
  Sulfasalazine
  Sulfathiazole
  Sulfisoxazole
  Syrosingopine (?)
  Tetracycline
  Thiotepa (?)
  Timolol (?)
  Urokinase

Visual Agnosia
  Benzathine Penicillin G
  Hydrabamine Penicillin V
  Potassium Penicillin G
  Potassium Penicillin V
  Potassium Phenethicillin
  Procaine Penicillin G

Visual Field Defects
  Acetophenazine
  Acetyldigitoxin
  Adrenal Cortex Injection
  Alcohol
  Aldosterone
  Alkavervir
  Allobarbital
  Aluminum Nicotinate (?)
  Aminosalicylate (?)
  Aminosalicylic Acid (?)
  Amobarbital
  Amodiaquine
  Antazoline
  Aprobarbital

Aspirin
Barbital
Betamethasone
Bromide
Bromisovalum
Brompheniramine
Butabarbital
Butalbital
Butallylonal
Butaperazine
Butethal
Calcitriol (?)
Caramiphen
Carbinoxamine
Carbon Dioxide
Carbromal
Carisoprodol
Carphenazine
Chloramphenicol
Chloroquine
Chlorpheniramine
Chlorpromazine
Chlorpropamide
Chlortetracycline
Cholecalciferol (?)
Clemastine
Clomiphene
Cobalt (?)
Cortisone
Cryptenamine
Cyclobarbital
Cyclopentobarbital
Demeclocycline
Deslanoside
Desoxycorticosterone
Dexamethasone
Dexbrompheniramine
Dexchlorpheniramine
Dextrothyroxine (?)
Diatrizoate Meglumine and
    Sodium
Diazoxide
Diethazine
Diethylcarbamazine

Digitalis
Digitoxin
Digoxin
Dimethindene
Diphenhydramine
Diphenylpyraline
Disulfiram
Doxycycline
Doxylamine
Emetine
Epinephrine
Ergocalciferol (?)
Ergonovine
Ergot
Ethambutol
Ethchlorvynol
Ethopropazine
Fludrocortisone
Fluorometholone
Fluphenazine
Fluprednisolone
Gitalin
Heptabarbital
Hexamethonium
Hexethal
Hexobarbital
Hydrocortisone
Hydroxychloroquine
Ibuprofen
Indomethacin (?)
Iodide and Iodine Solutions and
    Compounds
Isoniazid
Ketoprofen (?)
Lanatoside C
Levothyroxine (?)
Liothyroxine (?)
Liotrix (?)
Lithium Carbonate
Medrysone
Mephobarbital
Meprednisone
Meprobamate
Mesoridazine

Visual Field Defects (Cont'd)

Methacycline
Metharbital
Methdilazine
Methitural
Methohexital
Methotrimeprazine
Methyl Alcohol
Methyldopa
Methylprednisolone
Methysergide
Minocycline
Morphine (?)
Niacin (?)
Niacinamide (?)
Nicotinyl Alcohol (?)
Opium (?)
Oral Contraceptives
Ouabain
Oxygen
Oxytetracycline
Paraldehyde
Paramethadione
Paramethasone
Pentobarbital
Perazine
Periciazine
Perphenazine
Pheniramine
Phenobarbital
Piperacetazine
Prednisolone
Prednisone
Primidone
Probarbital
Prochlorperazine
Promazine
Promethazine
Propiomazine
Protoveratrines A and B
Pyrilamine
Quinacrine
Quinidine
Quinine

Radioactive Iodides
Secobarbital
Sodium Salicylate
Streptomycin
Sulfacetamide
Sulfachlorpyridazine
Sulfacytine
Sulfadiazine
Sulfadimethoxine
Sulfamerazine
Sulfameter
Sulfamethazine
Sulfamethizole
Sulfamethoxazole
Sulfamethoxypyridazine
Sulfanilamide
Sulfaphenazole
Sulfapyridine
Sulfasalazine
Sulfathiazole
Sulfisoxazole
Talbutal
Tetracycline
Thiamylal
Thiethylperazine
Thiopental
Thiopropazate
Thioproperazine
Thioridazine
Thyroglobulin (?)
Thyroid (?)
Tolbutamide
Triamcinolone
Trichloroethylene
Trifluoperazine
Triflupromazine
Trimeprazine
Trimethadione
Tripelennamine
Triprolidine
Tryparsamide
Veratrum Viride Alkaloids
Vinbarbital
Vitamin A

Vitamin D$_2$ (?)
Vitamin D$_3$ (?)

Visual Hallucinations
Acetophenazine
Acid Bismuth Sodium Tartrate
Alcohol
Allobarbital
Amantadine
Amitriptyline
Amobarbital
Amodiaquine
Amoxapine
Amphetamine
Amyl Nitrite
Antazoline
Aprobarbital
Aspirin
Atropine
Azatadine
Baclofen
Barbital
Belladonna
Benzathine Penicillin G
Benztropine
Biperiden
Bismuth Oxychloride
Bismuth Sodium Tartrate
Bismuth Sodium Thioglycollate
Bismuth Sodium Triglycollamate
Bismuth Subcarbonate
Bismuth Subsalicylate
Bromide
Brompheniramine
Butabarbital
Butalbital
Butallylonal
Butaperazine
Butethal
Calcitriol
Capreomycin (?)
Carbamazepine
Carbinoxamine
Carbon Dioxide

Carphenazine
Cefazolin
Cephalexin
Cephaloglycin
Cephaloridine
Cephalothin
Cephradine
Chloral Hydrate
Chlorcyclizine
Chloroquine
Chlorpheniramine
Chlorphenoxamine
Chlorpromazine
Chlortetracycline
Cholecalciferol
Cimetidine
Clemastine
Clomipramine
Clonidine
Cocaine
Cyclizine
Cyclobarbital
Cyclopentobarbital
Cyclopentolate
Cycloserine
Cycrimine
Cyproheptadine
Dantrolene
Demeclocycline
Desipramine
Dexbrompheniramine
Dexchlorpheniramine
Dextroamphetamine
Diethazine
Digitalis
Digoxin
Dimethindene
Diphenhydramine
Diphenylpyraline
Disulfiram
Doxepin
Doxycycline
Doxylamine
Droperidol

Visual Hallucinations (Cont'd)
  Ephedrine
  Ergocalciferol
  Ethchlorvynol
  Ethopropazine
  Fluphenazine
  Flurazepam
  Furosemide
  Glutethimide
  Glycerin
  Griseofulvin
  Haloperidol
  Hashish
  Heptabarbital
  Hexethal
  Hexobarbital
  Homatropine
  Hydrabamine Penicillin V
  Hydroxychloroquine
  Hydroxyurea
  Imipramine
  Indomethacin
  Iodide and Iodine Solutions and
    Compounds
  Isoniazid (?)
  Isosorbide
  Ketamine
  Levallorphan
  Levodopa
  LSD
  Lysergide
  Mannitol
  Marihuana
  Meclizine
  Mephentermine
  Mephobarbital
  Mescaline
  Mesoridazine
  Methacycline
  Methamphetamine
  Metharbital
  Methdilazine
  Methitural
  Methohexital
  Methotrimeprazine
  Methscopolamine
  Methyldopa
  Methylpentynol
  Methylphenidate
  Methyprylon
  Metoprolol (?)
  Minocycline
  Nalorphine
  Naloxone
  Nialamide
  Nitroglycerin (?)
  Nortriptyline
  Oxprenolol
  Oxyphenbutazone
  Oxytetracycline
  Paraldehyde
  Pargyline
  Pentazocine
  Pentobarbital
  Pentylenetetrazol
  Perazine
  Periciazine
  Perphenazine
  Phencyclidine
  Pheniramine
  Phenmetrazine
  Phenobarbital
  Phenylbutazone
  Phenytoin
  Piperacetazine
  Piperazine
  Potassium Penicillin G
  Potassium Penicillin V
  Potassium Phenethicillin
  Primidone
  Probarbital
  Procaine Penicillin G
  Prochlorperazine
  Procyclidine
  Promazine
  Promethazine
  Propiomazine
  Propranolol

Protriptyline
Psilocybin
Pyrilamine
Quinine
Radioactive Iodides
Scopolamine
Secobarbital
Sodium Salicylate
Sulfacetamide
Sulfachlorpyridazine
Sulfacytine
Sulfadiazine
Sulfadimethoxine
Sulfamerazine
Sulfameter
Sulfamethazine
Sulfamethizole
Sulfamethoxazole
Sulfamethoxypyridazine
Sulfanilamide
Sulfaphenazole
Sulfapyridine
Sulfasalazine
Sulfathiazole
Sulfisoxazole
Talbutal

Tetracycline
Tetrahydrocannabinol
THC
Thiamylal
Thiethylperazine
Thiopental
Thiopropazate
Thioproperazine
Thioridazine
Timolol
Trichloroethylene
Trifluoperazine
Trifluperidol
Triflupromazine
Trihexyphenidyl
Trimeprazine
Trimipramine
Tripelennamine
Triprolidine
Tropicamide
Urea
Valproate Sodium
Valproic Acid
Vinbarbital
Vitamin D_2
Vitamin D_3

Index